HUMAN TUMOURS IN SHORT TERM CULTURE

Techniques and Clinical Applications

HUMAN TUMOURS IN SHORT TERM CULTURE

Techniques and Clinical Applications

Edited by

P. P. DENDY

Department of Radiotherapeutics
University of Cambridge, England

1976

ACADEMIC PRESS
LONDON · NEW YORK · SAN FRANCISCO

A Subsidiary of Harcourt Brace Jovanovich, Publishers

ACADEMIC PRESS INC. (LONDON) LTD
24–28 Oval Road
London NW1

U.S. Edition published by
ACADEMIC PRESS INC.
111 Fifth Avenue
New York, New York 10003

Library of Congress Catalog Card Number: 75-19631
ISBN: 0-12-209850-1

Printed in England by
The Whitefriars Press Ltd., London and Tonbridge

LIST OF CONTRIBUTORS

Professor E. J. Ambrose, *Chester Beatty Research Institute, Fulham Road, London SW3.*

Dr G. Balconi, *Ist. di Richerche Farmacologiche, Mario Negri, Via Eritrea 62, Milano, Italy.*

Mrs F. R. Balkwill, *ICRF, Medical Oncology Unit, St Bartholomew's Hospital, West Smithfield, London EC1A 7BE.*

Dr D. I. Beeby, *Chester Beatty Research Institute, Fulham Road, London SW3.*

Dr R. J. Berry, *MRC Radiobiological Research Unit, Harwell, Didcot, Oxon.*

Professor P. K. Bondy, *Royal Marsden Hospital, Downs Road, Sutton, Surrey.*

Dr J. Boss, *Veterinary School, University of Bristol, Park Row, Bristol BS1 5LS.*

Mr M. V. Bright, *Newmarket General Hospital, Exning Road, Newmarket, Suffolk CB8 7JG.*

Dr A. J. Brockas, *Churchill Hospital Research Institute, Headington, Oxford OX3 7LJ.*

Professor D. Crowther, *Christie Hospital & Holt Radium Institute, Withington, Manchester M20 9BX.*

Miss O. M. Curling, *Williamson Laboratory, St Bartholomew's Hospital, London EC1A 7BE.*

Dr M. P. A. Dawson, *Department of Radiotherapeutics, University of Cambridge, Hills Road, Cambridge.*

Dr P. P. Dendy, *Department of Medical Physics, University of Aberdeen, Foresterhill, Aberdeen, Scotland.*

Dr John Dickson, *Cancer Research Unit, University Department of Clinical Biochemistry, Royal Victoria Infirmary, Newcastle upon Tyne NE1 4LP.*

Dr L. Donaldson, *Department of Anatomy, Saint Salvator's College, St Andrews KY16 9TS, Fife, Scotland.*

v

Dr D. M. Easty, *Chester Beatty Research Institute, Fulham Road, London SW3.*

Dr G. C. Easty, *Chester Beatty Research Institute, Fulham Road, London SW3.*

Dr L. H. Eijgenstein, *Pathologisch-Anatomisch Laboratory, University of Amsterdam, Wilhelmina Gasthuis, Eerste Helmerstraat 104, Amsterdam (Oud-West), Holland.*

Dr M. J. Embleton, *Cancer Research Campaign Laboratories, University of Nottingham, Nottingham NG7 2RD.*

Dr E. Erba, *Ist. di Ricerche Farmacologiche, Mario Negri, Via Eritrea 62, Milano, Italy.*

Professor J. F. Fowler, *Gray Laboratory, Mount Vernon Hospital, Northwood, Middlesex HA6 2RN.*

Dr R. I. Freshney, *Royal Beatson Memorial Hospital, The Beatson Institute for Cancer Research, 132 Hill Street, Glasgow G3 6UD.*

Dr J-C. Gazet, *Chester Beatty Research Institute, Fulham Road, London SW3.*

Dr R. C. Hallowes, *Department of Pathology, Imperial Cancer Research Fund, Lincoln's Inn Fields, London WC2A 3PX.*
Dr Bridget Hill, *ICRF Laboratories, PO Box 123, Lincoln's Inn Fields, London WC2A 3PX.*

Dr G. M. Hodges, *Department of Cellular Pathology, ICRF, Lincoln's Inn Fields, London WC2A 3PX.*

Miss D. J. Honess, *Department of Radiotherapeutics, University of Cambridge, Hills Road, Cambridge.*

Mr C. N. Hudson, *Williamson Laboratory, St Bartholomew's Hospital, London EC1A 7BE.*

Dr M. Kaufmann, *Institut fur Experimentelle Pathologie Deutsche, Krebsforschungszentrum, 69 Heidelberg 1, Kirschnerstrasse 6, Germany.*

Dr J. C. Klein, *Radiobiological Institute TNO, Lange Kleiweg 151, Rijswijk ZH, The Netherlands.*

Dr E. I. Kohorn, *School of Medicine, Yale University, 333 Cedar Street, New Haven, Connecticut 06510,USA.*

Dr A. H. Laing, *Radiotherapy Department, Churchill Hospital, Headington, Oxford OX3 7LJ.*

Professor L. F. Lamerton, *Biophysics Department, Institute for*

Cancer Research, Royal Cancer Hospital, Clifton Avenue, Belmont, Sutton, Surrey SM2 5PX.

Dr L. Levin, *Department of Obstetrics & Gynaecology, Williamson Laboratory, St Bartholomew's Hospital, London EC1A 7BE.*

Dr Doreen Lewis, *Department of Pathology, Imperial Cancer Research Fund, Lincoln's Inn Fields, London WC2A 3PX.*

Professor H. G. Limburg, *University of the Saarland, Medical School, Department of Obstetrics & Gynaecology, Homburg-Saar, West Germany.*

Dr V. Littlewood, *Department of Anatomy, Saint Salvator's College, St Andrews KY16 9TS, Fife, Scotland.*

Miss J. E. McHardy, *Williamson Laboratory, St Bartholomew's Hospital, London EC1A 7BE.*

Dr C. Macnally, *Gray Laboratory, Mount Vernon Hospital, Northwood, Middlesex HA6 2RN.*

Dr J. R. W. Masters, *Department of Clinical Surgery, The Royal Infirmary, Edinburgh, Scotland.*

Dr. J. Mattern, *Institut fur Experimentelle Pathologie Deutsche, Krebsforschungszentrum, 69 Heidelberg 1, Kirschnerstrasse 6, Germany.*

Dr J. Mehrishi, *Department of Radiotherapeutics, University of Cambridge, Hills Road, Cambridge.*

Professor J. S. Mitchell, *Department of Radiotherapeutics, University of Cambridge, Hills Road, Cambridge.*

Dr M. Moore, *Paterson Laboratories, Christie Hospital & Holt Radium Institute, Manchester M20 9BX.*

Dr L. Morasca, *Ist. di Ricerche Farmacologiche, Mario Negri, Via Eritrea 62, Milano, Italy.*

Dr A. Munro Neville, *Chester Beatty Research Institute, Fulham Road, London SW3.*

Dr R. T. D. Oliver, *ICRF, Medical Oncology Unit, St Bartholomew's Hospital, West Smithfield, London EC1A 7BE.*

Dr L. N. Owen, *School of Veterinary Medicine, Madingley Road, Cambridge.*

Dr A. R. Poole, *Strangeways Research Laboratory, Wort's Causeway, Cambridge.*

Dr F. J. A. Prop, *Pathologisch-Anatomisch Laboratory, University of*

Amsterdam, Wilhelmina Gasthuis, Eerste Helmerstraat 104, Amsterdam (Oud-West), Holland.

Dr G. C. B. Prop-Arnold, *Pathologisch-Anatomisch Laboratory, University of Amsterdam, Wilhelmina Gasthuis, Eerste Helmerstraat 104, Amsterdam (Oud-West), Holland.*

Dr A. C. Riches, *Department of Anatomy, Saint Salvator's College, St Andrews KY16 9TS, Fife, Scotland.*

Dr A. Richters, *Department of Pathology, University of Southern California, School of Medicine, 2025 Zonal Avenue, Los Angeles, California 90033, USA.*

Mr R. E. Robinson, *Addenbrooke's Hospital, Hills Road, Cambridge.*

Dr A. Schleich, *Deutsches Krebsforschungzentrum, Institut Zellforschung, D 69 Heidelberg 1, Kirschnerstrasse 6, West Germany.*

Dr R. Sherwin, *Department of Pathology, University of Southern California, School of Medicine, 2025 Zonal Avenue, Los Angeles, California 90033, USA.*

Dr P. A. M. Shipman, *Department of Anatomy, Saint Salvator's College, St Andrews KY16 9TS, Fife, Scotland.*

Dr E. Sidebottom, *Sir William Dunn School of Pathology, Oxford.*

Dr L. A. Smets, *Netherlands Cancer Institute, Sarphatistraat 108, Amsterdam, Holland.*

Dr M. G. P. Stoker, *ICRF Laboratories, PO Box 123, Lincoln's Inn Fields, London WC2A 3PX.*

Dr M. Suzangar, *Cancer Research Unit, University Department of Clinical Biochemistry, Royal Victoria Infirmary, Newcastle upon Tyne NE1 4LP.*

Dr G. H. Thomas, *Department of Anatomy, Saint Salvator's College, St Andrews KY16 9TS, Fife, Scotland.*

Dr P. R. Twentyman, *Academic Department of Radiotherapy, Middlesex Hospital Medical School, London W1.*

Dr M. Volm, *Institut fur Experimentelle Pathologie Deutsche, Krebsforschungszentrum, 69 Heidelberg 1, Kirschnerstrasse 6, Germany.*

Dr B. M. Vose, *Paterson Laboratories, Christie Hospital & Holt Radium Institute, Manchester M20 9BX.*

Dr H. Warenius, *Radiotherapy Department, Addenbrooke's Hospital, Hills Road, Cambridge.*

Miss D. M. A. Warner, *Department of Radiotherapeutics, University of Cambridge, Hills Road, Cambridge.*

Dr K. Wayss, *Institut fur Experimentelle Pathologie Deutsche, Krebsforschungszentrum, 69 Heidelberg 1, Kirschnerstrasse 6, Germany.*

Dr John Wells, *CEGB, Berkeley Nuclear Laboratories, Berkeley, Gloucestershire.*

Dr T. K. Wheeler, *Radiotherapy Department, Addenbrooke's Hospital, Hills Road, Cambridge.*

Dr F. Whitehouse, *Department of Microbiology, The University of Michigan, Ann Arbor, Michigan, USA 48104.*

Dr G. J. Wiepjes, *Pathologisch-Anatomisch Laboratory, University of Amsterdam, Wilhelmina Gasthuis, Eerste Helmerstraat 104, Amsterdam (Oud-West), Holland.*

Dr G. Wiernik, *Churchill Hospital Research Institute, Headington, Oxford OX3 7LJ.*

Miss Anne Wilson, *Department of Pathology, Weston Park Hospital, Sheffield.*

Professor Et. Wolff, *Laboratoire d'Embryologie Experimentale, 49 bis Avenue de la Belle Gabrielle, 94 Nogent sur Marne, France.*

Miss J. E. M. Wright, *Department of Radiotherapeutics, University of Cambridge, Hills Road, Cambridge.*

Dr G. P. Wüst, *Medizinische Klinik und Poliklinik der Westfalischen Wilhelms University, 4400 Munster/W, Weatring 3, Germany.*

PREFACE

This book is based on the proceedings of a meeting on "Clinical applications of short term cultures of human tumour biopsy specimens" held in Cambridge, England on Thursday and Friday 26–27 September 1974. The meeting was dedicated to Professor J. S. Mitchell, F.R.S., Regius Professor of Physics in the University of Cambridge and Head of the Department of Radiotherapeutics in his 65th year in recognition of a lifetime's work in cancer research.

Rather than look back over Professor Mitchell's career, it was thought to be more in accordance with his wishes to look forward to a new development in cancer research in which he has shown great interest during the past eight years. It is widely recognised that the systems most frequently used to study the cancer problem, notably established cell lines and tumours propagated in animals, have severe limitations as models for human cancer. Short term cultures of human biopsy specimens provide an alternative approach to the problem of malignant disease in man. The subject is relatively new and it is the purpose of this book to set down what is already known; to identify the technical difficulties which presently limit progress; and to discuss some of the clinical problems which the model may help to solve.

Each section begins with a review of one particular aspect of the subject. This is followed by a number of shorter contributions which illustrate current progress. Where appropriate, a latter part of each section is an edited review, based on the opinions of several contributors, emphasising the most important problems which need to be answered.

The book will be of interest to persons in a wide range of disciplines. First it is directed to histopathologists who are in the best possible position to receive human tumour material. Accurate histological diagnosis is essential to the management of malignant disease but this book opens up a whole new range of *dynamic* studies for which precious human tumour biospy material may be used.

Secondly it is intended for cell biologists, particularly those who have a strong interest in the techniques of tissue culture. This book pinpoints numerous difficult technical problems which must be resolved before we can have really appropriate and satisfactory methods of short term culture of human tumour cells. But it also gives an insight of the great prizes to be won when the right methods have been perfected.

Finally it is directed at clinicians. All too often it seems that the clinician and the cell biologist are approaching the cancer problem from totally different viewpoints using quite incompatible scales of values. This book considers in detail the problems and difficulties of clinical evaluation of predictive tests.

By emphasising the clinical applications of short term cultures of human tumours, it is hoped to show that in this subject clinicians and cell biologists can and indeed must join together if the work is to be brought to its logical conclusion, i.e. improved treatment of cancer.

I would like to acknowledge with thanks the help of Mrs Ann Dendy with the preparation of the final typescript and Miss Margaret Pole and Mr Paul Craske with the preparation of the illustrative material.

This work was supported by the Cell Tissue and Organ Culture Study Group of the Co-ordinating Committee for Human Tumour Investigation.

P. P. DENDY
January 1976

CONTENTS

Chapter 1

METHODS AVAILABLE FOR
IN VITRO STUDIES

(Moderator:G. Easty)

1. An Overview of Tissue Culture Procedures in Tumour Biopsy Studies

G. M. Hodges

INTRODUCTION

I have been asked that this introductory paper should present a general survey of tissue culture systems together with a discussion of the advantages and disadvantages of these systems for *in vitro* studies of human tumour biopsy specimens.

With these objectives in mind we may, as we peer down on the map of tumour tissue culture consider Alice, who, in her Adventures in Wonderland, asked the Cheshire-Cat, "Would you tell me, please, which way I ought to go from here?". Replied the Cat, "That depends a good deal on where you want to get to". Said Alice, "I don't much care where—so long as I get *somewhere*". Doubtless, this comment must, at present, be often echoed by those working with tumour biopsy material *in vitro* attempting to define those properties of human tumour cells and tissues which are relevant to the management of malignant disease—the clearly defined objective of the clinician.

Before reviewing tissue culture procedures, we should indicate the kind of information required by the clinician, namely prognosis and response to treatment. One of the major problems of the clinician, beside that of detecting and diagnosing cancer, is of correctly classifying patients for therapy. This requires meaningful information on tumour-host interaction and on the type and level of local and systemic response of the patient to the tumour. Arising from this stems the need for test systems capable of predicting the clinical response of an individual patient with cancer, to a given therapy. Numerous *in vitro* tumour tissue culture studies have been made since almost the inception of the technique in an attempt to provide information on the behavioural characteristics of human tumours and, more recently, of their response to therapeutic agents—the two basic questions of the clinician (for further discussion see in Ambrose *et al.* 1967; Katsuta, 1968; Cline, 1971; Sjögren, 1973; Garattini and Franchi, 1973; Herberman and Gaylord, 1973; Sherbet, 1974).

1. EVALUATION OF TUMOUR CELL CHARACTERISTIC *IN VITRO*

Various parameters have been used to characterise the tumour cell *in vitro* (Table 1) and involve a variety of techniques making different

TABLE 1

Parameters for Tumour Cell Characterisation

Behavioural	
cell kinetics	Baserga, 1971; Lala, 1971; Malaise *et al.* 1973
cell shape, size, nucleolar number	Barker and Sanford, 1970
cell surface characterisation	Burger, 1971; Emmelot, 1973; Easty, 1974
cell movement and interaction	Abercrombie, 1970; Weiss, 1972; Auersperg and Finnegan, 1974
growth pattern *in vitro*	Ambrose *et al.* 1967; Izsak *et al.* 1968; Katsuta, 1968; Auersperg and Finnegan, 1974; Sanford, 1974
Biochemical	Potter, 1969; Borek, 1971; 1972; Nigam and Cantero, 1972; 1973
Cytochemical	Burstone, 1962; Melnick, 1971; Poole, 1973; Shnitka and Seligman, 1973
Genetical	Fialkow, 1973; Simnett, 1974
Histophysical	Hall *et al.* 1974; Russ, 1974
Immunological	Hellström and Hellström, 1971; Heppner, 1973; Sinkovics, 1973
Structural	Willis, 1967; Jordan and Williams, 1971; Carr and Underwood, 1974
Transplantability	Sanford, 1965

demands on tissue culture methodology. The information obtained from *in vitro* tumour studies is limited and reflects deficiencies emanating not only from the procedure of tissue culture, but also from the techniques of analysis available. Practical aspects of these problems can be expected to be discussed in later chapters.

2. TISSUE CULTURE SYSTEMS

Tissue culture procedures can be classified into five separate systems based on two different morphological approaches, namely those of cell culture and of tissue or organ culture (Fedoroff, 1967). In cell culture, the cells are no longer organised into tissues and form the bases of the monolayer, suspension or explant culture techniques—

monolayer culture referring to a single layer of cells growing on a surface; suspension culture denoting a type of culture in which cells multiply while suspended in medium; explant culture describing the initiation of a cell culture from an excised fragment of a tissue or an organ. In contrast, tissue or organ culture, which includes the histotypic and organotypic culture techniques, denotes the maintenance or growth of tissues *in vitro* in a way that will allow differentiation and preservation of the architecture and/or function. Histoculture is distinguished from organotypic culture in that very thin slices of tissues are cultured *in vitro* to provide a method allowing direct microscopic visualisation of different cellular components maintained within a tissue framework, an approach not generally possible with the usually thicker organ culture explants. Several reviews discuss the application of these different tissue culture systems to *in vitro* studies of tumour tissues (*see,* Ambrose *et al.* 1967; Wolff, 1970; Auersperg and Finnegan, 1974).

A potential complication of *in vitro* tumour biopsy studies is that the biopsy specimen may not be a truly representative sample of the tumour and its study could lead to misleading conclusions. Tumour tissue culture may, at its very inception, therefore be hampered by biopsy sampling problems. These can be of particular significance in the study of solid tumours though less so, for example, in studies of hematologic neoplasia. Several reasons can be enumerated for the possible failure of an *in vitro* tumour biopsy culture:

(a) There may be extensive necrosis, possibly accentuated by clinical excision and pre-treatments.

(b) The tumour may contain non-representative or inert portions, either of intercellular substances such as collagen or osteoid or, these areas may be largely secretion as in some mucinous adenocarcinomas.

(c) There may be an absence of tumour material in the particular tissue specimen, or, the proportion of living tumour cells may be too little, and difficult to obtain for culture procedures.

A further complication is the potential heterogeneity of the cell population in a tumour sample with its possible mixture of different normal and neoplastic components. From this extends the need firstly, of tissue culture procedures which will allow growth of the full spectrum of the cell population in the tumour; secondly, of marker systems, which will distinguish normal and neoplastic cells; and thirdly, of cell separation techniques (Table 2) which can lead to the selection of each cell population essential for certain analytical approaches.

TABLE 2

Cell Separation Techniques

Differential sedimentation ⎫	
Isopycnic sedimentation ⎪	
Velocity sedimentation ⎬	*see* Shortman, 1972; Harwood, 1974
Centrifugal elutriation ⎪	
Electrophoresis ⎭	
Differential attachment	Rabinowitz, 1973; Edelman, 1973
Sequential enzyme treatment	Prop and Wiepjes, 1973
Selective media	Puck and Kao, 1967; Posner, Nove and Sato, 1971; Waymouth, 1972, 1974
Single cell cloning:	Ham, 1974
Capillary techniques ⎫	
Microdrop techniques ⎪	
Dilution plating ⎬	*see* Kruse and Patterson, 1973
Microtest plate ⎪	
Soft agar ⎭	

Factors Affecting In Vitro *Culture of Tissues*

A variety of different factors can influence the growth and function of cells in culture and can lead to cell instability and modified cell relationships (*see,* Rothblat and Cristofalo, 1972; McLimans, 1973; Auersperg and Finnegan, 1974; Taylor, 1974; Waymouth, 1974). Thus, composition of the culture medium, type of substrate, separation procedure, density and type of cell population are among some of the factors which could influence *in vitro* life of the tumour biopsy specimen and modify the behavioural characteristics of its cellular constituents. Probably the most critical *in vitro* variable is the medium, irrespective of the tissue culture system used. The need for media tailored for a specific purpose and a specific tissue is well documented in the literature (*see,* e.g. Taylor, 1974; Waymouth, 1972, 1974). In *in vitro* tumour therapy studies the metabolic activity of the neoplastic cells should be closely similar to that *in vivo*. Precisely controlled and reproducible conditions need to be established to permit meaningful extrapolation of observations from the *in vitro* test system to the clinical situation.

Substrates of a wide variety have been used in tissue culture systems including the use of glass, plastic, agar, Sephadex beads, polyester film and cellulose acetate membranes (see Kruse and Patterson, 1973; Maroudas, 1973). Numerous experimental studies show that cells can demonstrate varying affinities for different substrata, and that the biological expression of cells can be modified in relation to the particular substrate with which they are in contact (Wolff and Marin, 1960; Harris, 1964; Hauschka, 1972; Rappaport, 1972; Taylor, 1974; Weiss *et al.* 1975). Mixed populations of epithelial and fibroblast cells (from mouse mammary adeno-carcinoma) have been separated by their differential affinities to substrates—the neoplastic epithelial cell showing a strong affinity for plastic surfaces while poorly adhering to borosilicate glass surfaces (Riddle, personal communication; *see,* Steinberg, 1970).

Proteases, in particular trypsin, are widely used in tissue culture procedures. Although cellular viability is not affected to any great extent, an extensive literature shows that certain properties of the cell may be modified following protease treatment (*see,* Hodges *et al.* 1973a). In both cell and organ culture systems (Burger, 1970; Hodges *et al.* 1973b; Hodges and Muir, 1975), protease stimulation of cellular proliferation and increased DNA synthesis, for example, has been demonstrated (Fig. 1). While many of the observed changes may be transient and reversed after a period of time in culture, the possible selective effect of proteolytic activity on cell behaviour must be considered as another variable which can influence *in vitro* observations.

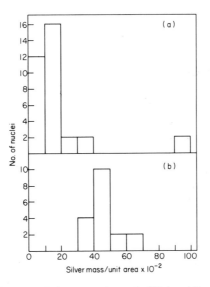

Fig. 1. Increased rate of incorporation of ^{3}H-thymidine, (1 μCi/ml for 24 h; 0·1 mg/ml colchicine for 4 h prior to fixation) in protease-treated bladder organ cultures (b), compared to untreated controls (a) (96 h *in vitro*). Quantitative X-ray microanalysis of mass of developed silver over individual nuclei (Hodges and Muir, 1975a).

The removal of a tissue from its *in vivo* environment must inevitably provoke biological changes and these changes may be further accentuated by the act of *in vitro* culture. There is, however, relatively little information on the structural and metabolic differences that occur in cells as a consequence of the tissue culture environment. Changes in the enzyme patterns of cells have been demonstrated following *in vitro* culture, some being reversible on reimplantation of the cells into syngeneric hosts, while others have appeared irreversible (*see,* Wilson, 1973).

It is obvious from the selected examples above, which by no means exhaust the list of factors influencing tissue culture systems, that the behaviour of a tissue *in vitro* may not only reflect the intrinsic properties of a given tissue, but may also reflect properties which are the result of the experimental procedure. This raises a critical problem in relation to *in vitro* tumour test systems and concerns the relevance of elegantly construed analyses of tumour cell behaviour and reaction *in vitro* with external agents to actual behaviour of these cells in the *in vivo* situation.

3. AN APPRAISAL OF TISSUE CULTURE SYSTEMS

Practical aspects of the advantages and disadvantages of the different tissue culture systems defined earlier can be expected to be discussed in subsequent chapters.

Monolayer and explant culture systems are of benefit in that cells may be easily examined in detail microscopically. Explant cultures, being primary cultures of excised tissue fragments can, initially, maintain some of the characteristic morphology of the tissue and include a selection of different cell types in the outgrowth. Both monolayer and explant culture systems have been widely used in the study of chemotherapeutic drugs, in radio- and immuno-biology and in chromosome studies, while some attempts have been made to use the explant system as a supplementary diagnostic technique in the identification of tumours. The particular advantage of the monolayer and suspension culture systems is that they provide methods for the production of large quantities of replicate cultures of cells, an essential requirement for a variety of quantitative metabolic and behavioural studies. Furthermore, use of these systems allows populations of cells to be derived from a single cell leading to more uniform experimental conditions.

A possible criticism of cell culture, inherent in its definition, is that the cells are no longer organised into tissues. Various studies have shown that many *in vivo* characteristics are lost when cells from tissues grow out into monolayers which can lead to a breakdown in cell to cell relationships and to a modified response to external stimuli.

A considerable degree of cell selection can occur during the establishment of a cell culture system, the result of a variety of factors some of which were discussed in the previous section. Alteration of cell density and cell contacts in such cultures are further factors which can influence the sensitivity and activity both of the test and control systems (see reviews, e.g. Auersperg and Finnegan, 1974; Sanford, 1974; Taylor, 1974; Waymouth, 1974).

In the organotypic culture system, many of the cell types may be maintained *in vitro* within an intact and characteristic tissue architecture and may show typical functional features of the *in vivo* material (*see,* e.g. Thomas, 1970). Thus, the tissue or organ culture approach provides an *in vitro* system which has potentially close and

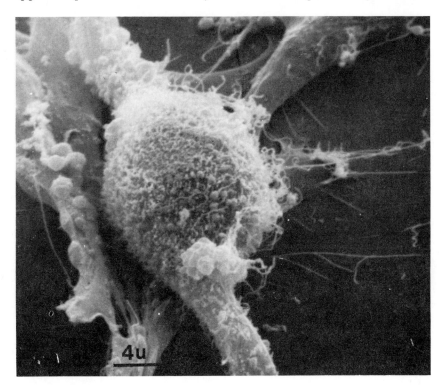

Fig. 2. SEM micrograph of COM 5 cell (Franks and Henzell, 1970) in early prophase with profuse microprocesses and small blebs.

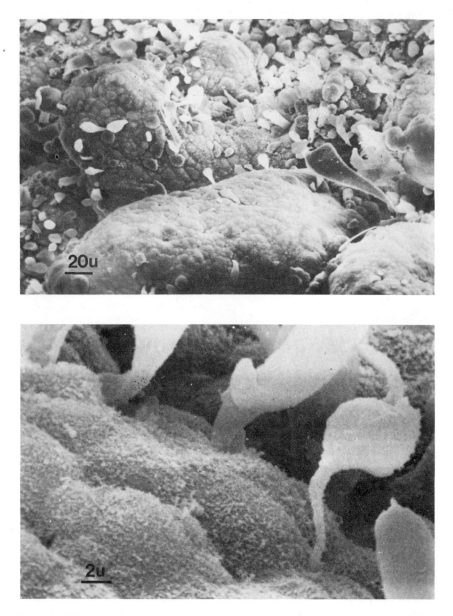

Fig. 3a,b. SEM micrograph of papillary transitional cell carcinoma of human bladder. Detail of surface showing cellular pleomorphism.

promising affinities with the *in vivo* situation though the complexity of the system makes the analysis of the results that much more difficult.

A general feature is that irrespective of the system employed, tissue culture systems suffer at present from failure of specific cell types to survive, from loss of functional characteristics in many of those cells that are maintained *in vitro* and by a general absence of easily defined markers to distinguish normal and neoplastic cells. These are some of the areas in which more research is needed (see Fedoroff, 1974).

4. A POTENTIAL TUMOUR CELL MARKER SYSTEM?

The entry of scanning electron microscopy (SEM) into biomedical research has given rise to a burgeoning literature (*see,* Jones *et al.* 1974 for bibliography) providing evidence of the considerable potential of this instrument. Its morphological applications and its non-destructive X-ray microanalytical capabilities provide histophysical techniques which should be able to make valuable contributions to cell characterisation studies.

Fine structural evaluation of large areas can readily be undertaken providing data on cell and tissue topography (*see,* e.g. Jordan and Williams, 1971; Hodges, *et al.* 1973; Revel, 1974) (Figs 2 and 3) difficult to obtain by light or transmission electron microscopy. Attempts have been made to relate changes in the surface structure of cells to known stages in the cell cycle based not only on cell shape but on such selected features as presence of blebs, ruffles and microprocesses which may help to distinguish cells in the G_1, S or G_2 periods (Porter *et al.* 1973).

Combined X-ray spectroscopy and morphological analysis allows chemical characterisation of specimens to be combined with structural topography. Areas of application of such an analytical approach include the localisation of natural elements present in a tissue; the detection of elements present as the result of pathological conditions; and the identification of sites of specific chemical activity using markers (Hall *et al.* 1974). Such markers could be elemental precipitates produced by staining reactions (DeNee *et al.* 1974); metal-tagged macromolecules (Hodges and Muir, 1974a); or, silver grains in autoradiograms (Hodges and Muir, 1974b, 1975a and b) (Fig. 1).

With these examples it is possible to envisage practical application of such analytical approaches to already existing tumour tissue culture systems, in particular to explant, histo- and organo-typic cultures.

REFERENCES

Abercrombie, M. (1970). *In vitro*, *6*, 128-142.

Ambrose, E. J., Easty, D. M. and Wylie, J. A. H. (1967). "The Cancer Cell *in vitro*". Butterworths, London.

Auersperg, N. and Finnegan, C. V. (1974). The differentiation and organisation of tumours *in vitro*. In "Neoplasia and Cell Differentiation" (G. V. Sherbet, ed.), pp. 279-318. Karger, Basel.

Barker, B. E. and Sanford, K. K. (1970). *J. natl. Cancer Inst.* *44*, 39-63.

Baserga, R. (1971). "The Cell Cycle and Cancer". Marcel Dekker, New York.

Borek, E. (1971). *Cancer Res.* *31*, 591-721.

Borek, E. and Kerr, S. J. (1972). *Adv. Can. Res.* *15*, 163-190.

Burger, M. M. (1971). Cell surfaces in neoplastic transformation. *In* "Current Topics in Cellular Regulation", Vol. 3, 135-193. Academic Press, New York and London.

Burstone, M. (1962). "Enzyme Histochemistry and Its Application in the Study of Neoplasma". Academic Press, New York and London.

Carr, I. and Underwood, J. C. E. (1974). *Int. Rev. Cytol.* *37*, 329-347.

Cline, M. J. (1971). Cancer chemotherapy. *In* "Major Problems in Internal Medicine", Vol. 1. W. B. Saunders Co., Philadelphia, London, Toronto.

DeNee, P. B., Abraham, J. L. and Willard, P. A. (1974). *SEM/IITRI*, *7*, 259-266.

Easty, G. C. (1974). Cell surfaces in neoplasia. *In* "Neoplasia and Cell Differentiation" (G. V. Sherbet, ed.), pp. 189-233. Karger, Basel.

Edelman, G. M. (1973). Non-enzymatic dissociations. B. Specific cell fractionation on chemically derivatised surfaces. *In* "Tissue Culture, Methods and Applications" (P. F. Kruse, Jr. and M. K. Patterson, Jr., eds.), pp. 29-36. Academic Press, New York and London.

Emmelot, P. (1973). *Europ. J. Cancer*, *9*, 319-333.

Fedoroff, S. (1967). *J. natl. Cancer Inst.* *38*, 607-611.

Fedoroff, S. (1974). *J. natl. Cancer Inst.* *53*, 1479-1480.

Fialkow, P. J. (1974). *J. clin. Path.* *27*, Suppl. 7, 11-15.

Franks, L. M. and Henzell, S. (1970). *Europ. J. Cancer* *6*, 357-364.

Garattini, S. and Franchi, G. (1973). "Chemotherapy of Cancer Dissemination and Metastasis". Raven Press, New York.

Hall, T., Echlin, P. and Kaufmann, R. (1974). "Microprobe Analysis as Applied to Cells and Tissues". Academic Press, London and New York.

Ham, R. G. (1974). *J. natl. Cancer Inst.* *53*, 1459-1463.

Harris, A. (1973). *Exptl. Cell Res.* *77*, 285-297.

Harris, M. (1964). "Cell Culture and Somatic Variation". Holt, New York.

Harwood, R. (1974). *Int. Rev. Cytol.* *38*, 369-403.

Hauschka, S. (1972). Cultivation of muscle tissue. *In* "Growth, Nutrition and Metabolism of Cells in Culture" (G. H. Rothblat and V. J. Cristofalo, eds.), pp. 67-130. Academic Press, New York and London.

Hellström, I. and Hellström, K. E. (1971). Colony inhibition and cytotoxicity assays. *In* "*In vitro* Methods in Cell-mediated Immunity" (B. B. Bloom and P. R. Glade, eds.), pp. 409-414. Academic Press, New York and London.

Heppner, G. H. (1973). Colony inhibition and microcytotoxicity assay methods for measuring cell-mediated and associated antibody immunity *in vitro*. *In* "Methods in Cancer Research" (H. Busch, ed.), Vol. 8, 3-32. Academic Press, New York and London.

Herberman, R. B. and Gaylord, C. E. (1973). *Nat. Cancer Inst. Monog. 37.*

Hodges, G. M., Livingstone, D. C. and Franks, L. M. (1973a). *J. Cell Sci. 12,* 887-902.

Hodges, G. M., Muir, M. D. and Spacey, G. D. (1973b). *SEM/IITRI, 6,* 589-596.

Hodges, G. M. and Muir, M. D. (1974a). X-ray spectroscopy in the scanning electron microscope study of cell and tissue culture material. *In* "Microprobe Analysis as Applied to Cells and Tissues" (T. Hall, P. Echlin and R. Kaufmann, eds.), pp. 277-291. Academic Press, London and New York.

Hodges, G. M. and Muir, M. D. (1974b). *Nature, Lond. 247,* 383-385.

Hodges, G. M. and Muir, M. D. (1975a). Quantitative evaluation of autoradiographs by X-ray spectroscopy. In press.

Hodges, G. M. and Muir, M. D. (1975b). Scanning electron microscope autoradiography. *In* "Principles and Techniques of Scanning Electron Microscopy", Van Nostrand Reinhold Co., New York. In press.

Izsak, F. Ch., Gotlieb-Stematsky, T., Eylan, E. and Gazith, A. (1968). *Europ. J. Cancer, 4,* 375-381.

Jones, S. J., Bailey, E. and Boyde, A. (1974). *SEM/IITRI, 7,* 835-849.

Jordan, J. A. and Williams, A. E. (1971). *J. Obst. Gynaecol. 78,* 940-946.

Katsuta, H. (1968). "Cancer Cells in Culture". University Park Press, Baltimore.

Kruse, P. F., Jr. and Patterson, M. K., Jr. (1973). "Tissue Culture: Methods and Applications". Academic Press, New York and London.

Lala, P. K. (1971). Studies on tumour cell population kinetics. *In* "Methods in Cancer Research" (H. Busch, ed.). Academic Press, New York and London.

Malaise, E. P., Chavaudra, N. and Tubiana, M. (1973). *Europ. J. Cancer, 9,* 305-312.

Maroudas, N. G. (1973). *Nature, Lond. 244,* 353-354.

McLimans, W. F. (1973). Cancer and the cultured cell. *In* "Perspectives in Cancer Research and Treatment" (G. P. Murphy, ed.), pp. 237-255. Alan R. Liss Inc., New York.

Melnick, P. J. (1971). "Cytoenzymology and Isozymes of Cultured Cells". Fischer, Stuttgart.

Nigam, V. N. and Cantero, A. (1972). *Adv. in Cancer Res. 16,* 1-96.

Nigam, V. N. and Cantero, A. (1973). *Adv. in Cancer Res. 17,* 1-80.

Poole, A. R. (1973). Tumour lysosomal enzymes and invasive growth. *In* "Lysosomes in Biology and Pathology" (J. T. Dingle, ed.), *3,* 83. North Holland, Amsterdam.

Porter, K., Prescott, D. and Frye, J. (1973). *J. Cell Biol. 57,* 815-836.

Posner, M., Nove, J. and Sato, G. (1971). Selection procedures for mammalian cells in monolayer culture. *In vitro, 6,* 253-256.

Potter, V. R., Watanabe, M., Pitot, H. C. and Morris, H. P. (1969). *Cancer Res. 29,* 55-78.

Prop, F. J. A. and Wiepjes, G. J. (1973). Sequential enzyme treatment of mouse mammary gland. *In* "Tissue Culture: Methods and Application" (P. F. Kruse, Jr. and M. K. Patterson, Jr., eds.), pp. 21-24. Academic Press, New York and London.

Puck, T. and Kao, F. T. (1967). *Proc. natl. Acad. Sci. U.S.A. 58,* 1227-1234.

Rabinowitz, Y. (1973). Non-enzymatic dissociations. A. Leukocyte cell separation on glass. *In* "Tissue Culture: Methods and Applications" (P. F. Kruse, Jr.

and M. K. Patterson, Jr., eds.), pp. 25-29. Academic Press, New York and London.

Rappaport, C. (1972). Some aspects of the growth of mammalian cells on glass surfaces. *In* "The Chemistry of Biosurfaces" (M. L. Hair, ed.), Vol. 2, 449-487.

Revel, J. P. (1974). *SEM/IITRI, 7,* 541-548.

Rothblat, G. H. and Cristofalo, V. J. (1972). "Growth, Nutrition and Metabolism of Cells in Culture", Vols 1 and 2. Academic Press, New York and London.

Russ, J. C. (1974). *J. Submicr. Cytol. 6,* 55-79.

Sanford, K. K. (1965). *Int. Rev. Cytol. 18,* 249-311.

Sanford, K. K. (1974). *J. natl. Cancer Inst. 53,* 1481-1485.

Sherbet, G. V. (1974). "Neoplasia and Cell Differentiation". S. Karger, Basel.

Shortman, K. (1972). *Ann. Rev. Biophys. Bioeng. 1,* 93-120.

Shnitka, T. K. and Seligman, A. M. (1973). Ultrastructural cytochemistry of enzymes and some applications. *In* "Methods in Cancer Research" (H. Busch, ed.), Vol. 10, 37-84. Academic Press, New York and London.

Simnett, J. D. (1974). Nuclear differentiation in the development of normal and neoplastic tissues. *In* "Neoplasia and Cell Differentiation" (G. V. Sherbet, ed.), pp. 1-26. Karger, Basel.

Sinkovics, J. G. (1973). Monitoring *in vitro* of cell-mediated immune reactions to tumours. *In* "Methods in Cancer Research" (H. Busch, ed.), Vol. 8, 107-175. Academic Press, New York and London.

Sjögren, H. O. (1973). Blocking and unblocking of cell-mediated tumour immunity. *In* "Methods in Cancer Research", Vol. 10, 19-34. Academic Press, New York and London.

Steinberg, M. S. (1970). *J. exp. Zool. 173,* 395-434.

Taylor, W. G. (1974). *J. natl. Cancer Inst. 53,* 1449-1457.

Thomas, J. A. (1970). "Organ Culture". Academic Press, New York and London.

Waymouth, C. (1972). Construction of tissue culture media. *In* "Growth, Nutrition and Metabolism of Cells in Culture" (G. H. Rothblat and V. J. Cristofalo, eds.), pp. 11-47. Academic Press, New York and London.

Waymouth, C. (1974). *J. natl. Cancer Inst. 53,* 1443-1448.

Weiss, L. (1972). Interactions between normal and malignant cells. *In* "The Chemistry of Biosurfaces" (M. L. Hair, ed.), *2,* 377-447.

Weiss, L., Poste, G., MacKearnin, A. and Willett, K. (1975). *J. Cell Biol. 64,* 135-145.

Willis, R. J. (1967). "Pathology of Tumours". 4th edn. Butterworths, London.

Wilson, P. D. (1973). *Cancer Res. 33,* 375-382.

Wolff, E. and Marin, L. (1960). *C.R. Acad. Sci. 250,* 609-611.

DISCUSSION

G. Easty said changes may take place when tumours are cultured so that their properties do not reflect those which they possess *in vivo*. This is one of the greatest problems faced by anyone attempting to use these techniques for screening for the effect of drugs.

Hodges suggested that within the experimental context of an *in vitro* system, when one examines the control and the treated system the results are no doubt valid. But this is a very artificial and closely defined system and if one wishes to relate it to the *in vivo* situation then the problems which are provoked by the choice of media, substrate and hormonal complements, etc., have to be re-examined.

Berry said the selective attachment of cells to cells in fresh explants is very important and in a number of fresh human tumour explants they looked at, attachment of epithelial tumour cells was not achieved to plastic surfaces but was achieved to fibroblasts explanted at the same time. Cells grow on fibroblasts acting as a "feeder layer" when they will not grow on any other surfaces, but this changes when cells have been continually cultured for several passages.

Morasca said that cell detachment from the tumour was also important. When fragments are prepared for explant culture, epithelial cells sometimes detach from the connective tissue and go into the washing medium. A culture made with washing medium gives almost pure epithelial cells. Hodges added that Lasfargues (1973) has described a "spilling" technique which allows him to obtain a higher yield of epithelial cells.

In reply to Mehrishi who suggested that 3% trypsin might cause unnecessary loss of material from the cell surface, Hodges said they had found this concentration of trypsin was necessary for the separation of epithelium from stroma in adult bladder tissues. She agreed that the concentration could be deleterious for many culture systems.

Freshney asked if the ascorbic acid requirement related to epithelial cells surviving within the explant or was another example of the dependence of collagen synthesis on ascorbic acid in organ cultures. Hodges said it is correlated to the dependence of collagen synthesis on ascorbic acid. In simple terms the adequate maintenance of the stroma in turn allows adequate maintenance of the epithelial layer.

Boss suggested that methods might be used which favour epithelial cells at the expense of fibroblasts, for example the relative amounts of calcium phosphate or the pH, to distinguish a tumour cell which is epithelial in origin from stromal cells which are not.

Dickson asked if more sophisticated methods—cell selection techniques, microspectrofluorimetry, scanning electron microscopy—could add to the methods already available for looking at sensitivity to drugs in patients. Hodges favoured the scanning electron microscopy microanalytical techniques because they can make observations on the short term culture.

Lamerton and G. Easty said it would be extremely valuable if the scanning electron microscope appearance and the phase of the cell cycle particularly G_0 phase could be correlated. Hodges added that the changes in morphology in relation to the cell cycle observed by Knutton *et al.* (1974) for mastocytoma cells in suspension culture differed from those described by Porter *et al.* (1973) for monolayer cultures of Chinese hamster ovary cells.

REFERENCES

Knutton, S., Sumner, M. C. B., Pasternak, C. A. (1974). Proc. 8th Int. Cong. Electron Micro. Canberra 2, 362.

Lasfargues, E. Y. (1973). *In* "Tissue Culture Methods and Applications" (P. F. Kruse, Jr. and M. K. Patterson, Jr., eds.), p. 45. Academic Press, New York and London.

Porter, K. R., Prescott, D. and Frye, J. (1973). *J. Cell Biol.* 57, 815.

2. Methodology for Human Tumour Biopsy Specimens

A. Introduction

1. TISSUE CULTURE METHODOLOGY

Numerous facets of the growth of human tumour biopsies in short term culture will be considered in the chapters which follow. Each of them requires methodology suited to that specific problem and the evidence gained is valuable to our better understanding of *in vitro* and *in vivo* growth of tumour cells.

However, by far the greatest emphasis is on some form of predictive test, the results of which can be useful for the management of patients with cancer. With particular reference to predictive studies of drug sensitivity for example, the culture methods must be relevant to the clinical situation. There are many highly sophisticated culture techniques which may represent the closest we can get to perfection in technology for measuring drug sensitivity in culture, but if they take 3 months to complete they are useless in a clinical type of test. Some of the questions which need to be answered and observations on the way they influence the choice of a suitable culture method are summarised below.

2. THREE DIMENSIONAL STRUCTURE

What part should the tissue architecture play in the performance of a culture to measure drug sensitivity? Is it feasible, and is it relevant to measure drug sensitivity of cells dispersed in monolayer when these cells occur as a solid matrix in the tumour? Cell to cell contact is lost when cells are dispersed in monolayer culture and the cell density or degree of crowding is extremely difficult to control in primary cultures of human tumour biopsies. There are many advantages in retaining cell/cell contact and many feel this is the only way to get a representative sample of the tumour into culture. However, there are considerable problems in the organ culture or slice culture type of system which have not yet been resolved. Also one important clinical problem is the prevention of distant metastases. This is particularly important for mammary carcinoma and carcinoma of the bronchus and gives much greater relevance to the behaviour of single cells or small groups of cells.

3. TUMOUR CELL IDENTIFICATION

The need for marker systems which will distinguish normal and neoplastic cells has already been mentioned and extensive references to work on parameters for tumour cell characterisation are given in Table 1 (page 4).

From a practical view-point a method is required which, beside being reliable, can be applied fairly easily to a relatively large number of specimens. Some methods which might be satisfactory are summarised below and many are considered in greater detail in later chapters.

(a) Morphological appearance—an organ culture or the outgrowth from a section can be compared with the original histology.

(b) Growth behaviour—studies in monolayers by time lapse cinematography; invasion studies; growth in semi-solid media, in suspension, or in immunosuppressed animals; density limitation of growth and/or contact inhibition.

(c) Tumour cells frequently have anomalous karyotypes or abnormal DNA values.

(d) Biochemical properties—correlation of the pattern of enzyme activity with the biochemical report; comparison of glycolysis or respiration; differences in cell surface properties; membrane pumps.

(e) Miscellaneous—antigenic tests; high level of reverse transcriptase and identification of the viral genome (*if* model for virus transformed cells, e.g. BHK21 is applicable to spontaneous human tumours); concanavalin A agglutination tests.

4. HETEROGENEITY OF THE SAMPLE

If the tissue is used to prepare a cell suspension then aliquots of that suspension can be assumed to be truly replicate cultures although very heterogeneous within each sample. Each organ culture sample or slice is a specimen with a character all its own and the statistical variation between replicate samples is relatively high. This may not be an insurmountable problem when using cytological, morphological, autoradiographic, and histological methods to study the behaviour of single cells provided that the tumour cells can be identified and their relative proportions are approximately the same as in the original biopsy. But it must be practicable to expand into a clinical type of test which will embrace a large number of drugs, perhaps as many as 15. Each drug will have to be tested at a range of concentrations and to a limited extent drug combinations will have to be used so the number of samples required could be well over 100. To provide a clinical test which meets all these requirements, precludes the use of cytological, morphological, autoradiographic and histological observations. First, because they are performed by experts who are hard to find and require a relatively long training to be able to analyse the sample. Secondly, the time taken and the subjectivity of the analysis is too great.

If methods are used which are biochemical or at least capable of objective automation, this problem can be solved but the question of sample heterogeneity with organ or slice cultures is then of paramount importance.

5. SURVIVAL AND SELECTION

It has been known since the earliest days of tissue culture that when dispersed cells are put into culture not all of them survive. Is it fair to say that those cells which survive are representative of the total tumour? If we measure the drug sensitivity are we measuring the sensitivity of tumour cells or are we measuring the sensitivity of tissue culture cells? This will undoubtedly be related to the proximity of the analysis to the time of explantation but as soon as the tumour is explanted and dispersed into single cells, a population which may not be representative of the total tumour is automatically selected.

6. PROLIFERATION RATE

An estimate of the total doubling time of the tumour mass in culture will be different, on some occasions being shorter than *in vivo* when the cells take to culture, in some cases longer if the cells do not take particularly well. Part of this difference may be due to a different rate of cell cycling *in vitro*. Will the chemosensitivity of a cell be altered if its cell cycle time changes? In addition a different compartment of the cells may be participating in the proliferation. In solid tumours *in vivo* the percentage of tumour cells which are participating in proliferation as opposed to those which are resting or in G_0 is very variable but typical figures range from 25% to 40% (Tubiana, 1971). In tissue culture very little work has been done but the proliferating pool of cells is sometimes very much higher and we have no idea if this correlates with *in vivo* or not. What we have to establish is does this matter? Is there a basic difference between a cell which proliferates in culture and a cell which proliferates *in vivo*? Are the 60% non-proliferating G_0 cells *in vivo* really any different or do they happen to be in G_0 because of their geographical location in the tumour? Far more work is required on the kinetics of tumour cell growth in short term culture and its relevance to the *in vivo* situation.

7. CELL SEPARATION

The presence of a heterogeneous population in a tumour biopsy immediately suggests the possibility of tumour cell separation. Methods available for cell separation have already been summarised in Table 2 (page 6). With particular reference to the separation of tumour and normal cells a number of promising techniques—gradient separation, isokinetic zonal centrifugation, unit gravity sedimentation have already been used successfully to separate HeLa cells from fibroblasts mixed together in the first instance.

Selective adhesion can also be mentioned as a method with some possibilities. There may be sufficient differential adhesion between malignant cells and fibroblasts that by successive replating at intervals of only a few hours, one can deplete the fibroblastic population and enrich the malignant population. Use of modified culture media or a particular pH have also been suggested (see page 15). Biological parameters which might be used for separating cells include chalones—if there is a fibroblastic chalone this might be the way to inhibit growth of the fibroblastic fraction of a tumour in culture. Hormones could perhaps also be used but this might be unwise if the culture is to be used subsequently for drug sensitivity tests.

One of these methods, or more than one in sequence, might give a substantial enrichment of the tumour cell population but little work has been done on this problem.

8. CHOICE OF DRUG CONCENTRATION AND ASSAY METHOD

Both of these points are discussed in detail elsewhere. Suffice to say that the former should be related to the concentration attained by the drug in the tumour *in vivo,* although far too little work of precision has been done on this. The assay method may have to be biochemical if it is to be effective in a clinical test. Compounds added for assay must not interact synergistically with any of the drugs tested and the assay should relate as closely as possible to the capacity of the cells, including the G_0 cells, for indefinite replication after drug treatment.

REFERENCE

Tubiana, M. (1971). *Br. J. Radiol. 44,* 325.

B. MONOLAYER CULTURES

(*i*) R. I. Freshney

1. PREPARATION OF PRIMARY CELL CULTURES

Principle
Human solid tumours, particularly those from breast, lung and gut, often contain a high proportion of fibrous stroma which makes conventional trypsin disaggregation rather difficult. We have found that collagenase will disaggregate such tumours and, moreover, viable cells may still be recovered even after prolonged exposure to the enzyme (up to 5 days; Freshney, 1972). Collagenase can be used in regular culture medium and is apparently not inhibited by serum.

A further advantage of the collagenase method is that the stromal cells are dissociated first and, if the exposure time is chosen carefully, a stage may be selected when small clumps of epithelial cells, more resistant to collagenase, can be separated by their rate of sedimentation from the more freely dispersed fibroblasts.

It has been suggested that intermittent treatment of cultures with collagenase, after monolayer has formed, favours the selection of epithelial cells (Lasfargues, 1971). We have found that some cells from human tumour samples will adhere in the presence of collagenase and, morphologically at least, appear to be different from the cultures derived from a total disaggregate.

Protocol
(1) Tumour biopsy collected in SF12/PSKF and freed of obvious contamination with fatty, fibrous or necrotic tissue. Transported to

tissue culture laboratory. If any delay involved at this stage, store at 4° C.

(2) Transfer to DBSS in petri dish, and rinse.

(3) Transfer again to fresh DBSS and chop to about 2 mm pieces.

(4) Transfer pieces by pipette (always wet the inside of the pipette first), using a wide tipped 10 ml pipette to a universal container.

(5) Allow pieces to settle, discard supernatant, add 15 ml fresh DBSS.

(6) Repeat (5) three times.

(7) Re-suspend pieces in last DBSS wash and transfer to culture vessels: about 50-100 pieces in one F25 flask and about 10-20 in a second.

(8) Allow to settle and discard supernatant.

(9) Add 4·5 ml SF12/20/PSG to each flask and 0·5 ml collagenase.

(10) Place at 37° C for from 24 hr to 5 days. Disaggregation will become evident by the "smearing" of the fragments and the appearance of smaller fragments and free cells on gently shaking the bottle.

(11) When the bulk of the fragments break down on gentle agitation, pipette the suspension up and down and transfer to 15 ml DBSS in a universal container. If this suspension is allowed to stand for about 10-15 min the remaining undissociated clumps of cells will settle to the bottom and may be separated from the bulk of the suspension. The sediment may then be washed and allowed to settle again several times to remove single cells. The washings can be added to the supernatant suspension from the first sedimentation.

(12) Spin down the supernatant suspension at 200 g for 5 min.

(13) Re-suspend the sediment from (11) in 2-5 ml medium (depending on the yield) and inoculate an F25 flask.

(14) Re-suspend the pellet from (12) in 6 ml medium. Take 10 ml of this and dilute to 5 ml with medium. Inoculate both suspensions separately into F25 flasks. The cells may be counted at this stage, though it is difficult to predict the optimum concentration for survival. As a rough guide they should be between 5×10^4/ml and 5×10^5/ml, though differences in viability and potential culture survival make these figures unreliable.

(15) Flasks should be checked after 24 hr for pH changes and the medium changed in high density samples if necessary. In general the culture from the sedimenting clumps in (11) will contain a higher proportion of epithelial cells than the suspension.

REFERENCES

Freshney, R. I. (1972). *Lancet*, Sept. 2, p. 488.
Lasfargues, E. Y. (1971). Human Mammary Tumours. *In* "Tissue Culture, Methods and Application" (P. Kruse and M. K. Patterson, eds.), p. 45. Academic Press, New York and London.

REAGENTS AND MATERIALS

SF12   Ham's F12 medium supplemented with Eagle's MEM amino acids, 10X folic acid, and lacking thymidine and hypoxanthine.

SF12/PSKF   SF12 with a high antibiotic concentration:
    250 units/ml penicillin
    250 μg/ml streptomycin
    100 μg/ml Kanamycin or 50 μg/ml gentamycin
    2·5 μg/ml Amphotericin B.

BSS   Hank's balanced salt solution without bicarbonate.

DBSS   Hank's balanced salt solution as above with antibiotics as in SF12/PSKF.

SF12/20/PSG   SF12 supplemented with 20% selected foetal bovine serum and antibiotics:
    50 units/ml penicillin
    100 μg/ml streptomycin
    50 μg/ml gentamycin or 100 μg/ml Kanamycin.

Collagenase   Worthington CLS grade 2000 units/ml in BSS, final concentration in medium 200 units/ml.

F25   Falcon 25 cm^2 disposable plastic flask (Code 3012).

2. MEASUREMENT OF CYTOTOXICITY OF ANTI-NEOPLASTIC DRUGS IN MONOLAYER CULTURES

Principle

This method has been developed with HeLa cells for ultimate use with human tumour material. It relies on the measurement of residual protein synthetic capacity after drug removal as an index of survival. If a prolonged recovery period is employed then the assay will measure the inhibition of proliferative ability rather than the immediate effects of cytotoxicity.

Protocol   Short Assay (Cytotoxicity)

(1) Trypsinise monolayer culture in exponential phase of growth.
(2) Dilute in medium to give 2×10^4 cells/ml.
(3) Inoculate microtitration tray(s), 0·2 ml/well.
(4) Place in humid incubator at 36·5°C with 5% CO_2 gas phase.

Plates should be contained in plastic "sandwich box" (see Fig. 1, p. 38) swabbed out previously with 70% EtOH and having a layer of cellulose wadding in the bottom, saturated with sterile BSS.

(5) After 48 hr drugs may be added to the left-hand side of the plate and diluted serially across the plate. It is best to avoid the outer row of wells all round the plate, since they tend to grow less well than the rest of the plate; they should, however, contain cells at an equivalent or higher cell concentration and not simply be left empty. Hence each dilution series will be A2-A9, B2-B9, etc; wells 10 and 11 are left free of drug to act as controls.

(6) After 24 hr at 36·5°C the drugs are removed and the wells washed three times with BSS containing 10% calf serum. Care must be taken with any addition or removal that cells are not dislodged from the monolayer.

(7) After washing free of drugs, add 0·1 ml fresh medium to each well and return plate to incubator for 4 hr.

(8) After 4 hr recovery, add 0·1 ml ^{3}H-4,5-leucine 20 μCi/ml, to each well and return to incubator for 3 hr.

(9) Remove medium slowly by suction (avoid dislodging cells) and wash plate gently with BSS at 37°C.

(10) Add methanol directly to BSS wash, decant, and replace with fresh methanol. Fix for 10 min, remove methanol and air dry (this helps monolayer to stick).

(11) Place plate on ice, add 10% TCA, ice cold, to all wells (a gentle stream from a wash bottle directed onto the side of each well). Repeat 3 times, 5 min each wash.

(12) Wash off remaining TCA with methanol and dry.

(13) Add 0·1 ml N NaOH to each well and leave overnight at room temperature to dissolve protein.

(14) Transfer the contents of each well to separate scintillation vials with plastic inserts.

(15) Acidify with 0·1 ml 1·1 N HCl and add 2 ml scintillation fluid.

(16) Count on scintillation counter.

(17) Calculate percentage inhibition within each row relative to the control, plot against drug concentration and derive ID_{50} (drug concentration causing 50% inhibition).

REAGENTS AND MATERIALS

Trypsin   0·25% Bacto trypsin (1:250) in isotonic citrate-saline.

Medium   Ham's F12 supplemented with Eagle's MEM amino acids, 10X folic acid concentration and lacking thymidine and hypoxanthine.

BSS   Hank's BSS without bicarbonate or glucose.

^{3}*H-4,5-leucine*   Radiochemical Centre.

TCA   Trichloracetic Acid, Analar, BDH, 10% w/v.

Scintillation Fluid   Toluene based with triton X.

Microtitration trays   Falcon (Becton-Dickinson)
         Limbro (Biocult, Flow)
         Nuclan
         Dynatech.

(*ii*) P. P. Dendy
(based on methods of Limburg and co-workers)

1. CULTURE OF A SOLID SPECIMEN

(a) Specimens which cannot be collected or cultured immediately are placed in a balanced salt solution at pH 7·2 and stored at 4° C. We find no evidence of loss of *in vitro* growth ability provided specimens are cultured within 24 hr.

(b) The specimen is transferred using sterile instruments to a petri dish and suitable tumour is carefully selected. This is placed in a small centrifuge tube and chopped finely with curved scissors.

(c) 0·2% trypsin is then added to this mash which is transferred to a conical flask containing a PTFE coated magnetic flea. The solution is agitated fairly vigorously on a magnetic stirrer for 20 min at 37° C and the supernatant is poured through a gauze filter. The filtrate is centrifuged and re-suspended in feeding medium comprising 90 parts 199 medium + 10 parts foetal calf serum + 5 parts 5% lactalbumin hydrolysate + bicarbonate to pH 7·2.

(d) A small aliquot is placed on a haemocytometer and examined under the microscope. The cell concentration is counted and a small quantity of trypan blue is added to check for viability. The bulk is set aside to await further fractions.

(e) More trypsin is added to the residual tissue and stages c and d are repeated until all the cells have been released. Suitable fractions are then pooled, diluted to 3×10^5 cells/ml and 24 tubes are seeded with 1 ml each.

(f) The tubes are placed in a perspex rack so that each tube is inclined at about 8° to the horizontal. Silicone bungs are used to seal the tubes, which are then labelled and placed in the incubator. Screw topped tubes are not satisfactory because some of them are not quite airtight and the pH of the culture medium becomes too alkaline.

2. ASCITES AND PLEURAL FLUIDS

(a) Fluid specimens are collected in sterile Lanes bottles. 25,000 units/litre heparin is added to reduce clotting.

(b) The fluid is poured into 250 cc centrifuge tubes and spun at 1500 rpm. The cell pellet is re-suspended in feeding medium, examined under the haemocytometer and seeded at 3×10^5 viable cells/ml into tubes.

3. A DRUG TEST

Satisfactory monolayers, suitable for drug testing are usually obtained after 2-5 days in culture.

(a) Drugs are selected and appropriate labels are written.

(b) Water soluble drugs are diluted by sequential methods using plastic syringes and pipette holders according to a specified schedule.

(c) Water insoluble and non-sterile drugs are first dissolved in a small quantity of absolute alcohol using a glass syringe. The alcohol is subsequently diluted at least 1000 : 1 and is not toxic at this concentration.

(d) Initial dilutions are made in balanced salt solution at pH 7·2. The final dilution is made into an equal volume of feeding medium and Hanks balanced salt solution.

4. MEASUREMENT OF ^{125}IODODEOXYURIDINE UPTAKE

(a) After 24 hr exposure to drugs, cells are returned to 50% drug free medium for 24 hr.

(b) The tubes are then given full feeding medium containing 0·06 μCi/ml ^{125}Iododeoxyuridine for 24 hr, before being washed three times in saline and re-fed.

(c) At this stage there appears to be firmly attached label adsorbed either to the glass or to the cells.

(d) 24 hr later it has been released into the medium so the cells can be washed once more, re-fed and the stable bound activity can be counted in a sodium iodide crystal well counter.

5. ESTIMATE OF CELL NUMBERS

It is useful to know at the end of the test how many cells were present during assay of ^{125}Iododeoxyuridine uptake. This is also a check for overcrowding. The following procedure gives a suspension of single cells—essential for automatic counting—from the majority of specimens. Unfortunately it does impair viability.

(a) The feeding medium is replaced by 1 ml of 0·02% versene.

(b) After 2 min 1 ml of 0·2% trypsin and 1 drop ($\sim$0·05 ml) of 5% trypsin is added. The pH is carefully adjusted with bicarbonate.

(c) When all the cells are detached, 8 ml saline is added and the suspension is pipetted vigorously at least 50 times.

(d) Cell numbers are measured with a Coulter counter.

6. MICROCULTURE OF SMALL SOLID SPECIMENS

(a) The procedure follows that for larger solids except that the tissue is trypsinised in a 10 ml conical flask with a magnetic flea only $\frac{1}{2}$ cm long. 0·1 ml only of tumour cell suspension (3×10^4 cells) is seeded into each well of a microtiter tray and the tray is covered with parafilm.

(b) After exposure to drug for 24 hr the wells are re-fed with drug free medium for 24 hr and then fresh medium containing 1 μCi/ml ^{3}H thymidine is added.

(c) 24 hr later the cultures are fixed in 25% acetic acid in ethanol for 15 min followed by 70% ethanol for 5 min.

(d) The wells are punched out, mounted cells upward on gelatinised slides, autoradiographed with Ilford K2 liquid emulsion, stored for 3 days, developed, fixed and examined under the microscope.

7. STORAGE IN LIQUID NITROGEN

Storage of disaggregated tumour cells in liquid nitrogen before the cells have been cultured, and their recovery in a viable state is difficult. We have been unsuccessful using a number of methods which work well after the cells have been grown *in vitro*. The following procedure has been successful.

(a) Make a cell suspension in feeding medium at about 2×10^6 cells/ml and cool to $0°$C in ice cold water. Add 10% dimethyl sulphoxide and quickly transfer to 1 ml ampoules.

(b) Place the ampoules in a pre-cooled box made of expanded polystyrene and lined with cotton wool. The polystyrene should be about 2-3 cm thick.

(c) Put the box in the vapour phase of a liquid nitrogen container and allow to cool slowly overnight. Store the ampoules immersed in liquid nitrogen.

(d) To recover the cells, the rate at which they are warmed to $0°C$ is relatively unimportant but the dimethyl sulphoxide *must be diluted out slowly* with constant gentle mixing before addition of further medium. A suggested procedure is to add to 1 ml of cell suspension 0·25 ml, 0·25 ml, 0·5 ml, 1·0 ml, 2·0 ml and 4·0 ml medium with thorough mixing after each addition.

(e) Centrifuge, re-suspend in feeding medium, count and estimate viability in the usual way and seed into test tubes.

Using this method we have obtained 75% viability and good subsequent monolayer growth for tumour cell suspensions frozen directly after biopsy trypsinisation and stored for 2 weeks at liquid nitrogen temperature.

(*iii*) G. J. Wiepjes and F. J. A. Prop

SEQUENTIAL ENZYMATIC DIGESTION FOR MAMMARY TUMOURS

The procedure is an adaptation of the principle of sequential enzyme treatment published earlier (Wiepjes and Prop, 1970; Prop and Wiepjes, 1973) to provide a high cell yield from the majority of human mammary tumours and successful cultures in most cases.

(1) The sooner after re-section or biopsy the tissue is obtained, the better the results. Excess adipose and connective tissue are removed.

(2) The tumour is cut into thin slices using forceps and a surgical blade (No. 11). To reduce cell damage it is essential to make cutting movements, not merely to apply pressure. Very hard scirrhous tumours are sliced using a tissue sectioner of the McIlwain type. This causes more cell damage but saves time and the time factor is important.

(3) The slices are rapidly rinsed in two changes of a calcium and magnesium free balanced salt solution (CMF) (NaCl 8·00, KCl 0·30, $NaH_2PO_4.H_2O$ 0·05, KH_2PO_4 0·025, $NaHCO_3$ 1·00, glucose 2·00 g/litre) containing 1000 U/ml penicillin-Na and 0·5 mg/ml streptomycin sulphate.

(4) Subsequently the slices are cut into small cubes approximately $\frac{1}{2}$ mm long using crossed scalpels with No. 11 blades, again taking care to cut and not press, to minimise mechanical damage.

(5) The diced tumour is added to 25 ml CMF including antibiotics as above in an Erlenmeyer vial and stirred gently on a gyrotary shaker (70 rpm, $\frac{3}{4}''$ rotation) at 36° C for 30 min.

(6) The CMF with debris and blood elements is pipetted off and replaced by 15-30 ml CMF containing 250 U/ml collagenase (Worthington, code: CLS)*, 0·1% hyaluronidase (Sigma type I) and 4% demineralised bovine albumin (Poviet Producten N.V.). The tissue is digested for 3 hr on the gyrotary shaker at 36° C.

(7) The supernatant fluid is then replaced by 15-30 ml pronase 1·5% (CalBiochem, B grade) in medium 199 and digestion on the gyrotary shaker continues for one hour at 36° C.

(8) Twice the fluid volume of ice-cold human serum is added to stop enzyme action. The cells are then spun down at 200 g for 5 min. The supernatant is discarded and the cell pellet is very gently re-suspended in at least 20 ml of culture medium (0·5% lactalbumin hydrolysate, 20% human male serum in Hanks (BSS). Re-suspension is followed by filtration through a No. 1 sintered glass filter (pore width 90-150 μm). The filtrate contains single cells and small cell clumps. These are washed twice in culture medium by centrifugation and re-suspension performed as described above. Dye exclusion tests using Erythrosin B at a final concentration of 0·036% give an estimate of the viable percentage of cells.

(9) The cell concentration is measured with a Coulter counter or a Fuchs-Rosenthal cytometer and the final required concentration is obtained by dilution of the suspension with culture medium. If all preceding operations have been performed under normal aseptic conditions, there is no need to add antibiotics to the cultures. These cultures will adhere well to glass and plastic tissue culture vessels.

(10) Medium should be renewed when the pH drops below 7·0 as shown by the phenol red indicator and in any event at least once a week. Cultures in good condition and of moderate cell densities will require medium renewal two or three times a week. Very dense cultures require daily renewal.

Although it is known that collagenase requires the presence of calcium and magnesium ions for its activity (Lasfargues and Moore, 1971) it should be noted that during the collagenase step a calcium and magnesium free medium is used. Results are definitely better with the method described than when using calcium and magnesium

* We are presently working out a modified procedure for the more purified CLS 3.

containing media in the first steps of the procedure. Probably sufficient amounts of calcium and magnesium are left to guarantee collagenase activity while the low level of these ions helps to preserve cell integrity.

Sometimes, mainly after dissection with the tissue sectioner, a mucous gel develops in which the cells are trapped during the procedure. Treatment with 0·04% DNA-ase—3 drops in 20 ml medium—(Worthington, code D) will dissolve this gel.

Cell yields vary considerably depending on the cell-richness of the tumour and the amount of tissue available. Viability measured by dye exclusion is often about 80% but only about 30% of the cells adhere to the culture vessel bottom and those which remain in suspension finally prove to be non-viable.

REFERENCES

Lasfargues, E. Y., Moore, D. H. (1971). *In vitro*, 7, 21.

Prop, F. J. A., Wiepjes, G. J. (1973). *In* "Tissue Culture Methods and Applications" (P. F. Kruse and M. K. Patterson, eds.), p. 21. Academic Press, New York and London.

Wiepjes, G. J., Prop, F. J. A. (1970). *Exptl. Cell Res. 61*, 451.

C. CELL SUSPENSION CULTURES

(*i*) J. Mattern

1. PREPARATION OF CELL SUSPENSION

(a) Solid tumours were removed under sterile conditions, reduced to small pieces which were suspended in a Hanks solution and drawn several times through the capillary of a pipette.

(b) The resulting cell suspensions were filtered through gauze and centrifuged for 5 min at 200 g. After decanting the Hanks solution and re-suspending the sediment in TCM-199, the suspensions were adjusted to a specific cell count (5×10^5 cells/ml, measured using a Neubauer counting chamber).

2. TEST PROCEDURE

(a) The cell suspensions were divided into aliquots of 0·9 ml, put into test tubes with cytostatic drugs, and preincubated by shaking at $37°$ C in a waterbath for 2 hr.

(b) The appropriate radioactive precursor (^{3}H thymidine, ^{3}H uridine, ^{3}H deoxyuridine) was then added to a final concentration of 2·5 μCi per ml medium.

(c) At certain defined intervals, 100 μl aliquots of the cell suspensions were removed from the tubes, pipetted on to filter paper discs and dried in a stream of warm air. The acid soluble radioactive material was removed by extraction twice for 30 min with 5% ice cold trichloroacetic acid. The discs were washed with ethanol/ether (1:1) for 20 min, after which the total incorporated radioactivity was measured in a liquid scintillation-spectrometer.

(ii) G. Wüst

Fresh human tumour material straight from theatre is cultured in a manner similar to that of Rajewsky (1966) (see Wüst and Matthes, 1970).

(1) A mechanical chopper is used to cut pieces off the tumour 0·5 cm long and 400 μ thick. Each test comprises 10-15 such slices in Eagles basal medium.

(2) In vitro doses of chemotherapeutic agents are obtained by finding the body fluid concentration when a therapeutic dose is administered in vivo. Concentrations equal to 1/10X, 10X, 50X, and 100X this figure are tested in vitro.

(3) The chemotherapeutic agent and either ^{3}H thymidine or ^{3}H uridine at 5 μCi/ml are added to the medium containing tumour pieces.

(4) The medium is enriched with 5% CO_2 in oxygen for 10 min at 4° C and the cultures are then incubated for several hours in a shaking thermostat.

(5) For studies on the effect of hyperthermia, incubations are at 37·0° C, 39·0° C and 41·0° C.

(6) Tritium counts are made in a Packard Tri Carb liquid scintillation spectrometer (model 3003) and expressed in counts per min per mg tumour dry weight.

REFERENCES

Rajewsky, M. F. (1966). Biophysik, 3, 65.
Wüst, G. P., and Matthes, K. J. (1970). Z. Krebsforsch. 73, 204.

D. FREE-FLOATING SLICE CULTURE

John A. Dickson and Mohammad Suzangar

(1) The tumour is transported from the operating theatre to the laboratory in an ice-container and is maintained at this temperature until placed in culture. Sterile technique is adhered to throughout the establishment of the cultures.

(2) A frozen section is performed on the specimen to confirm the diagnosis of malignancy. The tumour is placed in a Petri dish and washed with Rinaldini Saline (Rinaldini, 1959) containing penicillin (100 units/ml), streptomycin (100 μg/ml) and Mycostatin (100 units/ml). Necrotic material and surrounding normal tissue are carefully dissected free from the tumour before it is sectioned. This is an important step, since although the stroma of tumours usually incorporates only slight amounts of labelled precursors, the normal tissue of origin of the neoplasm, e.g. intestinal mucosa, can take up significant amounts of nucleosides (Wolberg, 1969).

(3) The tumour is diced into thin slices less than 1 cu mm in size using cataract knives or scalpel blades. The sections are then allocated at random into aliquots of approximately 100 mg to minimize the effects of tumour heterogeneity.

(4) For culture, 100 mg tissue is placed in 3 ml Waymouth medium MB 752/1, supplemented with 10% pooled human AB serum, in 5 cm diameter plastic Petri dishes (Esco grade A; Esco Rubber Ltd., London) and placed in a CO_2 incubator (gas phase 5% CO_2 in air, humidity 100%) at 37·5° C. The method is described as "free-floating" slice culture, the fragments being suspended without support in the nutrient medium. Cytotoxic drugs and isotopic precursors are added to the medium in 0·1 ml aqueous solution. The cultures are maintained without change of medium for 24 hr. The effect of a cytotoxic drug or other agent on metabolism over this culture period is then assessed over 6 hr. For this, the slices are washed in warm Rinaldini saline and transferred to fresh medium containing isotopic (^{14}C-labelled at 0·5 μCi/ml initial concentration) thymidine, uridine or leucine but no drug and incubated for a further 6 hr; similarly, aliquots of the washed tumour are placed in buffer and their respiration (O_2 uptake) or glycolysis (CO_2 production) measured by Warburg manometry over 6 hr at 37·5° C, again in the absence of drug.

This method of culture has evolved over a period of several years work with slices of human tumours. It has been found that the metabolism and response to cytotoxic drugs of free-floating tumour slices are similar to those of slices supported at a gas-liquid interface. Nor has the traditional organ culture gas mixture of 95% O_2/5% CO_2 proved superior to air/5% CO_2 for these short-term cultures. The value of 5% CO_2 in O_2 for organised cultures has also been questioned by other workers (see Dickson, 1970a).

After 24 hr in culture, O_2 uptake of the tumour slices was often less, and CO_2 production more, than in the fresh tumour; the change was usually about 30%. It was found that the extent of the change in respiration and glycolysis could be minimised by including 0·5% yeast ultrafiltrate (Oxoid Ltd., London), or the patient's own serum (10%), in the culture medium. Although these agents have been found to be of benefit in prolonging survival of human tumour fragments *in vitro* (see Wolff and Wolff, 1967, and Roller *et al.* 1966 respectively), the effect of their inclusion in the medium of free-floating short-term cultures was not consistent enough to warrant their routine use; the presence of these supplements did not alter the tumour response to drugs.

Minimal necrosis is observed in histological sections following culture, and the active tumour metabolism is reflected by nucleoside uptake obtained in autoradiographs at the end of 30 hr. Maintenance of active metabolism in tumours cultured by this method is probably a reflection of the predominantly glycolytic pattern of metabolism in human cancers (Aisenberg, 1961; Macbeth and Bekesi, 1962; Bickis and Henderson, 1966).

The amounts of tumour required for assay can be considerably reduced (to 25-50 mg) by the use of miniature culture vessels and micro-respirometers. The technique is a versatile one: in addition to studying the effects of various modalities (e.g. drugs, hyperthermia) on tumours by the parameters described, more sophisticated biochemical investigations are feasible. For examination of alternative metabolic pathways with differentially labelled glucose, for example, the tumour can be cultured in sealed units of the Filter-Well type that permit collection of radioactive CO_2 at the end of the experimental period (Dickson, 1970b). Thus, all three components of the culture system, the tissue, the medium and the gas phase are amenable to analysis.

REFERENCES

Aisenberg, A. C. (1962). "The Glycolysis and Respiration of Tumours". Academic Press, New York and London.

Bickis, I. J. and Henderson, I. W. D. (1966). *Cancer, 19,* 89.
Dickson, J. A. (1970*a*). *Lab. Practice, 19,* 912.
Dickson, J. A. (1970*b*). *Cancer Res. 30,* 2336.
Macbeth, R. A. and Bekesi, J. G. (1962). *Cancer Res. 22,* 244.
Rinaldini, L. M. J. (1959). *Exptl. Cell Res. 16,* 477.
Roller, M., Owen, S. P. and Heidelberger, C. (1966). *Cancer Res. 26,* 626.
Wolberg, W. (1969). *Cancer Res. 29,* 2137.
Wolff, E. M. and Wolff, E. T. (1967). *In* "Cell Differentiation", Ciba Symposium
    (A. V. S. de Reuck and J. Knight, eds.), p. 208. Churchill, London.

E. ORGAN CULTURE

(*i*) L. Morasca

1. COLLECTION OF TISSUE

To avoid cell death and bacterial contamination either of which would prevent cultures being established the surgeon must follow several rules:

(a) Extremes of temperature including electro-coagulation or the use of hot sterile instruments must be avoided since cancer cells will certainly die above 42° C and below 0° C.

(b) The use of antiseptics and detergents on surgical equipment or gloves which come in contact with the tissue must be carefully avoided.

(c) The concept of sterility should be re-evaluated. Because the human body is well equipped to counteract quite a large number of non-pathogen contaminants, a surgeon needs only to have a pathogen free low saprofite area. For tissue culture samples absolute sterility is essential. Thus tissue to be collected should be touched only with fresh instruments kept sterile on a table until the last minute. The tissue must be placed immediately in a closed container of appropriate size.

(d) The first dissection of the specimen must be performed immediately by a trained tissue culture technician. Fragments of 10 x 5 mm must be taken from areas of different consistency and colour and stored each in a 30 ml screw-cap test tube containing 199 TC medium without serum or bicarbonate, supplemented with 50 μg/ml Gentamycin.

(e) Transportation to the tissue culture laboratory should be immediate keeping the tissue at room temperature.

2. PREPARATION OF CULTURES

(a) The different samples collected must be checked for typical cancer areas.

(b) The fragments containing cancer cells are dissected into smaller areas in an effort to separate grossly different tissues.

(c) From each batch of fragments, representative samples are squashed in acetic orcine. This last step permits comparison of the aspects seen in the frozen preparations with the actual structures present in the different batches of fragments.

(d) The fragments are cut between two sharp blades in explants 1 mm in size. They are then ready for implantation in Rose's chambers (Rose *et al.* 1958).

(e) The assembly of these chambers is performed as described by Morasca *et al.* (1973). A coverslip is glued with a drop of paraffin jelly on the bottom retaining plate and three explants are laid in the centre. A strip of perforated cellophane 5 mm wide (Microbiological Associates, Bethesda, Maryland, U.S.A.) sterilised by autoclaving in Hank's BSS is then laid across the coverslip covering the fragments. The two edges of the cellophane strip must reach the border of the chamber to permit a silicone gasket to hold the strip firmly in place. The gasket is covered by a second coverslip and by the retaining plate. The four screws are inserted and tightened until a syringe needle can be inserted through the silicone gasket. The screws are then further tightened, bearing in mind that the two retaining plates will buckle if too tight, except in the case of the modified Rose Chambers or the short plates of our infusion chamber (Morasca and Rainisio, 1966; Rose *et al.* 1970).

(f) Culture medium is injected by a syringe through the silicone gasket of the chamber using the needle already inserted as an air vent. The culture medium is 199 buffered by Hepes, fortified by 20% calf serum and protected from contaminants by 10 μg/ml of Gentamicin.

(g) One standard experiment requires about 100 Rose chambers. These chambers are checked daily for outgrowing cells by low power phase contrast microscopy.

(h) When migrating cells are observed the coverslip of the chamber is marked on the outside by a spring-mounted rubber stamp leaving an ink circle around the area of interest.

(i) A photograph is taken, a number is given to the chamber, and culture medium is immediately replaced by fresh medium containing one of the drug concentrations to be studied.

(j) The field or fields chosen initially are photographed at different time intervals during treatment or recovery. The photographic records are contact printed from 35 mm film and directly compared.

(k) It is possible to evaluate the response of different cell types to the same treatment, detecting the toxicity both as a morphological alteration (cytotoxic endpoint), or as a lethal effect (lethal endpoint). The latter effect is the most relevant when cell killing agents are studied and can be studied for a long time after treatment simply by putting the cells back in fresh growth medium. This procedure allows evaluation of delayed toxicity, as well as unsuspected recovery of heavily damaged cells.

REFERENCES

Morasca, L. and Rainisio, L. (1966). *Experientia, 22,* 337.
Morasca, L. and Balconi, G. (1973). *Europ. J. Cancer, 9,* 301.
Rose, G. G., Pomerat, L. M., Shindler, T. P. and Trunnel, J. B. (1958). *J. Bioph. Bioch. Cytol. 4,* 761.
Rose, G. G., Kumegawa, M., Nikai, H., Bracho, M. and Cattoni, M. (1970). *Microvascular Res. 2,* 24.

(*ii*) R. C. Hallowes

1. HUMAN ORGAN CULTURE

(a) The cancerous area was dissected free from fat, non-involved breast and any surgical trauma. It was cut into slabs about 15 mm × 10 mm × 1·2 mm thick and these were mounted in 7% ion agar on the specimen holder of a Sorvall TC-2 tissue sectioner. Slices 200-250 μm thick were cut and floated out into medium 199 in a petri dish placed on top of an X-ray viewing box.

(b) Individual slices were placed on top of stainless steel grids in plastic Repli boxes (Sterelin P103). Medium, with or without hormones, was added to each compartment so that the slices were interfaced between medium and the incubator atmosphere (95% oxygen and 5% carbon dioxide).

(c) After 20 hr culture, 2 μCi/ml ^{3}H-thymidine was added. Four hours later the slices were removed, washed in medium, blotted dry and weighed. They were homogenised, the DNA precipitated, collected and counted by scintillation.

2. CULTURE OF RAT BREAST CANCER

(a) The tumour was removed aseptically from the rat, rinsed with medium 199 to remove blood etc., and cut into 1-2 mm cubes using opposed scalpels. These cubes were mechanically chopped into 200 μm pieces and suspended in medium 199 plus 5% foetal calf serum (growth medium) to which collagenase (2 mg/ml) and hyaluronidase (1 mg/ml) were added.

(b) The pieces were digested for up to 90 min at 37°C, centrifuged at 100 g for 5 min and re-suspended in growth medium. The use of trypsin in the digestive mixture was avoided as this appeared to increase the number of fibroblasts produced and/or decrease the number of viable epithelial cells.

(c) The suspension was re-centrifuged at 100 g for 5 min and the cells and micro explants suspended in a volume of growth medium so that 0·1 ml of suspension could be added to each 30 mm plastic dish. A 1·5 cm diameter tumour yielded sufficient cells to plate 150 dishes. The volume per dish was made up to 2 ml by adding growth medium with or without added hormones.

(d) The medium was changed at 24 and 48 hr. At 67 hr, 0·2 μCi/ml ^{3}H-thymidine was added to each dish.

(e) At 69 hr the medium was removed, the cultures washed with warm 199 and all medium removed. The cultures were dissolved by 1N NaOH, DNA isolated and the radioactivity and total DNA determined.

3. HUMAN HISTOCULTURE—METHOD OF SHERWIN AND RICHTERS

(a) The growing edge of the carcinoma was selected and thin wedges of tissue prepared using opposed scalpels.

(b) Wedges with areas 2-3 cells thick were carefully placed on the lower glass of a Rose chamber and covered with sterile dialysis tubing.

(c) The chamber was assembled but was not tightened until the dialysis tubing had been stretched to hold and to compress slightly the histocultures.

(d) The chamber was filled with medium and this was changed once per week.

4. HUMAN HISTOCULTURE—METHOD OF HALLOWES AND LEWIS

(a) The growing edge of the carcinoma was selected and slices 200 μm thick were cut mechanically.

(b) These were transferred to either collagen-coated 30 mm plastic dishes or collagen-coated cover glasses. Collagen coating is necessary to ensure prolonged attachment of the slices to the culture surface.

(c) Sufficient medium was added so that surface tension kept the slices in contact with the collagen. Twenty-four hours later more medium was added and after a further 24 hr the full medium volume was added.

(d) Cultures were examined after 5 days and daily thereafter; those liberating fibroblasts were removed. Some histocultures did not release epithelial cells for up to 10-14 days.

(iii) D. I. Beeby

(1) After surgical removal from the patient each biopsy specimen was transported to the laboratory in medium 199.

(2) It was dissected by scalpel under sterile conditions into slices about 1 mm thick by 3-5 mm diameter. Two of these were fixed in 10% formal saline for subsequent histological examination. A further two were placed on cardice and stored at $-80°$ C for future pentose shunt dehydrogenase estimation.

(3) Several slices were cultured by a method based on that described by Trowell (1959). Slices were placed directly on stainless steel grids without interposing lens paper, agar slabs, etc., at the interface of Trowell's T8 medium and a gas phase of 95% oxygen and 5% carbon dioxide in plastic petri dishes 5 cm in diameter.

(4) Trowell's T8 was selected as being one of the simplest chemically defined synthetic media. To this was added insulin, glutamine and antibiotics.

(5) To ensure a standard gas phase surrounding all samples in one experiment, all the petri dishes were sealed inside a single modified plastic sandwich box (Fig. 1). All cultures were gassed for 10 min at the outset. The 72-hr cultures were regassed for 10 min at 24-hr intervals.

(6) Each experiment comprised 5 or 6 culture dishes with one grid per dish and 3 explants on a grid. We used 5 ml of medium per dish, and to all but one control dish, added 50 μl of a specific hormone solution. The hormones used were oestradiol 17β, testosterone, and tamoxifen a triphenylethylene compound with antioestrogenic properties donated by ICI Ltd., each in ethanolic solution, and MRC sheep prolactin in 0·9% saline. The final concentration of

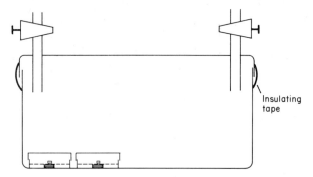

Fig. 1. Modified sandwich box used to provide the correct atmosphere of CO_2 and oxygen for tumour cultures.

hormones used in most experiments was 3 μg/ml of oestradiol, testosterone, or tamoxifen; or 1 μgm/ml of prolactin.

(7) Five experiments were conducted to determine the effects of differing concentrations of hormones on cultured tumours in which oestradiol and testosterone were each used in concentrations of 3, 0·3, and 0·03 μgm/ml, and prolactin of 1, 0·1, and 0·01 μgm/ml. We added an amount of alcohol to the control dishes and those containing prolactin, equivalent to that added in the other hormone solutions.

(iv) A. C. Riches

ORGAN CULTURE OF HUMAN BENIGN PROSTATIC HYPERPLASIA

The method is based on the technique introduced by Trowell (1954, 1959). Explants were prepared from the biopsy specimen which was transported dry in a sterile container in crushed ice.

(1) The tissue was first trimmed into small blocks and slices of about 3-5 mm square and 1 mm deep were cut using a sterile disposable scalpel.

(2) Small explants of tissue were placed on a square of millipore filter which was supported on a stainless steel grid.

(3) Eagles Minimum Essential Medium (3 ml) supplemented with 10% calf serum was added to 30 mm Petri dishes which were contained in a 90 mm Petri dish.

(4) The dishes were then gassed in a McIntosh and Fildes jar with 95% oxygen and 5% carbon dioxide and cultured at 37° C.

REFERENCES

Trowell, O. A. (1954). *Exp. Cell Res. 6*, 246.
Trowell, O. A. (1959). *Exp. Cell Res. 16*, 118.

(*v*) G. M. Hodges

1. TISSUE

Tumour specimen is

(a) Placed in a sterile Petri dish containing Hank's balanced salt solution.

(b) Cut into small explants approximately 1-2 mm^2.

(c) Transferred onto membrane filter squares either

    (i) cellulose acetate—Millipore RA 1·2 μ pore size

    (ii) polycarbonate plastic—Nucleopore NO 0·4 μ pore size

    (iii) cellophane (Visking)

2. CULTURE SYSTEM (BASED ON TROWELL, 1954)

Tumour/membrane assemblies are either

(a) Placed on expanded stainless steel grid platforms standing in small dishes containing 5 ml of medium. The medium is previously added to the dish up to the level of the platform. The small dishes are enclosed in Petri dishes containing surgical lint previously moistened with sterile double distilled water, or

(b) Placed over 3-4 mm holes punched in flat expanded stainless steel grids lying in small Anumbra optical glass dishes containing 2 ml of medium. (This system can be used for cinematography).

3. CULTURE MEDIUM (BASED ON MELCHER AND HODGES, 1968)

Waymouth's MB 752/1 medium supplemented with

    0·45 g/ml ferrous sulphate

    300 g/ml ascorbic acid

    1·0 g/ml hydrocortisone sodium succinate

    10% calf serum

    100 units/ml penicillin/streptomycin

4. GAS PHASE

5% carbon dioxide in air.

5. CONDITIONS OF INCUBATION

Culture incubated at 36·5° C in sealed, humidified chambers. Medium and gas phase renewed every three days.

REFERENCES

Melcher, A. H. and Hodges, G. M. (1968). *Nature, Lond. 219*, 301.
Trowell, O. A. (1954). *Exp. Cell Res. 6*, 246.

F. Techniques of Organotypic Culture

Et. Wolff

The techniques employed for the culture of human tumours derive from those developed for cultures of mouse and rat tumours. Initially, the mesonephros was used as nutrient substrate, acting as intermediary between the medium and the tumour. In later studies, dialysing membranes were interposed between the mesonephros and the tumour. Still later, living embryonic organs were replaced, first by dialysates then by active fractions of these dialysates.

It should be pointed out that the basic medium used in all these experiments, as in those concerning organ cultures, is a nutrient medium which contains either embryo extract and serum or serum alone. Living embryonic organs are used as aliments when they are in direct contact with the cancerous tissues; in addition, they provide growth-promoting substances. Extracts of normal tissues, dialysates of these extracts, and various fractions prepared from them provide the tumours with substances indispensable for their growth. In their absence, the culture media, although adequate for normal embryonic organs, are insufficient despite their rich nutrient capacity for the survival and development of tumours.

1. CULTURES OF HUMAN TUMOURS ON MESONEPHROS

The following medium has been developed by us (Et. Wolff and Em. Wolff, 1960):

1% agar in Gey's solution	10 vol
Horse serum	4 vol
Embryo extract diluted at 50% in Tyrode's solution	4 vol
Penicillin and various other antibiotics	several drops

Fragments of the tumour are placed on the medium next to fragments of the mesonephros of roughly similar dimensions (0·1 to 0·2-mm cube). They form a mosaic of small polygons which generally fuse with one another.

An improvement in the technique consists of spreading a piece of the vitelline membrane of a non-incubated chicken egg over the medium. The mosaic of tumour and mesonephros fragments is deposited on the membrane. The latter is then folded over the explants so as to envelop them in a kind of bag. The vitelline membrane thus serves as an intermediary between the medium and the explants on the one hand and the explants and the atmosphere on the other. It plays no part in the nutrition of the culture, but facilitates exchanges, allows the explants to spread out more thinly over a larger area, and promotes their fusion.

2. CULTURES ON MESONEPHROS WITH INTERPOSITION OF A VITELLINE MEMBRANE OR A DIALYSIS MEMBRANE (ET. WOLFF AND EM. WOLFF, 1961).

A logical development of the aforementioned technique was to determine whether the living mesonephros was necessary for the culture of tumours. Must the tumours be in direct contact with the embryonic tissue or can they be sustained by the substances produced by the mesonephros which diffuse across the filtering membrane?

The same technique as before was used, but this time only the fragments of mesonephros were placed in the "bag" formed by the folded vitelline membrane. The tumour fragments were placed on top, thus being separated from the mesonephros by the membrane. The latter was then folded a second time over the tumour explants. Thus the two sorts of explants were separated by a fold of membrane. Although the pores of the membrane allowed large molecules to pass, no structural elements could cross: only substances in solution or fine suspension could filter through the pores.

Thus the tumour fragments were able to use dissolved substances derived from the culture medium and, equally, diffusable substances exuded from mesonephros. Both categories of substances have been found to be indispensable for the culture.

In certain experiments, the vitelline membrane was replaced by dialysing membranes (cellophane, Visking tubing) for which the upper limits of permeability are known (mol wt 15,000) (Et. Wolff and Em. Wolff, 1966).

In subsequent experiments, we replaced the embryonic organs by dialysates of yeast or of liver from young chickens (Em. Wolff *et al.* 1966). These experiments were suggested by the preceding step, in which tumour explants were nourished by diffusion across a membrane. It should be noted that in such media embryo extract and serum were always present (under certain conditions, however, only the scrum was retained).

3. WITH DIALYSATES

(a) *With yeast dialysate*

Having found that mesonephros extract was toxic, we decided to use an extract of an acetone powder of brewers yeast and, subsequently, the dialysate of this extract (Et. Wolff *et al.* 1965).

The composition of the culture medium was as follows:

1% agar in Gey's solution	11 vol
Horse serum	4 vol
Extract of eight and a half-day chick embryo diluted 50% in	
Tyrode's solution	4 vol
Yeast extract	1 vol

The yeast extract is prepared in the following way: yeast (aerobic, Fould-Springer) is treated with 10 vol of acetone at $0°$ C. The suspension is disrupted in a blender capable of breaking the nuclei and filtered through paper. The residue is left to dry and the fine powder obtained is re-suspended in Tyrode's solution and incubated for 3 hr at $37°$ C. After centrifugation at 1000 g for 15 min, the supernatant is sterilised by filtration through millipore membranes. It is this preparation which is used in the cultures.

The control media are prepared with the same ingredients minus the yeast extract. The explants used initially were tumour nodules previously cultured for several months on a dialysing membrane and derived, respectively, from the 107th passage of tumour strain Z 200 and the 60th passage of tumour strain Z 516.

4. WITH DIALYSATE OF MESONEPHROS FROM CHICK EMBRYO OF LIVER FROM YOUNG CHICKEN (EM. WOLFF *ET AL.* 1967).

(a) *Dialysate of mesonephros from chick embryo*

Cultures grown on a crude extract of 8-10 day mesonephros decline rapidly because of the toxicity of the extract. However, the dialysate was found to be favourable for the tumour culture. It is prepared from a homogenate in Tyrode's solution of 8-10 day mesonephros. The dialysis is carried out, as for yeast extracts, against distilled water, using Visking tubing. The dialysate is reduced by rotary evaporation to the initial volume of the mesonephros homogenate.

(b) *Dialysate of liver from young chicken (Croisille et al. 1967)*

At first, dialysates were prepared in the same manner from homogenates of livers from 8 to 10 day embryos. However, on account of the considerable number of embryos required to prepare these extracts, tests were performed to determine whether dialysates of liver from 3 month old chickens gave the same results. These were found to be just as active as the extracts of embryonic organs, and for this reason they have been used regularly ever since.

(c) *Preparation of the dialysate of liver homogenate*

Fifty grams of liver from 3 month old chickens is suspended in 90 ml of a 1:1 dilution of Tyrode's solution with distilled water and homogenised in a blender (type H 451, Equipements Industriels, Paris) at 40,000 rpm for $2\frac{1}{2}$ min. The homogenate is dialysed in tubes of Visking cellulose (Union Carbide, Chicago) at 4° C against a large volume of distilled water. The dialysate is concentrated to 90 ml by rotary evaporation in vacuo.

(d) *Properties of the dialysates*

To determine the approximate size of the pores of the dialysis tubes, we have used solutions of substances of known molecular weight. Cytochrome c (mol wt 16,500) does not cross the membrane; lysozyme (mol wt 14,380) is at the limit of retention, whereas ribonuclease (mol wt 12,700) passes easily. Thus we can assert that the dialysates of liver, mesonephros, and brewers yeast contain only substances with a molecular weight lower than 15,000. All molecules with a molecular weight higher than 15,000, and, in consequence, large protein molecules are retained in the dialysis bag.

Fractionation of the dialysates showed that the same active fraction could be recovered from both brewers' yeast and chicken liver. It was rich in ninhydrin positive substances, among which were numerous amino acids. In addition polypeptides, ultraviolet absorbing substances and fluorescent and coloured material were detected (Croisille *et al.* 1967). Subsequent studies in which the active fraction was replaced by prepared solutions of amino acids (Smith *et al.* 1971) have shown that cysteine, methionine, arginine, leucine and lysine are essential for tumour growth.

REFERENCES

Croisille, Y., Mason, J., Wolff, Em. and Wolff, Et. (1967). *Europ. J. Cancer, 3,* 371.

Smith, J., Wolff, Em. and Wolff, Et. (1971). *C.R. Acad. Sci. 272,* 1465.

Wolff, Em., Croisille, Y., Mason, J. and Wolff, Et. (1966). *C.R. Acad. Sci. 262,* 2120.

Wolff, Em., Croisille, Y., Mason, J. and Wolff, Et. (1967). *C.R. Acad. Sci. 265,* 2157.

Wolff, Et. and Wolff, Em. (1960). *C.R. Acad. Sci. 250,* 4076.

Wolff, Et. and Wolff, Em. (1961). *J. Embryol. exp. Morph. 9,* 678.

Wolff, Et. and Wolff, Em. (1966). *Europ. J. Cancer, 2,* 93.

Wolff, Et., Wolff, Em. and Croisille, Y. (1965). *C.R. Acad. Sci. 260,* 2359.

3. Cellular Dynamics of Human Breast Carcinoma

E. J. Ambrose and Dorothy M. Easty

1. INTRODUCTION

Human breast carcinomas have proved to be difficult to study in explant or monolayer culture due to the problem of identifying the various cell types found in the mixture after dispersing the biopsy specimens. With a view to relating the character of the cells to their expected biological behaviour, we have investigated some distinct cell types obtained from these tumours by culturing them simultaneously in three different systems. These methods are a new type of organ culture (D. Easty and G. Easty, 1974), a microexplant culture method (Ambrose, G. Easty and Tchao, in course of publication) and wounded edge cultures of confluent monolayers (Levine *et al.* 1965; Dulbecco and Stoker, 1970). The behaviour of cells in these three systems has been recorded by time lapse filming and by histology or cytology combined with autoradiography.

2. ORGAN CULTURE METHOD

The method is illustrated diagrammatically in Fig. 1 (a and b). A normal tissue has been used as a substratum in which to investigate the invasive or non-invasive character of cells, when placed on the surface. By the selection of intact membranous tissues such as the chick chorioallantoic membrane, the rat omentum, chick amniotic membrane etc., the normal tissue surface is obtained in an undamaged state.

Culture of the chorioallantoic membrane from 12-day embryonated hen eggs

The shell covering the egg airspace was sterilised with ethanol and removed. The circle of shell membrane with attached chorioallantoic membrane (CAM) thus exposed was cut round the edge with scissors and removed. The egg contents were gently decanted leaving the CAM attached to the shell, from which it was carefully removed with

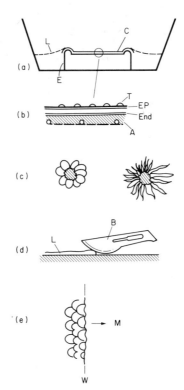

Fig. 1(a). Organ culture technique for the maintenance of intact membranous tissues. E, expanded metal grid; C, chick chorioallantoic membrane (CAM); L, surface of liquid culture medium.

(b) Detail of the CAM in organ culture. Ep, epithelial layer; End, endothelial layer; T, tumour cells from suspension now attached to the surface of the epithelium of the CAM; A, agar coating of expanded metal grid.

(c) Technique of microexplant culture of primary tumours. *Left,* Fragment of epithelial tissue (shaded) now resting on plastic surface. Epithelial cells are spreading out to form a microexplant. *Right,* Similar fragment of connective tissue with fibroblasts spreading out to form a microexplant.

(d) Method for preparing wounded edge cultures from confluent monolayer of cell lines, as seen in section. L, confluent layer of cells; B, curved scalpel blade being drawn across the surface in a direction perpendicular to the paper.

(e) Appearance of wounded edge culture seen in plan → M general direction of cell migration.

blunt forceps and allowed to slide, ectoderm upwards, into Hepes buffered medium in a dish. The membrane was cut into circles 20-25 mm diameter, which were lifted using 2 pairs of forceps on to agar-coated expanded metal culture grids. The tissue was then gently pulled into place without undue stretching, so that there were no folds.

Culture methods

These were a modification of the method of Trowell (1959) where tissue to be cultivated was supported on a stainless steel grid of expanded metal mesh at the interphase between the liquid culture medium and the gas phase. The grids were circular with a flat central well and a ridged edge to retain the cell suspensions added. The grids were dipped in molten 2% agar (Difco Bacto Agar) in Simm's saline solution and then placed in culture medium, which was Dulbecco's Eagle's medium and 10% foetal calf serum in 10% CO_2 in air, or medium 199 buffered to pH 7·4 with Hepes + 10% foetal calf serum in air.

Cell suspensions of the non-malignant or malignant cells used for study were prepared from confluent monolayers either with trypsin or versene, and a suspension placed on the surface of the membranous normal tissue as shown in Fig. 1b. Cultures were subsequently fixed at 24 and 48 hr in Carnoy and sectioned for histological studies. The method for time lapse filming of the living tissues is described by Ambrose and D. Easty (1973), and a more recent development to observe "optical sections" of the intact folded chick chorioallantoic membrane by Ambrose and D. Easty (in course of publication).

3. MICROEXPLANT CULTURE

This method of culture is used for primary cultures from human biopsy specimens. The techniques generally used for dispersing tissues, as for example by trypsin treatment, are intended to produce a suspension consisting mainly of single cells. When such suspensions are placed in culture vessels, particularly in the case of breast carcinoma specimens, a highly complex mixture of cells generally spreads on the surface of the vessel. When fragments of about 1 cm^3 are prepared for standard explant cultures, a similar mixed group of cells generally migrates from the centre. In the technique of micro-explant culture (Ambrose, G. Easty and Tchao, in course of publication) a technique is deliberately employed to produce fragments of about 30-100 cells instead of single cells. These fragments, being so small, often arise from small regions of the tumour which are homogeneous in cell type, in some cases coming from tumour tissue, in others from connective tissue, normal epithelium, etc. When placed in a culture vessel, the fragments produce microexplants some of which are homogeneous in cell type as shown in Fig. 1c. The cell types can therefore be characterised according both to their cell morphology and social behaviour.

Preparation of enzyme solution

An enzyme mixture consisting of collagenase (Sigma from Cl. histolyticum Type 1) at a final concentration of 0·2 mg/ml and hyaluronidase (BDH testis hyaluronidase) at a final concentration of 0·2 mg/ml is made up in MEM-HEPES or 199-HEPES buffer.

The enzyme solution is sterilised by filtering through a millipore filter. This solution is divided into 20 ml portions in sterile universal bottles. It may then be stored in the refrigerator for a few weeks. For a particular biopsy, one universal bottle is withdrawn and antibiotic added.

Preparation of Tissue Fragments

The piece of human tissue is placed in 199 synthetic culture medium as soon as possible after operation. It can then be safely left for up to 24 hr. 199 medium is placed in a sterile dish and the tissue placed in this dish. One piece 1 cm³ in size is removed. This is washed with fresh culture medium from a pipette while held in forceps. This is transferred to a second dish containing about 5 ml of synthetic medium. The fragment is chopped up into small pieces of 1 mm diameter using crossed scalpel blades and the fragments are then transferred to the enzyme solution. The top is screwed down lightly and left overnight in the incubator at 37° C; after 18 hr the bottle is taken out and gently shaken; many large fragments will break up. They can be further dispersed by very slow movement in a wide Pasteur pipette for 5-10 min. The suspension is decanted off leaving the large fragments. The suspension is centrifuged at speed 1 (Bench centrifuge) for 5-10 min. The supernatant is decanted off. The packed cells are re-suspended by gentle pipetting in culture media for washing, then recentrifuged and redecanted. They are finally re-suspended in 15 ml of culture medium. 5 ml is placed in each culture bottle and gassed. After 24 hr the medium is changed very gently to remove debris. The original large fragments remaining in the bottom of the bottle of the enzyme solution can also be used. They can be washed with culture media and prepared in the same way as the fine fragment suspension; sometimes they do better than the fine suspension.

4. WOUNDED EDGE CULTURES

Confluent monolayers, which are reasonably homogeneous in cell type, can sometimes be obtained from first or second cultures of the microexplant cultures of human breast carcinoma cells. Very occasionally cell lines can also be obtained. Wounded edge cultures can readily be prepared by scraping the surface lightly with a curved scalpel blade, Fig. 1 (d and e).

In the case both of the primary microexplant cultures and the wounded edge cultures the migration of cells from a densely packed group can be recorded by time lapse filming. Autoradiography of cultures, after labelling with tritium labelled thymidine, uridine and proline, has also proved to be of some help for cell characterisation with the microexplant cultures (Ambrose and Stephen, in course of publication).

5. RESULTS OBTAINED WITH BIOPSY SPECIMENS

(a) *Fibroblasts in Human Breast Carcinoma Cultures*

In one or two sub-cultures from patients' biopsies a moderately uniform population of cells which resembled human embryonic fibroblasts in morphology was obtained. In one instance a cell line was established. Various tests were carried out on this line. The cells showed considerable labelling with proline sometimes just outside the cell border, suggesting collagen synthesis. They were completely resistant up to the highest concentration currently used for drug sensitivity tests in the case of melphalan, methotrexate and vinblastine. Fibroblasts are already known to be highly resistant to anti-tumour drugs.

In the organ culture test, the cells were found to spread smoothly on the surface of the chick chorioallantoic membrane, without invasion (Fig. 2a). They showed strong mutual adhesiveness and tended to form cell masses. One such mass was filmed in "optical section". The boundary between the fibroblasts and epithelium of the chick chorioallantoic membrane remained extremely sharp indicating no damage to or penetration of the normal epithelium (Fig. 2b). A histological section is shown in Fig. 3.

The cells were also set up in wounded edge culture when they migrated uniformly and in extremely elongated form. In the packed layer they had the spindle-shaped form (Fig. 2c). All the data supported the view that these cells were non-malignant and were probably proliferating fibroblasts.

Microexplants of this type are often seen after 1-2 days in primary microexplant cultures of human breast carcinoma cells. They evolve into the characteristic fan-like form as shown in Fig. 4a.

HTSTC–3

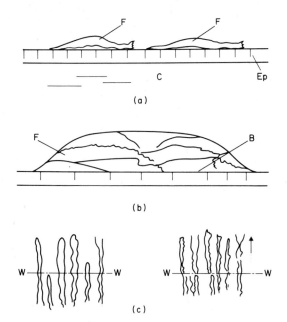

Fig. 2. Behaviour of fibroblast cell line obtained from a primary culture of human breast carcinoma.

(a) Behaviour of isolated cells when placed on the CAM in organ culture as shown in Fig. 1(b) and observed by "optical sections" in time lapse films. C, connective tissue; Ep, epithelial layer; F, fibroblasts spreading by ruffled membrane activity.

(b) Similar view of a large mass of fibroblasts on the CAM. F, mass of fibroblasts; B, sharp boundary between fibroblasts and epithelium of the CAM.

(c) Behaviour of the human fibroblast line in wounded edge culture w-w wound. *Left,* Aligned cells before wounding; *right,* After wounding showing a migration of aligned cells perpendicular to the wound.

(b) *Epithelial cells from human breast carcinoma biopsies.*

The epithelial cells show individual characteristics for different cells, Fig. 4 (b-d):

(*i*) Close contacted epithelial sheets. These closely resemble normal epithelium of cultures from various normal embryonic and adult tissues. They maintain the epithelial morphology as the microexplant evolves.

(*ii*) Loose contacted epithelial sheet. Although these cells do not overlap, the cell-cell contacts at the borders are not continuous. Such cultures evolve into spreading cells which closely resemble the lamellar form of fibroblasts. Of particular interest are the cells which

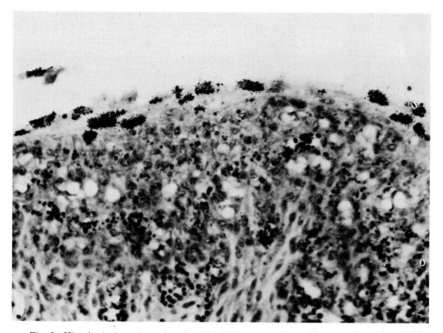

Fig. 3. Histological section showing the behaviour of the human fibroblast cell line obtained from a breast carcinoma on CAM. The well spread out fibroblasts have been previously labelled with thymidine and can be seen to be well spread without penetrating the epithelium after 24 hr in culture. (×420).

eventually separate from the main mass. Time lapse filming shows that these cells have acquired *two heads*. Lamellar ruffled membranes occur at each end of the cell which stretch the cell into its elongated form. This is in contrast to fibroblasts in which the head region provides the spreading membrane for considerable periods, with little active movement in the tail region. Sometimes the elongated epithelial cells stretch themselves so much that they do themselves "an injury" and lose some cytoplasm. Epithelial cells in this form can easily be confused with fibroblasts. However, the slow labelling of the nucleolus with uridine and the low proline labelling help in the recognition of the cells. They are generally sensitive to drugs.

(*iii*) Trigonal cells with polypodia. These cells can readily be distinguished from normal epithelium and from fibroblasts. They show loss of contact inhibition and the polypodia overlap. Preliminary indications have suggested that these cells may be the type occurring in metastases. When present in primary biopsy they may represent the really dangerous cells.

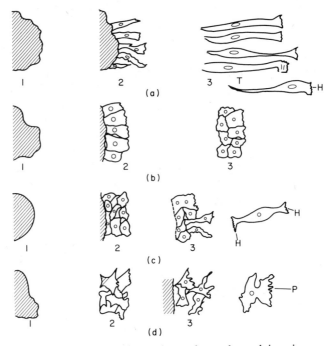

Fig. 4. Migration of cells in various microexplants observed in primary cultures of human breast carcinoma. 1-2-3 stages of evolution of the microexplant.

(a) *Top*, Fibroblasts migrating 1-2-3-. In 3 the familiar spindle shape with leading head (H) showing ruffled membranes, and trailing tail (T) can be seen.

(b) *Upper middle*, Normal appearance of epithelium with continuous cell-cell contacts except on leading edge.

(c) *Lower middle*, Abnormal epithelium showing gaps in cell-cell contacts in early stages of migration (2). Later (3) leading cells elongate. Some become detached and look remarkably like fibroblasts when seen without time lapse. In time lapse they can be seen as *double*-headed cells (H) which frequently reverse their direction of locomotion.

(d) *Bottom*, Anaplastic cells showing trigonal form with surface polypodia (P) and cell-cell overlap. Such cells have been seen in cultures of metastases of carcinomas.

Cell lines of human breast carcinomas provided by Professor Lasfargues (HBT3, HBT39 and HBT20) have also been tested in the organ culture system (Figs 5 and 6). One of these (HBT39) has been filmed. Unfortunately, the characterisation of the cells as breast carcinoma is a little uncertain in the case of the first two. All three lines invaded the CAM.

The characteristic polypodia are extremely clearly seen in the case of the HBT39 tumour. They can be observed to penetrate progressively between the normal cells and so lead to invasion by the tumour (Fig. 7).

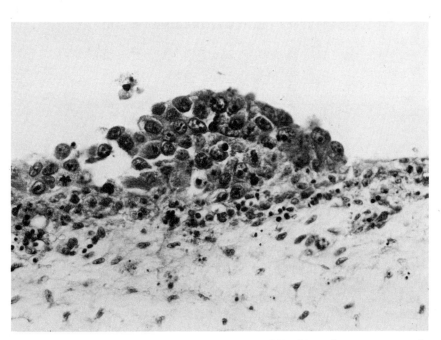

Fig. 5. Histological section showing the behaviour of HBT39 carcinoma tumour on the CAM. The invasion of the tumour cells as far as the bottom of the epithelial layer can be seen. 24 hr in culture (×420).

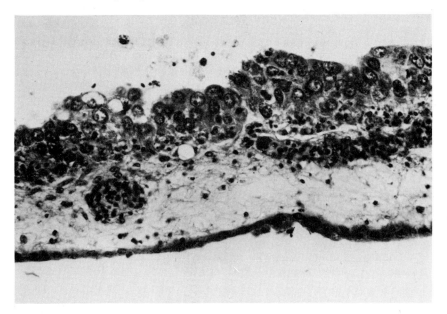

Fig. 6. Histological section showing the behaviour of human breast carcinoma cell line HBT20 on CAM. The invasion as far as the bottom of the epithelial layer can be clearly seen. 24 hr in culture. (×420).

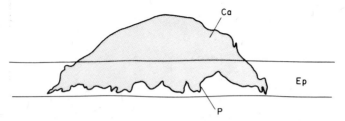

Fig. 7. Behaviour of a human carcinoma cell line (HBT39) on the CAM seen in "optical section" by time lapse filming. Ep, epithelium of CAM; Ca, single carcinoma cell. The invading region of the carcinoma shows intense polypodial activity (P).

CONCLUSION

A systematic study of the various cell types found in human breast carcinomas is of importance both for diagnostic studies and for interpretation of drug tests, tests with cytotoxic lymphocytes, etc. In order to characterise the highly malignant cells, a comparison between the cell types found in primary tumours and in metastases is particularly useful.

ACKNOWLEDGMENTS

This investigation was supported by grants to the Chester Beatty Research Institute (Institute of Cancer Research: Royal Cancer Hospital) from the Medical Research Council and the Cancer Campaign for Research.

REFERENCES

Ambrose, E. J. and Easty, D. M. (1973). *Differentiation*, 1, 277.

Ambrose, E. J., Easty, G. C. and Tchao, R. In press.

Ambrose, E. J. and Easty, D. M. In press. Time Lapse Filming of Cellular Interactions in Organ Culture. III: The role of Cell Shape.

Ambrose, E. J. and Stephen, J. In press.

Ambrose, E. J. and Stephen, J. (in press). Cellular Dynamics of Human Tumours. II: Breast Carcinomas.

Dulbecco, R. and Stoker, M. G. P. (1970). *Proc. Nat. Acad. Sci. U.S.A. 66*, 204.

Easty, D. M. and Easty, G. C. (1974). *Brit. J. Cancer, 29*, 36.

Levine, E. M., Becher, Y., Boone, C. W. and Earle, H. (1965). *Proc. Nat. Acad. Sci. U.S.A. 53*, 350.

Trowell, O. A. (1959). *Exptl. Cell Res. 16*, 118.

4. Use of an Organ Culture System to Demonstrate Various Types of Malignant Growth

A. Schleich

Any explantation of surgical specimens into tissue culture is to some extent a gamble because we do not know whether the composition of the cell population *in vitro* still represents the original tumour *in vivo*. During removal from the living organism and establishment *in vitro*, a selection takes place and we do not know which parts of the tumour cell population survived, neither do we know to what extent the lost cells were essential for the malignant potential of the tumour. In other words, apart from histological sections we know very little about the malignancy of this particular cell population in culture, originating from a particular human tumour.

Lack of reliable *in vitro* proof of malignant invasiveness has worried many investigators and we also joined the line hoping to find a biological method to study this problem. These experiments have been done in co-operation with M. Frick and A. Mayer (1974).

After a series of unsuccessful attempts we finally found human decidua graviditatis from the first trimenon to be an ideal receptor tissue. We cut the decidua into cubes approximately 1 mm^2, soaked them in medium and rotated them in Erlenmeyer flasks in the New Brunswick Shaker at 60 rpm and at 37° C (Moscona, 1961). The medium contained 79% Eagles basal medium, 1% Glutamine 20% foetal calf serum and antibiotics. Forty-eight hours later the decidua cubes looked healthy and the epithelia were unchanged. The muscular cells around the arterioli and the typical decidua cells showed no signs of disintegration. No growth, as far as mitotic activity was concerned, could be detected. There was migration consistent with wound healing along some cutting edges.

Confrontation with dissociated cells from other origins, the invasiveness of which was to be tested, followed 48 hr after first setting up the decidua cubes. 1·5 million trypsinised cells/ml were added to the medium containing the cubes. Specimens were fixed 2, 4 and 6 days following confrontation. The histological procedures were standard fixation in Bouin, embedding in paraffin, sectioning and staining with haematoxylin/eosin.

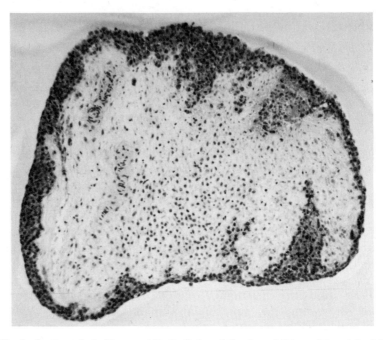

Fig. 1. Section of decidua graviditatis 6 days following addition of trypsinised HeLa cells. x90, H-E stain. Note the wedgeshaped concentric invasion of tumour cells to the centre of the section.

This system is extremely flexible. The receptor tissue can be modified by pre-treatment, for example by hormones, radiation or chemotherapeutic agents. A wide range of different types of aggressor cells can be tested, and additionally these aggressor cells can be modified by chemical, physical, immunological or any other factors.

Three examples of manifestations of malignant invasiveness by human tumour strains, grown *in vitro* will now be given.

(1) The adenocarcinoma of the cervix HeLa, isolated in 1952 in G. O. Gey's laboratory, Baltimore (Gey *et al.* 1962).

(2) Strain AFi, a fibrosarcoma of the humerus, isolated in 1938 also in G. O. Gey's laboratory.

(3) A human lymphoid cell strain transformed *in vitro* according to Chang (1971).

The strains HeLa and AFi definitely originated from human tumours, the lymphoid strain is a striking example of a malignant transformation of normal human lymphocytes *in vitro*.

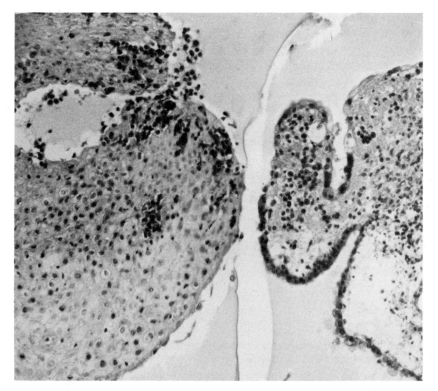

Fig. 2. Section of decidua graviditatis 6 days following additiòn of spontaneously transformed human lymphocytes. x150, H-E stain. To the left, clumps of invading lymphoblastoid cells. Invasion starts from an open gap in the normal tissue. To the right heavily degenerated normal tissue. The epithelial membrane detaches from the disintegrating stroma.

As soon as trypsinised HeLa cells are added to the medium containing the decidua cubes, many of them tend to form solid spherical aggregates, which float in the medium until they attach to the decidua surface or until they are trapped in a lacuna. So we have a two phase invasion; first aggregation of the tumour cells and second, attachment to the decidua-tissue and invasion (Fig. 1).

Though the fibrosarcoma has now been grown in tissue culture for 36 years, it has not lost the property of a highly destructive sarcoma. The cells infiltrate individually causing degeneration wherever they appear.

The third type of infiltration is similar to the sarcoma, but differs in its origin. This lymphoid strain underwent a spontaneous transformation *in vitro,* probably due to an Epstein-Barr-Genome in

3*

the original lymphocytes of the healthy donor. Histologically it has very much the appearance of a lymphosarcoma (Fig. 2). Time lapse cinematography can be used to demonstrate the rapid movement of the lymphoblastoid cells into the decidua tissue.

One possible use of this model as a test system could be to follow the effect of chemotherapeutics upon the surface and, in close relation to the surface conditions, upon the migration capacities of tumour cells, preferably of leukaemic cells, into the normal tissue. On the other hand we hopefully continue our efforts to extend the experiments to a broader spectrum of human tumour specimens.

REFERENCES

Chang, R. S., Hsieh, M. and Blankenship, W. (1971). *J. Natl. Cancer Inst. 47.* 469.

Gey, G. O., Coffman, W. D. and Kubicek, M. T. (1962). *Cancer Res. 12*, 264.

Moscona, A. A. (1961). *Exptl. Cell Res. 22*, 455.

Schleich, A., Frick, M. and Mayer, A. (1974). *Z. Krebsforsch. 82*, 247.

DISCUSSION

Poole suggested doing this work with acid treated serum taking the pH down to about 3·5. This should inactivate α-2 macroglobulin, an inhibitor of proteinases and might have an effect on invasiveness.

GENERAL DISCUSSION

Boss reported experience they have had with smears. In some types of carcinoma for example of the bladder, it is relevant to prognosis certainly and to any attempt to classify the tumour for practical purposes, to understand the extent to which the cell population deviates from the normal diploid in its karyotype. This does not necessarily involve karyotyping because the difference may be such that simple DNA content is sufficient information for a large sample of cells. For tumour which smears easily all is well, but it is important that for ordinary microdensitometry the nucleus is flat, i.e. that it is entirely within focus with a lens of fairly high numerical aperture. When it is not possible to smear or spread cells, it may be helpful to use short term tissue cultures with cells spreading themselves on a transparent medium or plastic thereby becoming suitable for microdensitometry. This is relatively undemanding because as soon as a few hundred cells have spread out, provided they are from the tumour and not from stroma, one can fix the whole mount and proceed.

G. Easty noted the allusion to whether the cells were malignant. This is a problem about which there are daily discussions. We do a number of experiments elegantly but except for organ cultures do we always know what we are looking at?

Owen asked if these different tumour cells growing in tissue culture had been put into nude mice and to what extent the question of malignancy can be answered in this way. G. Easty said that this was a cyclic problem—positive growth in nude mice can be taken as an indication of malignancy but is not proof. A number of long established human tumour lines have been put into nude mice, but they do not all give rise to tumours even when as many as 30×10^6 cells per mouse, five million cells per site are injected. This may mean some well known human tumour strains are not malignant, or alternatively the biochemical and metabolic environment provided in the mouse is not adequate for the growth of these tumour cells. Not everything that is labelled "human tumour" or even labelled "tumour" may be tumour even though it may be HeLa!

Freshney said one problem of the nude mouse type experiment is that even assuming implantation of the human tumour in the mouse is successful it takes a long time to grow. It will be at best many weeks before there is a detectable nodule and when using tissue cultures for clinically orientated work, the clinician is not going to wait for a couple of months while the nature of the material is investigated. Any test that is used in a study like this must give an answer in days and not weeks or months. G. Easty agreed adding that the vast majority of primary tumours used by Detré and Gazet (1973) and at the Chester Beatty are very slow growing and certainly do not all grow. Some, like colonic tumours, grow particularly well and fairly quickly but for others, like tumours of the breast, the proportion of the number which maintain and possibly increase in size is low and growth is slow.

Kohorn said there are now several tumour cell lines available in culture which if re-injected into immunologically protected sites, do reproduce the architecture of the original tumour. (For example one of the endometrial carcinomas (Kuramoto *et al.* 1972).) Moreover, they have similar chemical and biological properties as far as can be assessed. Although the yield is low and the work involved is tremendous, it may be worthwhile to make an effort with each particular neoplasm of a particular histological type if the end results obtained are justified by the clinical situation.

Hudson suggested that immune deprived mice might be used as a control for the material which had been prepared for *in vitro* experiments. This might later validate conclusions derived much earlier from a predictive test based on short term glass or plastic cultures.

Dickson expressed uncertainty about the significance of growth of tumour lines or tumours in nude mice or in any laboratory animal. They have transplanted a large series of human tumours into immuno-suppressed mice, rats, and hamsters (but not nude mice) as a bioassay following treatment of these tumours with cytotoxic drugs. In about 50% of cases human tumours of different types grow in these laboratory animals after no treatment with drugs. If they are treated with cytotoxic drugs, there is correlation between the inhibition of the biochemistry of the tumour in the presence of the drug and the inability to grow in mice, rats or hamsters in quite a high percentage of cases. This simply means that a tumour may or may not grow in a laboratory animal. Whether this has any relationship to the malignancy of the tumour in the human cannot be determined.

Twentyman referred to some of Harris's cell fusion experiments (Harris, 1970) in which he combined either mouse malignant cell lines or normal cell lines with cell lines known to be malignant. Normal cell lines can suppress the malignancy of the known malignant lines whereas other malignant lines do not. It is certainly possible to fuse human cells with mouse malignant cells, but whether this could be used as a test on the same basis as for malignant mouse lines is uncertain.

G. Easty said Tisdale and Phillips (1974) had worked with L strain cells which, although they do not give tumours when implanted into the original C_3H line, assuming that it is the same line, will give uncontrolled growth which metastasizes in nude mice. When these cells were fused with a highly malignant tumour from a mouse and some of the selected hybrid clones were put into nude mice, they did not grow. So both parent lines give histological tumours which will kill the nude mice but when the cells are fused to give a heterokaryon which is checked for chromosomes etc., this fused cell will not give a tumour. One has the possibility that elimination of some chromosomes, even when both parent cells are malignant, may destroy or reduce the capacity for malignant growth.

Sidebottom agreed that there is a difficulty here. The first extensive series of experiments which Klein *et al.* reported (1971) involved fusion of highly malignant cells with A9 cells (a sub-line of mouse L cells). We say this is a "non-malignant" cell line but what does that mean? A9 cells will give tumours so this may be rather like the situation just described. Certainly the malignancy of a highly malignant cell can be suppressed by a cell of low malignancy. But in a recent series of experiments about a dozen crosses were made between different highly malignant cells and in nearly every case except one a malignant cell resulted. The one exception is thought to be a special case and may provoke quite a lot of discussion. But the cell fusion experiments come back to the same difficulty of what is a non-malignant established cell line.

G. Easty asked if the autoradiographic work described by Hodges could be used to distinguish between the normal and malignant states of cells and if it could be quantitated. Hodges said this was only one example of a tagging system. A metal tagged macromolecular approach is perhaps better because it eliminates some autoradiographic problems. The advantage of this instrumentation is that large areas can be evaluated at a fine structural level. The SEM approach allows not only a scan of the superficial malignant surface but by doing fractures, one can also go inside a cell and look at the surface within a cell. This offers very large sampling areas which is of particular value in tagging studies and although it is a sophisticated approach, it can be linked to a computer system to provide independent quantitation.

Klein and Schleich both felt that any definition of malignancy would be to some extent, arbitrary, because there is a range of histological grades from normal to pseudo-normal and highly malignant. Schleich added that they have tested a series of so-called permanent normal strains using the criteria of destruction or damage of the receptor tissue and invasion and obtained a complete spectrum from highly malignant to non-malignant. S_3 strain cells for instance caused severe destruction of the adjacent tissue but not very much invasion. They stuck to the surface of the receptor tissue and piled up but they did not invade. So for all these permanent strains there was no clear-cut invasion and the main damage was an injury of the adjacent normal receptor tissue.

Morasca said this problem is very important for the animal models we are using and from which we learn most of our basic knowledge in terms of malignancy. It is very rare to have really malignant tumours in animals. Although all of them are able to kill the animal, very few can metastasize. But if tumours like Ehrlich or sarcoma 180 are injected into favourable sites, metastases can be induced, so the problem is very complex and we have no clear criteria. Rather it seems we require the clinician to say what he intends for malignancy.

Boss added that the question of malignancy is also complicated by the fact that if someone has a malignant growth, the malignancy for that person, and therefore for their medical attendant, depends not only on the growth but on the person's reaction to it. This may open up important work for short-term tissue culture. Clearly one can not only grow a patient's tumour, but can also compare its reaction with, say, the patient's serum or the patient's lymphocytes versus control serum or control lymphocytes. This type of approach would then enable one better to imitate the balance of factors which recur in the patient. It is not just one unopposed tumour in a passive field.

Limburg said they had studied the effect of a patient's serum on a monolayer culture of the patient's tumour cells. In cases where there was some immunological resistance the cultures would not grow, but where the immunological system was going down hill, the growth was pretty good. Easty added that *in vitro* techniques can be applied to analyse several aspects of the patient's immunological response and therefore define the whole immunological interaction between the host and its tumour.

Poole suggested further consideration should be given to the use of serum in these cultures. Ross *et al.* (1974) have found that platelets are responsible for the production of a serum factor during clotting that will stimulate the proliferation of smooth muscle cells *in vitro*. So if serum is used for growing cultures, we may get a differential growth stimulation either of malignant cells, which has not yet been reported, or of normal cell types. Thus factors may exist which would switch on the tumour cells or could switch on the normal cells contaminating the cultures, thereby making examination of the tumour cells more difficult. Perhaps we should think about not using serum all the time but consider using plasma.

Lamerton thought the problem faced at the moment in tissue culture work is the technical limitation that only a very small proportion of human tumours can be grown. The first requirement of research is to introduce some logical understanding of the precise conditions under which human tumour cells will grow *in vitro*. If one wishes to grow human tumours in clonal form, which may be the only way to do really quantitative measurements, one is very limited indeed with present techniques. Whitehouse said there were definite historical parallels with the field of microbiology. Details of metabolism in cultured tumour cells still have to be worked out; and the development of corresponding growth media similar to that in early microbiological studies had to be worked out, but there is no reason to suppose this cannot be done. The basic science aspect of clinical feasibility is very important but, at the same time, a continuing relationship must be maintained between the clinicians and the scientists to ensure increasingly significant data on which to base predictive diagnostic methods for more routine use.

G. Easty was disturbed about using cloning assays for evaluating immune responses of patients lymphocytes to their tumour cells. Hellström and Hellström (1971) reported results for some 150 tumours where the effects of the lymphocytes had been assessed by colony growth. If single cells can be plated out in this way and give rise to colonies, this must be equivalent to establishing cell lines from over 90% of the primary tumours which is completely contrary to everyone's experience.

Kohorn added that an interesting feature of the Hellströms' work, is that when they took fresh cultures which had just been established, or possibly just unfrozen, their results with cytotoxicity testing were much better than if they used cell lines. This has been reproduced by other people, including Kohorn's group.

Dendy mentioned two problems of particular interest clinically. First, a study of tumour material is really rather incomplete without a study of host material. Are there any tumour types where it would be feasible to get normal material for study? Secondly we would like to know if metastases behave like the primary tumour. Lamerton was cautious about the use of the term "normal tissue" in this context because the particular normal tissue most at risk will vary with the type of cytotoxic agent used. It is true that all therapy depends on a good differential response, but one has to understand a great deal about the mode of action of an agent before knowing which tissues really have to be compared.

Laing introduced further clinical aspects. First, the clinician is dealing with a dynamic situation. The position with regard to the tumour and the body response to the tumour at any one time, may be entirely different within a few days. This is seen in the clinical phase where tumour and body are lying quite nicely in symbiosis and suddenly something happens and the tumour runs away. Secondly, accepting that one must know which normal tissue to study, there are other problems even here. How does one define normal tissue in the body? If a piece of "normal colon" is taken close to a carcinoma of the colon, this may or may not be normal tissue because of the phenomenon of field change in the body and one may be dealing with just enough abnormal tissue to invalidate the findings. Finally, within this clinical context, what really matters is time. Patients do not remain static while laboratory reports are prepared, so if this work is to be at all useful clinically, it *must* be quick.

Berry felt that having defined by clinical criteria that there is a patient with a tumour, we must come back to the question of how the *in vitro* studies can be made relevant. The amount of work involved in this should be pointed out. In the first two years using a short term *in vitro* human tumour culture system in Oxford, 100 tumours were obtained and cultured. 30 actually grew, and of those 30 the largest series were two groups of 9 and 7 patients for whom there was adequate chemosensitivity testing to try and compare what happened to them clinically. Of those, 5 of one group and 2 of the other actually got the drugs tested *in vitro*, so there is a very small yield for a lot of work.

Dickson said the discussion was now focussing on the patient and the value of such tests to the patient, and the point raised by Boss regarding tumour/host relationship was very valid. Most systems we have today for assessing the response of tumours to drugs and other treatments, take no account of this. Systems are just becoming available for assessing the immune response but there are many factors (drug distribution, activation and metabolism, drug dosage level) which will never be accessible to evaluation outside the human body. For example, a tumour may be sensitive and be shown to be sensitive *in vitro* to say, fluorouracil, but unless the appropriate concentration can be introduced into the tumour the only effect is to create a population of resistant cells. Another important factor is the total host burden of cancer cells because tumour specimens are often from near terminal patients. No matter what one does for these patients it will not be possible to save them, because it has been shown that even if the tumour is sensitive to a drug, when the tumour cell burden is too great it is not possible to kill the tumour without killing the animal (Martin *et al.* 1962; Goldin, 1973).

Many of these problems appertain not only to purely *in vitro* systems. The clinician also has the problem of assessing whether or not a drug has had an effect on a tumour. For example, he cannot assess tumour cell kill unless there is something like a 50% decrease in the size of the tumour. Mention must be made of the Willcox phenomenon—the serious under-estimation of tumour cell kill when assessment is based solely on tumour volume measurements (Skipper, 1971). As many as 99% of the cells in a tumour can be killed without detection, simply because there is very rapid overgrowth of resistant tumour cells after giving the drug (Johnson and Wolberg, 1971). In other words we are not concerned with the cells killed by giving a drug on the basis of predictive *in vitro* tests, but the cells left behind. So there are many problems here, both *in vitro* and from the host (*in vivo*) point of view.

REFERENCES

Detré, S. I. and Gazet, J.-C. (1973). *Brit. J. Cancer, 28*, 412.

Goldin, A. (1973). *In* "Chemotherapy of Cancer Dissemination and Metastasis" (S. Garattini and G. Franchi, eds.) p. 341. Raven Press, New York.

Harris, H. (1970). "Cell Fusion". Clarendon Press, Oxford.

Hellström, I. and Hellström, K. (1971). *In* "*In vitro* Methods in Cell Mediated Immunity" (B. Bloom and P. Glade, eds.) p. 409. Academic Press, New York and London.

Johnson, R. O. and Wolberg, W. (1971). *Cancer, 28*, 208.

Klein, G., Bregula, U., Wiender, F. and Harris, H. (1971). *J. Cell Sci. 8*, 659.

Kuramoto, H., Tamura, S. and Notake, Y. (1972). *Am. J. Obst. Gynaec. 114*, 1012.

Martin, D. S., Fugmann, R. A. and Hayworth, P. (1962). *J. Nat. Cancer Inst. 29*, 817.

Ross, R., Glomset, T., Kariya, B. and Harker, L. (1974). *Proc. Nat. Acad. Sci. U.S.A. 71*, 1207.

Skipper, H. E. (1971). *Nat. Cancer Inst. Monogr. 34*, 2.

Tisdale, M. J. and Phillips, B. J. (1974). *Exptl. Cell Res. 88*, 111.

Chapter 2

EVALUATION OF SHORT TERM CULTURES: IDENTIFICATION OF TUMOUR CELLS AND USE IN DIAGNOSIS

(Moderator: L. F. Lamerton)

1. Modern Developments in the Characterisation of Tumour Cells in Tissue Culture: Cell Kinetics and Biochemical Changes

L. A. Smets

INTRODUCTION

Primary cultures of tumour cells can be used to investigate various aspects of the tumour of origin in the hope of improving the management of this or related malignant diseases. A number of papers in this volume deal with sensitivity tests *in vitro* for chemo- or radiotherapy. Others deal with the assessment of response to hormones and of the immunological status of the patient.

In addition, primary cultures must be studied for the various parameters characterising their proliferation kinetics as an aid in the evaluation and prediction of chemo- and radiosensitivity of the tumour under study. Moreover, biochemical investigations of tumour cells or their components can be helpful in the further characterisation of the tissue. These aspects, viz. cell cycle analysis and biochemical characterisation, will be dealt with in this contribution with special reference to modern developments in the field. Moreover, some remarks will be made on the use of automated cytology in early diagnosis of cancer.

1. CELL CYCLE ANALYSIS

The cells of most renewing or growing tissues—whether in the steady state or not—can be divided into various compartments such as (a) proliferating cells, (b) resting cells capable of re-entering the cell cycle and (c) differentiating cells which are usually incapable of further division and therefore have a finite life-span. This scheme is a very simplified one derived from bone-marrow kinetics. Variations in the number of compartments as well as refinements in the transition capacities of various cell types can be made However, full analysis of all relevant parameters in a single biopsy specimen in tissue culture is impossible on a routine basis. Therefore, restriction must be made to those parameters which are *at least* to be measured in order to evaluate proliferation properties of the tissue studied. These parameters are:

(a) The rate of cell loss (as a continuous process or induced by therapy).

(b) The fractions of resting and proliferating cells.

(c) The length of the various cell cycle phases and the distribution of cells over these phases.

Cell loss in tissue cultures has to be estimated largely by indirect methods, since dead or dying cells are not rapidly removed from the cultures, except in sparse monolayers. Histological examination or the use of dyes excluded by living cells (i.e. trypan blue) can be useful in some cases. The most quantitative system is the assessment of cell viability by the potential to develop into a visible colony of cells when seeded as sparse, single cell suspensions (survival curves). However, plating efficiencies of cells from primary culture are often very low.

The discrimination between cells in resting phase and cells passing through the cell cycle is perhaps the most important parameter of cell kinetic studies related to the management of cancer (cell recruitment studies, the effect of split-dose irradiation, etc.). The available methods are mainly indirect, one being the killing of cycling cells by a cycle-specific drug or suicide by the uptake of tritiated thymidine of high specific activity. The non-cycling cells are then assayed by the viability tests described above. Non-cycling or slowly cycling cells can also be detected radioautographically as unlabelled cells in continuous labelling experiments (see below). Information as to the size of the pool of non-proliferating cells is also obtained from the discrepancy between the population doubling time and the average duration of cell cycle time (Brown, 1968).

In general, no direct methods are presently available for the discrimination of resting and cycling cells also denoted by Q (= quiescent) and P (= proliferating) cells. However, in model experiments with tissue culture cells, it has been demonstrated (Smets, 1973) that cells committed for division have a higher affinity of their DNA for fluorescent dyes such as acridine orange ("chromatin activation"). If reliable methods for a variety of cells become available, cytochemical techniques discriminating directly between resting and cycling cells might be developed.

The estimation of cell cycle length and its subdivisions (G_1, S, G_2 and M phase) is particularly important when studies of cell phase specific cytotoxic agents are contemplated (Fig. 1) and is almost

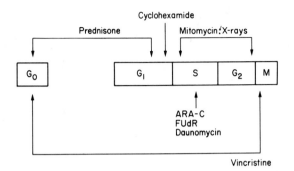

Fig. 1. Cell phase specificity of cytotoxic agents.

exclusively based on radioautographic techniques using tritiated thymidine (Cleaver, 1967). In *pulse-chase* experiments, the cells in S phase are labelled by a short exposure to the radioactive precursor and their passage through subsequent mitosis is measured in a number of preparations made after different time intervals (pulse labelled mitosis or PLM curve). The length of the cell cycle and of the cell cycle phases can be calculated from this curve.

Alternatively, the culture can be exposed continuously to tritiated thymidine and the curve relating the percentage of labelled cells with incubation time can be constructed. Though less precise than the pulse-chase method, the continuous labelling procedure has some practical advantages over the former technique in that:

(a) less individual points are required and the duration of the assay is shorter.

(b) the analysis of radioautographs is faster and more accurate.

(c) the method can be used when the mitotic index is very low.

(d) an estimate of the non-proliferating fraction is obtained from the size of the unlabelled fraction after an incubation time equal to, or longer than, the cell cycle time.

Figure 2 shows unpublished results (M. E. Lloyd and P. P. Dendy) for a culture of a human cystadenocarcinoma of the ovary which had been maintained *in vitro* for only 2 days before ^{3}H thymidine was added. Simple theory indicates that the percentage of cells labelled with ^{3}H thymidine should increase nearly linearly with time until there is a sharp discontinuity when all the cycling cells have passed through S phase. The duration of $G_2 + M + G_1$ can be estimated from the graph and the negative intercept on the time axis is comparable with ($\sim$) the duration of S phase. The percentage of cells

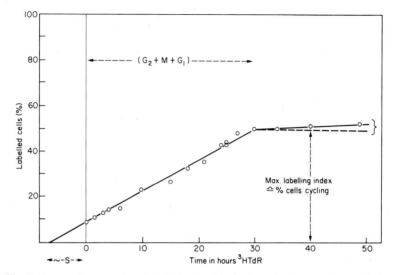

Fig. 2. Increase in percentage labelled cells with time in a short term culture of a human cystadenocarcinoma of the ovary during continuous exposure to ^{3}H thymidine.

Five different human tumour specimens, four of which were ovarian in origin and the fifth was a carcinoma of the colon, have been examined in this way. The maximum labelling index was very variable—ranging from 24% to 95%—but the values for intermitotic times derived from the graphs were very similar for each specimen, ranging from 34 hr to 38·5 hr.

cycling can also be estimated from the graph and this figure may be relevant to the *in vivo* situation.

A serious disadvantage of these and other radioautographic methods, is the need to obtain samples at different times, a pre-requisite often obstructed by the limited amount of biopsy material available. Moreover, proliferation conditions may change in the course of the experiment (48 hr!) and little information is obtained as to the number of cells present in the phases before and after DNA synthesis (G_0, G_1 and G_2) at any moment of the experiment.

An alternative method of cell cycle analysis is the determination of DNA per cell by cytophotometry. This technique, however, is very time-consuming since thousands of individual cells must be measured to obtain a histograph of sufficient accuracy for detailed analysis. However, in recent years, cytophotometers have been developed which can measure the DNA content of individual cells at a rate of about 500 cells per sec. (Göhde, 1973, Holm and Cram, 1973). The samples for these so called pulse-cytophotometers consist of fixed cells suspended in a solution of fluorescent DNA-stain such as acridine orange or ethidium bromide. The preparative technique is relatively simple depending on the tissue to be measured. For bone marrow samples, DNA histographs of 100,000 cells can be obtained within 1-2 hr following aspiration. A typical histograph for cells distributed through the various phases of the cell cycle and the synchronising effect of X-irradiation is shown in Fig. 3.

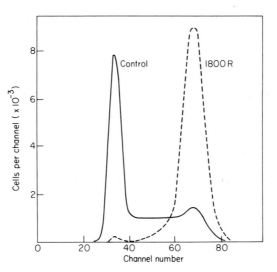

Fig. 3. Redrawn histograph plotted by the ICP11 impulse-cytophotometer. Solid graph: DNA per cell distribution of 50,000 SV-3T3 cells in log phase of growth showing cells in G_1 phase (channels 30-40), S phase (channels 35-63) and G_2 + M phase (channels 60-80). Dashed graph: idem of cells 24 hr after X-irradiation, note accumulation in G_2 phase. The channel number is proportional to the DNA per cell content of ethidium bromide stained cells.

The information obtained could be used for the choice of chemotherapy schemes. In addition, cytophotometric analysis allows for rapid characterisation of aneuploid tumour cells and gives direct information on distribution over the cell cycle phases (Fig. 4). This parameter, which is difficult to measure by radioautography, is of great value in studies on synchronisation of tumours and in the localisation of cytostatic activity in the cell cycle.

A serious disadvantage of pulse-cytophotometry is that the assay cannot take into consideration cell morphology. In consequence, the measurement does not discriminate between tumour and normal cells except in cases of tumour cell aneuploidy. Moreover, techniques for

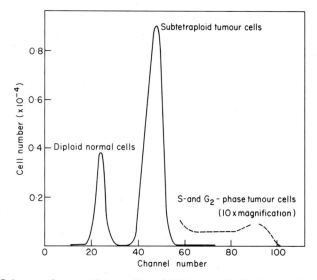

Fig. 4. Pulse-cytophotometric recording of DNA per cell distribution (represented by channel number) in the peripheral blood from a patient with lymphosarcoma with leukaemic transformation. The ratio between normal and tumour cells and the proliferative activity of tumour cells can be rapidly estimated in samples from blood, bone-marrow and tumour. The impulse-cytophotometer used was the IGP11 (Phywe AG, Gottingen).

the selective preparation of single cell suspensions are not yet available for all types of tumour biopsy.

2. BIOCHEMICAL PARAMETERS

The search for a specific biochemical defect or change as a marker of malignancy, has a very long history in fundamental cancer research. Numerous studies have been aimed at the discovery of a specific "cancer protein", a changed base sequence in DNA or RNA or a specific enzyme alteration characterising the malignant condition. These efforts have not resulted in any unifying or general concept of a biochemical parameter specifically characterising the malignant cells as compared with the normal ones.

More recently, however, some sophisticated and promising approaches in the search for biochemical parameters of malignancy have been initiated. These studies are based on the following considerations:

(a) Tissue culture studies have indicated that growth control is a sociological phenomenon which manifests itself during cell-to-cell contact. Consequently defective growth control in malignant cells is somehow a phenomenon of changed cell recognition.

(b) Cell recognition occurs at the cell outer membrane and surface glycoproteins and glycolipids are molecules specifically involved in cell recognition.

Therefore, biochemical studies have been started to investigate glycoproteins and glycolipids of the surface membrane of normal and malignant cells. These studies can be divided into two main categories: *expression of carbohydrates* and *structural changes in glycoproteins and glycolipids.*

A variety of plant agglutinins recognise specific sugar residues expressed at the cell surface. In transformed cells, the expression or the lateral mobility of molecules (glycoproteins) containing specific sugar residues is increased, so transformed cells are agglutinated by plant lectins such as concanavalin A or wheat germ agglutinin, whereas normal cells are not or to a much lower extent. The actual mechanism of increased agglutinability of tumour cells is still a matter of dispute (Nicolson, 1974). Studies with human tumour biopsies are limited or in the case of leukaemia the results are conflicting, so studies of this type are still in an experimental phase and not yet ready for the characterisation of human tumours in primary culture. Nevertheless, these plant lectins are important probes of the cell surface and will undoubtedly find their application in clinical studies, for instance in the assessment of (tumour specific) antigen expression (Smets and Broekhuysen-Davies, 1972).

Differences in the chemical composition of glycoproteins and glycolipids from the surface of transformed cells as compared with similar material from normal cells, have been reviewed recently (Emmelot, 1973). In particular, surface glycopeptides from virus-transformed cells differ from normal glycopeptides by an increase in the density of sialic acid residues. This biochemical change was detected by column chromatography as faster elution of the malignant component due to increased sialic acid density (Buck *et al.* 1971).

The assay is a relatively simple one. Tumour cells are incubated for some time in tissue culture medium containing radioactive fucose to label the glycoproteins. The surface material is solubilised by mild trypsination, exhaustively digested with pronase and eluted on columns. The elution profiles of control and malignant cell material are then compared. Fig. 5 shows the elution profiles for an acute myeloblastic leukaemia compared with the profile for normal

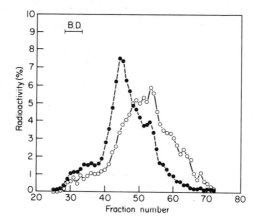

Fig. 5. Elution profiles of surface glycopeptides isolated from cells labelled in tissue culture with radioactive fucose for 48 hr. Surface material from human myeloblastic leukaemia cells labelled with ^{14}C-fucose (● — — — ●) was co-chromatographed with ^{3}H-fucose labelled surface material from control lymphocytes (○ — — — ○). B.D. = Blue dextran column marker.

lymphocytes. The difference disappears if the material is treated with neuraminidase indicating that these glycopeptides have a higher sialic acid density.

Of particular importance is the question whether such changes are of a general nature and not a feature of transformed cells in established cell cultures. This question has been extensively studied in the Departments of Experimental Cytology and Biochemistry of the Netherlands Cancer Institute (Van Beek *et al.* 1973 and in press). Our results up to now, summarised in Table 1, have led to the following conclusions: increased sialic acid density is found in all malignant cell lines studied, irrespective of their morphology, the malignant determinant (that is, viral, chemical or spontaneous) or the conditions of growth (that is, tissue culture, tumour cells *in vivo* or biopsy specimens *in vitro*). Moreover, it has been observed in animal as well as in human cells and is not caused by high cell density or blastoid transformation. Thus, the biochemical change meets most— if not all—criteria for a universal marker or malignancy.

The relevance of these observations for fundamental oncology seems obvious, but in the context of *in vitro* cultures, one wishes to know whether the assay is valuable for the diagnosis and the evaluation of primary cultures of human tumour cells. For the time being, any final conclusion will be far too premature. However, some

TABLE 1

Transformed and Malignant Cells Positive for a Structural Change in Surface Glycoprotein (Van Beek, Smets and Emmelot)

A. ANIMAL CELLS

Permanent cell line "in vitro"	*Tumour cells grown "in vivo"*
PG-BHK	
SV40-3T3	
3T3-F	
Mouse lymphosarcoma	lymphosarcoma (ascites)
Rat hepatoma	rat hepatoma (solid tumour)

Controls: normal mouse and hamster cells, regenerating and fetal rat liver cells.

B. HUMAN LEUKAEMIC CELLS

Permanent cell line "in vitro"	*Peripheral tumour cells in primary tissue culture*
lymphoblastic lymphoma	lymphosarcoma
Burkitt's lymphoma	chronic lymphocytic leukaemia
	chronic myelocytic leukaemia
	acute lymphocytic leukaemia
	acute myelocytic leukaemia
	acute myelomonocytic leukaemia
	acute promyelocytic leukaemia

Controls: normal and PHA-stimulated peripheral lymphocytes, infectious mononucleosis lymphocytes.

observations emphasise at least the potential value of glycoprotein analysis for diagnostic purposes.

(1) At the time of assay, the diagnosis of one of the donors was uncertain. He was suspected of leukaemia but infectious mononucleosis was not excluded. The biochemical assay indicated malignancy and in the further course of the disease, the patient developed the typical clinical picture of chronic myelocytic leukaemia of the juvenile type.

(2) Details of the elution profiles of glycopeptides from various cases of leukaemia displayed characteristic differences which, for instance, allowed the discrimination between acute and chronic myelocytic leukaemia by elution parameters only.

(3) Correlations between the elution patterns of surface glycopeptides and parameters of transformation *in vivo*, i.e. saturation density, agglutinability etc.) were suggested by experiments with established cell lines.

Thus, it may be that structural differences in surface glycopeptides are not only indicative for malignancy *per se*, but might be also related to the type of the disease and the degree of malignancy. If further research confirms this possibility, a potent analytical tool for the characterisation of primary cultures of biopsies will become available.

3. EARLY DIAGNOSIS

The ultra-rapid pulse-cytophotometric determination of cellular DNA content has been mentioned as an analytical tool in cell cycle analysis. It has been suggested that machines of this type could be used in the early detection of cancer by pre-screening of the population or of high-risk groups. Carcinoma of cervix, lung, stomach and bladder appear suitable cases for pre-screening by automated cytology.

The parameter to be studied by the pulse-cytophotometer is the presence of cells with more than diploid DNA content. Ancuploidy could be indicative for malignancy since even diploid tumour cells always contain a (small) fraction of cells with unusual DNA values. Moreover, increased DNA content could result from the presence of DNA synthesising tumour cells.

The main problem for the moment is to develop suitable techniques of sample preparation. These samples must be aselective or controlled selective (enrichment in suspected cells) and should not contain an excess of cell debris or non-relevant cells such as granulocytes. Serious progress in this area is not to be expected before these conditions have been met.

REFERENCES

Brown, J. M. (1968). *Exptl. Cell Res. 52,* 565.
Buck, C., Glick, M. and Warren, L. (1971). *Science, 172,* 169.
Cleaver, J. (1967). "Thymidine Metabolism and Cell Kinetics" (Frontiers in Biology, Vol. 6). North-Holland Publ. Co., Amsterdam.
Emmelot, P. (1973). *Eur. J. Cancer, 9,* 319.
Göhde, W. (1973). *In* "Fluorescence Techniques in Cell Biology" (A. Thaer and M. Sernetz, eds.), p. 79. Springer, Berlin.
Holm, D. and Cram, L. (1973). *Exptl. Cell Res. 80,* 105.
Nicolson, G. L. (1974). *Int. Rev. Cytol. 39,* 89. (G. H. Bourne and J. Danielli, eds.). Academic Press, New York and London.
Smets, L. and Broekhuysen-Davies, J. (1972). *J. Eur. Cancer, 8,* 541.
Smets, L. A. (1973). *Exptl. Cell Res. 79,* 239.
Van Beek, W. P., Smets, L. and Emmelot, P. (1973). *Cancer Res. 33,* 2913.
Van Beek, W. P., Smets, L. and Emmelot, P. (1975). *Nature, Lond., 253,* 457.

DISCUSSION

Lamerton emphasised both the importance and the difficulty of trying to determine the number of resting cells. The methods using phase specific agents will not really tell us at the moment which cells are resting. They may indicate that a certain proportion of cells are slowly dividing, but it is extremely difficult or even impossible, to distinguish slowly dividing cells from cells that have not yet been triggered into preparation for DNA synthesis or are arrested in certain parts of the cell cycle. If cytochemical methods can be developed to identify such cells they will be very important.

Smets said we should also try to discriminate between really resting G_0 cells and non-cycling cells. The required approach is to combine the methods he discussed with work on gradients, first separating cells in different phases of growth and then starting to measure biochemical and cytochemical differences on partially purified cells instead of on the mixture of cells, but this might take years to achieve. Lamerton supported this approach because of the difficulty with present techniques in working with a population which has a wide spread in cell cycle characteristics.

In reply to Brockas, who asked if the glycopeptide patterns from normal lymphocyte donors were reproducible, Smets said that if a sample was divided into 10 separate samples and they were all run on the columns there was no problem. As far as reproducibility for different human material is concerned, for most of the diagnoses they had two samples and in the case of chronic lymphatic leukaemia there were three samples and they all showed the same pattern. Reproducibility is also improved by always mixing control and test cells together and any procedure, trypsinisation, Pronase treatment, dialysis, lyophylisation or chromatography, is done together.

Asked if there were any differences between lymphocytes from normal donors or between normal lymphocytes and phytohaemaglutinin stimulated lymphocytes, Smets said only in the height of a peak. Horizontal differences are not seen.

Mehrishi said that recent work by Weiss and Hauschka (1970) using various strains of mice, and his own work on certain mammalian cells (Mehrishi, 1972) suggested that the net negative charge at the surface of cancer cells bears no functional relation to degree of malignancy.

Smets emphasised that they had studied sialic acid density in fucose-labelled, trypsin-sensitive material from the cell surface. It is likely that this has nothing to do with the total sialic acid which might be isolated from the cell under different conditions, or the total electronegative charge, since it represents only 25% of all glycoprotein and perhaps 10% of all sialic acids.

REFERENCES

Mehrishi, J. N. (1972). *In* "Progress in Biophysics and Molecular Biology", Vol. 25, (1). (J. A. V. Butler and D. Noble, eds.). Pergamon Press, Oxford.
Weiss, L. and Hauschka, T. S. (1970). *Int. J. Cancer*, 6, 270.

2. Advances in Morphological Identification of Cell Types in Primary Culture

L. Morasca, G. Balconi and E. Erba

In vitro testing of the activity of anticancer agents on human cancer biopsy material is often performed on the bulk tissue assuming that everything in the biopsy is cancer. Although we know there is often very little tumour in a biopsy, this may often be the only possible approach when short term assays are performed on surviving tissue. When a sub-culture method is applied, it becomes of primary importance to be able to recognise the different types of cells that are living in that culture. We have developed morphological methods to answer very basic questions like (a) do cancer cells survive *in vitro*? (b) are they more or less sensitive to the compound tested than stromatic fibroblasts or endothelial cells? Phase contrast microscopy provided a useful method to evaluate, for long periods of time, the behaviour of the same cultures before, during and after treatment with drugs.

Small explants (Morasca *et al.* 1972) or cells spilled from explants (Lasfargues, 1973) were cultured in Rose Chambers under perforated cellophane (Rose *et al.* 1958) using medium 199 + 20% calf serum and antibiotics.

Figure 1 shows a frozen section of a clear cell carcinoma of the ovary. Cells are of variable dimensions with irregular dense chromatin. One polynucleated structure which may be a giant cell or a cell aggregate, is surrounded by secretion and such figures were frequent for this specimen. The cells found in the culture of the same biopsy after five days *in vitro* appeared very similar to the tissue of origin. The giant cell of Fig. 2 with its several nuclei and the secretion droplets on one side, strongly resemble the polynucleated structure of Fig. 1. The same applies to the extremely irregular population of cells appearing in both preparations.

The second example is a serous carcinoma of the ovary which showed small clusters of cells surrounded by connective tissue in the section (Fig. 3). Three separate cultures were prepared. The spillage method gave clumps of practically pure epithelial cells in the washing

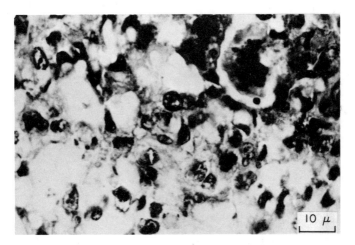

Fig. 1. Frozen section of a clear cell carcinoma of the ovary.

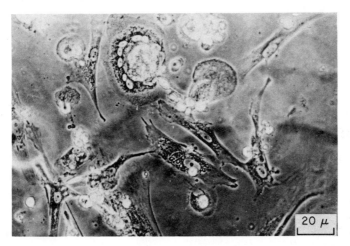

Fig. 2. Cells cultured from the biopsy shown in Fig. 1 after 5 days *in vitro*.

solution and these grew as clusters, or nests of cells, with an acinar-like structure strongly suggestive of tumour (Fig. 4). The explant method on the other hand gave mixed cultures containing variable amounts of stromal tissue. Finally, cells were also cultured from ascitic fluid and this culture was followed by time-lapse photography for its first few hours in culture (Fig. 5). Large single spherical cells settled on the base of the chamber together with many active lymphocytes. A number of cells were observed to collapse and

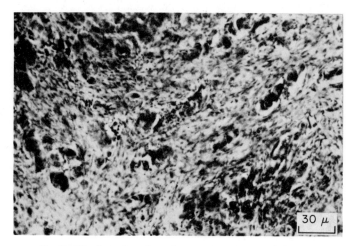

Fig. 3. Histological section of a serous carcinoma of the ovary.

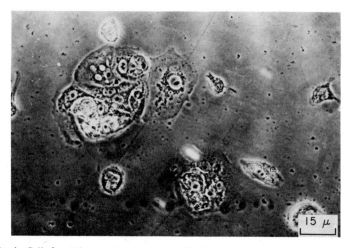

Fig. 4. Cells from the specimen shown in Fig. 3 cultured by the spillage technique.

it was noted that many lymphocytes immediately became active and formed rosettes around the dying cells. On subsequent days it was noted that the number of cells had decreased and although a culture had established by day 5, none of the cells was epithelial in shape (Fig. 6).

When cultures were prepared from a metastasis from an undifferentiated mammary carcinoma, although the histology showed a uniform pattern of epithelial cells surrounded by bundles

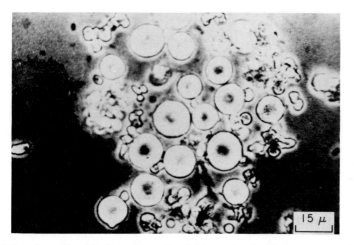

Fig. 5. Cells cultured for 2 hr from the ascites fluid associated with the specimen of Fig. 3.

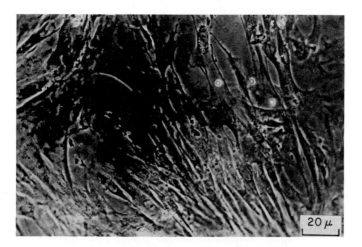

Fig. 6. The same cells as Fig. 5 after 5 days in culture.

of connective tissue, the outgrowths were very variable. One hundred cultures were prepared with two explants in each. Some showed typical polygonal, flat epithelial cells, very reminiscent of KB cells (Fig. 7a) while others showed a more acinar type structure (Fig. 7b) and yet a third class consisted of spindle-shaped epithelial cells (Fig. 7c) sometimes alone and sometimes as single elements in almost pure stromatic populations (Fig. 7d).

Four different biopsies from Ewing sarcomas have been cultured

HTSTC–4

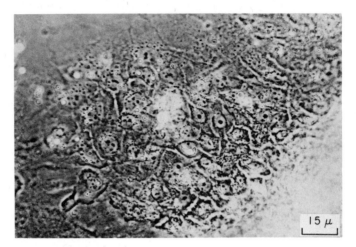

Fig. 7. Different cellular morphologies in cultures prepared from the same biopsy of a metastasis from an undifferentiated mammary tumour.

Fig. 7a. Polygonal, flat "KB-like" cells.

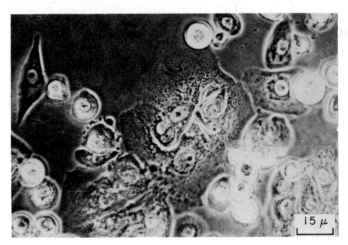

Fig. 7b. Acinar-like cells.

but it has never been possible to find on the day after culture the typically small rounded cells characteristic of this tumour. When cultures were obtained at 5 days they had the appearance of normal stroma.

A number of conclusions can be drawn: (a) We may obtain in culture morphological patterns clearly similar to the original tumour;

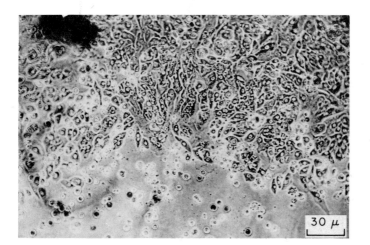

Fig. 7c. Spindle shaped epithelial cells.

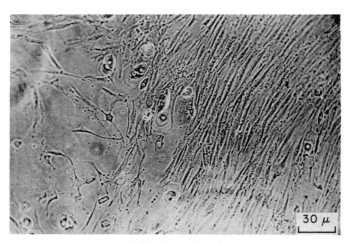

Fig. 7d. Stromatic cells.

(b) In other cases, however, a substantial amount of cell selection may take place and the proportion of the various cell types in the original biopsy may be drastically altered. Cells may die in culture for natural reasons like lymphocyte activity or, different cell populations may be present in different explants; (c) Some types of cells do not survive in our culture conditions. This suggests that some kinds of human cancer cells, in this case the Ewing sarcoma, may have specific metabolic needs that were not satisfied in the culture environment we provided. Further studies are required to learn which are the metabolic needs of this tumour. This point may become increasingly important in the future, leading to specific culture procedures for each type of tumour, and to a better knowledge of the metabolic needs of human cancer cells.

REFERENCES

Lasfargues, E. Y. (1973). *In* "Tissue Culture" (Kruse and Patterson, eds.), p. 45. Academic Press, New York and London.

Morasca, L., Balconi, G., De Nadai, F. and Dolfini, E. (1972). *Europ. J. Cancer,* *8,* 429.

Rose, G. G., Pomerat, L. M., Shindler, T. P. and Trunnel, J. B. (1958). *J. Bioph. Biochem. Cytol. 4,* 761.

3. Behaviour of Tumour Cells in Monolayer Culture

J. C. Klein

The sensitivities of tumours to chemotherapeutic drugs show large variations and tests of short duration that measure *in vitro* the sensitivity of individual tumours to particular drugs could be very helpful in the selection of the most effective therapy. However, because tumours contain not only tumour cells but also non-malignant connective tissue and blood-borne cells, one must question if the results really represent the effect of the drugs on the tumour cells. In other words, which cell types are active in tumour pieces and tumour cell suspensions and could be influenced by drug treatment? The following experiments were designed to learn something about the cells which are active when monolayer culture are initiated from "spontaneous" and certain transplantable tumours.

Tumour material was cut into pieces 1-2 mm^3 with a pair of scissors. Some of the pieces were attached with serum to the glass and medium was added some hours later. The rest of the material was treated with trypsin or collagenase and inoculated as a suspension. The cultures were inspected daily and classified for cell attachment, outgrowth and growth capacity.

Table 1 shows data for spontaneous tumours. Tumours are grouped according to their organ of origin because the location of the tumour influenced its structure, processing, and the outcome of the culture. For instance, mammary tumours contained a relatively high percentage of connective tissue, collagen and fibrocytes which trapped the tumour cells and made it difficult to obtain a good cell suspension. The cell yield of these suspensions was low, contained many fibroblasts and activity in culture was at first low. Although these tumour pieces showed some outgrowth on the day after inoculation, active growth of fibroblasts developed only after about a week and growth of epitheloid cells was even longer delayed.

On the other hand, it was very easy to make suspensions of brain tumours. The use of trypsin was hardly necessary and in some cases it was difficult to prepare pieces of tumour suitable for culture. In culture the cells were very active and on morphological criteria seemed to represent reliable tumour material.

TABLE 1

Behaviour in Primary Monolayer Culture of Tumour Cells and/or Tumour Pieces Derived from Spontaneous *Tumours*

| | TUMOUR | | | GROWTH | |
Organ	Tumour type	No.	Delay in days	Cell type
	HUMAN			
Breast	adeno carcinoma	8	11 (7-19)	fib/ep
Brain	astrocytoma	3	2 (1-3)	fib/ep
	mixed glioma	2	2	ep/fib
	meningoma	1	2	fib
Colon	adeno carcinoma	1	5*	fib/ep
Bladder	carcinoma	1	3*	ep/fib
	RAT			
Bladder	carcinoma	1	3*	fib/ep
Urether	squamous cell carcinoma	2	6*	ep/fib
Pituitary gland	adeno carcinoma	1	5	fib/ep
Bladder	normal	3	3 (2-4)	ep/fib

* Cultures plated from suspension showed good attachment for one day but then extensive cell death.

ep = epitheloid cells
fib = fibroblastic cells

    Colon, bladder and urether tumours could be processed easily, but we found a striking difference in growth between cells plated as suspensions and the tumour pieces. Cells freshly derived from the tumour attached well and the culture looked healthy next day, but thereafter most cells died and detached from the glass and only some fibroblasts survived. The comparable tumour pieces attached well and showed active cell growth in the outgrowth zone after 3-5 days. Suspensions made from detached pieces in these cultures did not show the cell deterioration found in freshly prepared suspensions. In all these cultures a mixture of cell types was found, dominated by probably normal fibroblasts.

    In Table 2 similar data are presented for transplantable tumours. The first three represent cultures derived from human tumours which grew in nude mice and the others were rat tumours transplantable in isologous animals. Active growth started much earlier than in the previous group, a higher percentage of the cells was active and relatively more typical tumour cells were present. Several of the cultures set up from cell suspensions were lost after a promising start in culture.

TABLE 2

Behaviour in Primary Monolayer Culture of Tumour Cells and/or Tumour Pieces Derived from Transplanted *Tumours*

	TUMOUR			GROWTH	
Organ	Tumour type	No.	Delay in days	Cell type
	HUMAN *via nude mice*				
Brain	mixed glioma	1	1	fib/nerve
Colon	adeno carcinoma	2	2, $<$ 4	ep/fib
	RAT *via isologous rat*				
Breast	fibroadenoma	1	1	fib
Brain	schwannoma	1	1	atypical
Bladder	carcinoma	3	3*	ep/fib
Urether	carcinoma	1	2*	ep/fib

* Cultures plated from suspension showed good attachment for one day but then extensive cell death.

ep = epitheloid cells
fib = fibroblastic cells

It is clear from this data that not all tumour cell suspensions are equivalent. The suspension of cells from spontaneous mammary tumours gave not only a very low yield but also a poor representation of the tumour. The other spontaneous tumours provided a much better yield, but again the non-malignant cells were generally more numerous than the tumour cells and the fibroblasts often grew better than the epitheloid tumour cells. Cell suspensions of brain tumours gave the best yield of spontaneous tumour cells in culture. Transplanted tumours provided better target material with a higher yield of active cells and relatively more tumour cells.

In conclusion, measurements of the effect of drugs on the metabolic activity of cell populations prepared in this way, especially from spontaneous tumour material, can be expected to be greatly influenced by the effect on the non-malignant cells present in the suspension.

4. Human Tumour Cell Identification in Short Term Monolayer Culture

J. E. M. Wright and P. P. Dendy

We have found that short term cultures prepared by the monolayer technique (see page 24) are particularly useful for studies designed to predict the *in vitro* sensitivity of a patient's tumour to chemotherapeutic agents (Dendy *et al.* 1970, and page 139).

A serious criticism of the method is that in nearly all tumour biopsies there is associated stroma which may contain normal cells and evidence is essential that the cells actually cultured are malignant. In practice, at the single cell level there are no criteria which can be used as unequivocal evidence of malignancy in the clinical sense, and the best one can hope to achieve is to show that the cultured cells are demonstrably abnormal. Development of a quantitative method is clearly desirable.

1. SIZE OF NUCLEOLUS RELATIVE TO SIZE OF NUCLEUS

Early work of Quensel (1928) and Karp (1932) suggested that nucleolar size could be used as an indication of malignancy. Quensel measured nucleolar diameters and found values of 1-1·5 μ for normal cell nucleoli and 2-4 μ for tumour cell nucleoli, with the occasional tumour cell nucleolus in the 6-9 μ range. The ratio of nucleolar to nuclear diameter was 0·16 for endothelial cells and 0·2-0·4 for tumour cells. An approach based on measurement of nucleolar and nuclear size would have two advantages. First, it would be simple and quick and secondly, would allow us to imitate the growth conditions used in the *in vitro* chemosensitivity test closely.

Coverslips in Leighton tubes were seeded with 5 x 10^5 cells/coverslip in 1 ml medium (90 parts medium 199, 10 parts foetal calf serum and 5 parts 5% lactalbumin hydrolysate adjusted with bicarbonate to pH 7·2). The cultures were grown for times ranging from 2 to 15 days, fixed in Susa for 8 min and stained with Heidenhains iron alum haematoxylin, to give sharply defined nuclear and nucleolar membranes. High-power photographs were prepared and a planimeter was used to measure nuclear and nucleolar areas.

TABLE 1

Summary of Results for Nucleolar Areas, Expressed as a Percentage of the Nucleoplasmic Area for Cells in Monolayer Culture

Specimen	Fluid (F) or Solid (S)	Diagnosis	Number of days in culture	RATIO $\dfrac{\text{nucleolar area}}{\text{nuclear sap area}}$ %
HEp		Established cell line, many years in culture		10·6 ± 0·5
L		Established cell line, many years in culture		28·8 ± 1·6
Human embryonic spleen	S	Normal tissue	4	11·5 ± 1·1
Human amnion	S	Normal tissue	12	13·6 ± 1·2
Normal ovary	S	Normal tissue	3	8·1 ± 0·4
Patient 1	F	Ca breast	8	9·1 ± 0·5
Patient 2	S	Ca stomach	5	9·3 ± 0·6
Patient 3	S	Eye melanoma	8	9·4 ± 0·4
Patient 4	S	Ca caecum	6	15·2 ± 0·8
Patient 5	F	Hepatoma	13	13·3 ± 0·8
Patient 6	S	Ovarian cystadenoma	8	6·3 ± 0·4
Patient 7	S	Benign ovarian neoplasm	3	10·6 ± 0·7
Patient 8	F	Ca ovary with secondary ascites	13	9·2 ± 0·5
Patient 9	F	Ca ovary with secondary ascites	14	11·0 ± 0·6
Dog 1	S	Myxofibrosarcoma	6	8·3 ± 0·5
Dog 2	S	Mammary tumour	3	14·4 ± 1·2
Dog 3	S	Mouth tumour	15	11·1 ± 0·9

The mean ratio

$$\frac{\text{nucleolar area}}{\text{nucleoplasmic area}} = \frac{n}{N\text{-}n} \times 100\%$$

was tabulated for two established cell lines, three normal human tissues, a wide range of human tumours and 3 dog tumours (Table 1).

The results are disappointing and provide no evidence for a method of tumour cell identification. A possible cause of this negative result is the known correlation between nucleolar size and the level of nucleolar metabolism (Edstrom, 1958). Metabolism in short term culture of human biopsies is very variable from one specimen to another, at least as measured by the progress of cells through the cell cycle, and difficult to control: this may be the reason for the inconsistency of the results. At this stage we must also of course, admit the possibility that the cells measured were actually normal.

2. CHROMOSOME NUMBERS IN KARYOTYPE

Abnormality in neoplastic cells is genetic and is transmitted vertically at each division to the daughters of the dividing cells. Thus the presence of a marker chromosome or chromosomes (Seif and Spriggs, 1967) provides the most stringent biological definition of neoplasia currently available, namely that of clonal proliferation of aneuploid cells (Kaplan, 1972).

Methods were therefore developed to study karyotype in our short-term monolayer cultures. The cells were incubated with 0·25 µgm/tube colcemid for 4 hr, returned to colcemid free medium for 24 hr; swollen in hypotonic saline solution comprising 1 part Hanks and 3 parts distilled water at 37° C for 20 min; fixed for 10 min in 25% acetic acid in ethanol; and stained with Giemsa.

Results are shown in Table 2. Very few cells could be scored unequivocally and a number of counts which might have been 45 or 47 have been recorded as 46.

The main conclusions are as follows:

(1) It is easy to obtain a detailed pattern for the distribution of chromosomes in established cell lines.

(2) For normal tissues, with the exception of the adult ovary (vide infra) all measurable cells had 46 chromosomes.

(3) For all the tumour specimens except one, several cells were found with chromosome numbers differing from 46.

This positive identification of cells with more or less than 46 chromosomes would probably be sufficient for diagnostic purposes.

TABLE 2

Distribution of Chromosome Numbers for Cultured Cells from Various Normal and Malignant Tissues

| | Human Cell Type | Number of cells at given chromosome number or within the indicated range | | |
		Less than 45	46 (±1)	more than 47
	Normal			
	Normal leucocytes		18	
	Amnion		4	
	Adult Ovary		14	*
	Embryonic skin and muscle (8 day culture)		17	
	Embryonic skin and muscle (107 day culture)		9	
	Tumour			
20/7/73(1)	Probably Ovarian		2	
10/8/73(3)	Ovarian Tumour	9	9	
7/9/73(1)	Pleural effusion		9	2
23/10/73(2)	Ovarian Tumour	5	5	
9/11/73(1)	Melanoma		11	8
7/11/73(1)	Ovarian Tumour	1	10	6
28/6/73(2)	Ascites Fluid	6	6	10
11/7/73(1)	Ovarian Tumour	6	10	3

* A few cells with definitely more than 46 chromosomes but exact number uncountable.

For fuller details on the tumour histologies see Table 3.

However, each result is the total yield of information from a systematic survey of two coverslips seeded with 10^6 cells and may be quite unrepresentative of the population as a whole. It is therefore unlikely that this method can give information on the nature of the cells responding to cytotoxic drugs, when the whole culture is treated with chemotherapeutic agents.

3. DNA MEASUREMENTS—INTERPHASE AND MITOTIC CELLS

A number of workers have already shown that in the majority of cases DNA values for tumour cells do differ from those for normal cells (Atkin and Richards, 1956, Freni James and Prop, 1971, Mundy, 1973, Pfitzer and Pape, 1973). After fixation, cells were therefore stained by the Feulgen reaction and the absorbance of individual nuclei was measured using a Deeley type scanning microdensitometer (Barr and Stroud).

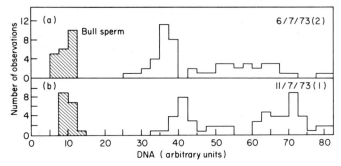

Fig. 1. DNA distributions for interphase cells in cultures of two tumour specimens. The distributions for bull sperm which was used as a biological standard are also shown. 6/7/73(2) was an advanced carcinoma of ovary. 11/7/73(1) was an advanced carcinoma of ovary.

Figure 1 shows two results when DNA values were measured for all cells. Interpretation is difficult, because when measurements are made on interphase cells, the spread of DNA values due to heterogeneity of the population cannot be separated from the spread caused by cells being in different phases of the cell cycle. The

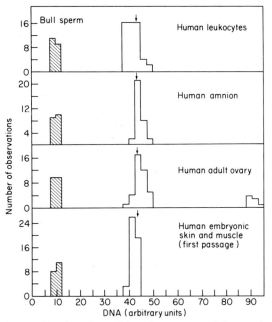

Fig. 2. Metaphase DNA values for cells in cultures prepared from various normal human tissues relative to a normalised mean bull sperm value of 10·0.

presence of tumour cells can be inferred from the extreme DNA values, but there are several DNA values in the middle which might correspond either to normal diploid cells mid-way through S phase, or tumour cells in either G_1 or G_0 phase. For work on the prediction of drug sensitivities, it is essential to know about the majority of the population, not just a few selected cells, so neither chromosome study nor DNA measurement on interphase cells is valid.

By combining the last two ideas and making DNA measurements only on metaphase cells, we have been more successful. Figure 2 shows metaphase DNA values for a wide variety of normal human cells. The intensity of Feulgen stain is not reproducible, being very sensitive to the exact hydrolysis conditions, and fades with storage. Therefore a slide carrying a smear of bull sperm was placed close to each experimental slide during staining and used as a biological standard. In each instance, the mean absorbance of 20 cells on the appropriate bull sperm slide has been normalised to 10·0 and DNA values for cultured cells have been adjusted accordingly. The best estimate for the ratio

$$\frac{\text{Human DNA/cell}}{\text{Bull DNA/cell}}$$

is about 1·05 (Sandritter, 1962) so for a

$$\frac{\text{Metaphase Human Cell (double diploid)}}{\text{Bull Sperm \quad (haploid)}}$$

the ratio is 4·2 and this figure has been arrowed on each diagram. All the distributions are narrow and have a mean DNA value close to 4·2. There were a few tetraploid cells in the culture of adult ovary (probably corresponding to the chromosome counts in excess of 46) but intermediate values were not obtained.

The distributions for several tumour specimens are shown in Fig. 3. They are generally quite different both from each other and from the distributions for normal cells.

The ratio of mean metaphase DNA value to the corresponding mean bull sperm value has been tabulated (Table 3) and the main features of these results can be summarised as follows:

(1) Apart from the 107 day culture of human embryonic skin and muscle, all the results for normal human cells lie between 4·10 and 4·57 with a mean at (4·35 ± 0·12).

(2) For the 9 malignant tumours all the ratios are either less than 4·0 or greater than 5·0 and well outside the range of ratios for normal cells.

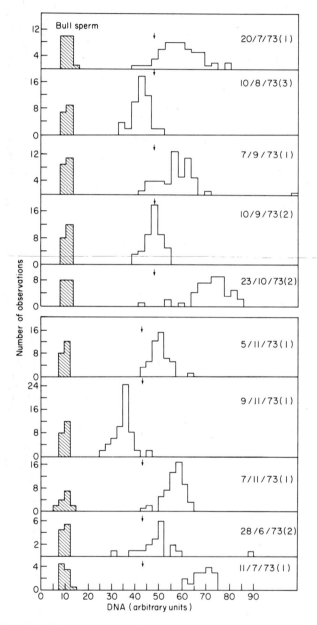

Fig. 3. Metaphase DNA distributions for 10 human tumour biopsy specimens relative to a normalised mean bull sperm value of 10.0. Expected ratio of 4.2 arrowed.
For histological identification see Table 3.

TABLE 3

Ratio of Mean Metaphase DNA Value to the Bull Sperm DNA Value for Various Cell Types Studied

Normal tissues		Cell metaphase DNA / Bull sperm DNA
Phytohaemoglutinnin stimulated human leucocytes		4·10
Human amnion		4·46
Human adult ovary		4·45
Human embryonic skin and muscle (8 day culture)		4·18
Human embryonic skin and muscle (76 day culture)		4·27
Human embryonic skin and muscle (107 day culture)		4·72
Tumour tissues		
20/7/73(1)	Omental biopsy of mainly differentiated malignant cells. Primary doubtful, possibly ovary	5·35
10/8/73(1)	Ovarian biopsy showing poorly differentiated mitotically active tumour cells	3·83
7/9/73(1)	Omental secondaries from cystadenocarcinoma of the ovary	5·13
10/9/73(2)	BENIGN ovarian dermoid cyst	4·32
23/10/73(2)	Pleural effusion from an old carcinoma of the breast	6·49
5/11/73(1)	Ascites Fluid from recurrent carcinoma of the ovary	5·06
9/11/73(1)	Amelanotic malignant melanoma of left calf mitotically active	3·50
2/11/73(1)	Biopsy of malignant ovarian tumour	5·63
28/6/73(2)	Ascites Fluid from poorly differentiated adenocarcinoma of the ovary	5·42
11/7/73(1)	Biopsy from papillary serous cystadeno carcinoma of the ovary	6·64

(3) The presence of a benign ovarian cyst is easily detected and opens up new possibilities of early diagnosis.

(4) With careful experimental technique the majority of metaphase cells are suitable for measurement and sampling errors should be small.

(5) The method is also sufficiently accurate for the proportion of normal dividing cells to be estimated. About 30% of the cells measured in the specimen 7/9/73 might have been normal, but the figure is usually a lot lower and may even be zero (11/7/72 (1)).

In conclusion, a method has been developed which gives useful information on the normality or otherwise, of dividing cells in short term monolayer cultures prepared from human biopsy specimens by our procedures. The method gives no information on the nature of non-dividing cells and this must be kept in mind when assays for the effects of drugs, radiation or other treatments on the cultures are developed.

REFERENCES

Atkin, N. B. and Richards, B. M. (1956). *Brit. J. Cancer, 10,* 769.
Dendy, P. P., Bozman, G. and Wheeler, T. K. (1970). *Lancet,* Jul. 11, 68.
Edstrom, J. E. and Eichner, J. (1958). *Nature, Lond. 181* 619.
Freni, S. C., James, J. and Prop, F. J. A. (1971). *Acta Cytologica, 15,* 154.
Kaplan, H. S. (1972). "Hodgkins Disease". Harvard Univ. Press, Cambridge, Mass.
Karp, H. (1932). *Zeit. Krebsforsch. 39,* 579.
Mundy, G. R. (1973). *Cancer, 32,* 61.
Pfitzer, R. and Pape, H. D. (1973). *Acta Cytologica, 17,* 19.
Quensel, U. (1928). *Acta Med. Scand. 68,* 458.
Sandritter, W. (1962). *In* "Introduction to Quantitative Cytochemistry" (G. L. Wied, ed.), p. 171. Academic Press, New York and London.
Seif, G. S. F. and Spriggs, A. I. (1967). *J. Nat. Cancer Inst. 39,* 557.

5. An Attempt to Discriminate between Sporadic and Hereditary Retinoblastoma by means of Tissue Culture

F. J. A. Prop, G. C. B. Prop-Arnold and L. H. Eijgenstein

Retinoblastoma is a rare, highly malignant tumour of the eye that occurs in young children; it is even sometimes found in the newborn. The tumour may occur sporadically but there is also a hereditary form which obeys Mendelian laws for dominant heredity. Slightly less than 50% of the offspring of such an affected parent will acquire the tumour; the deviation from 50% being due to imperfect penetration (Schappert-Kimmijser *et al.* 1966).

If the tumour occurs in children whose ancestors are not affected, it has been shown that a considerable proportion of these tumours are the first cases of a new hereditary line, whereas the remainder are truly sporadic and offspring are not endangered. Sometimes these tumours occur in both eyes and it has been shown that these are always hereditary. In the unilateral cases arising in a family for the first time, there is no way to predict whether the patient's offspring will be affected or not. It has been shown, however, that 20% of these cases are hereditary, whereas the offspring of the other 80% remain free of the tumour.

As there are no means to discriminate between the hereditary and the non-hereditary cases, except by looking for the tumour in the offspring, the children of *all* these patients have to be examined under general anaesthesia every three months from birth until well into school age. General anaesthesia so frequently in young children is never completely without risk. Moreover, this policy causes a lot of inconvenience for the patients and unnecessary mental strain from the anxiety that their progeny may become ill. It may often make them abandon the idea of marriage or having children. Since only 20% are at risk—of which less than half will get tumours—the policy would be quite unnecessary for 80% of the people if only the group at risk could be identified at an earlier stage.

For several years now a group in the Netherlands sponsored by the Netherlands Society for the Prevention of Blindness and subsidised by the "Koningin Wilhelmina Funds for the Fight against Cancer" has studied this problem experimentally in order to find methods to discriminate between the sporadic and the hereditary cases. We are co-ordinating this effort and although several modern and sophisticated disciplines and techniques are involved, only with tissue culture have we any prospect of a solution at the moment.

The tumour is rather rare so we see only about 10 cases per annum in Holland, and we are very lucky to have collaboration with all eye clinics in Holland and also clinics in Essen (W. Germany), Ghent and Brussels (Belgium). In this way we hope to get sufficient evidence to be statistically valid within a reasonable time.

In culturing the retinoblastoma, we tried several different techniques and different media and we were old-fashioned enough (a consequence probably of early studies with Albert Fischer many years ago) also to use the plasma clot method in Carrel flasks. This proved to be a lucky choice and we are now using this method routinely in this investigation.

Large series of pictures were taken for all cultures, mostly with phase contrast, of every aspect that seemed interesting. The cultures grew well and from one case to another the main cell type in culture could be anything from purely epithelial (Fig. 1) to purely fibro-

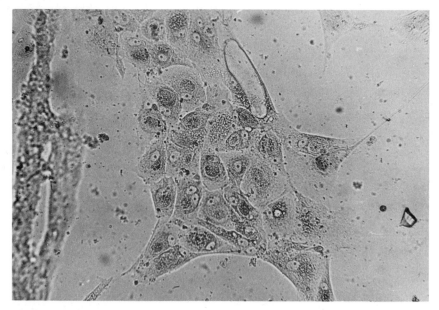

Fig. 1. Well contact inhibited epithelial type outgrowth from a retinoblastoma in a plasma clot (phase contrast 100X).

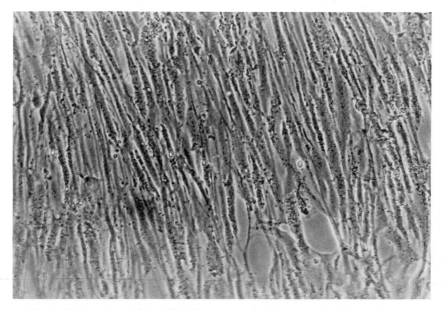

Fig. 2. Well contact inhibited fibroblastic outgrowth from a retinoblastoma in a plasma clot (phase contrast 100X).

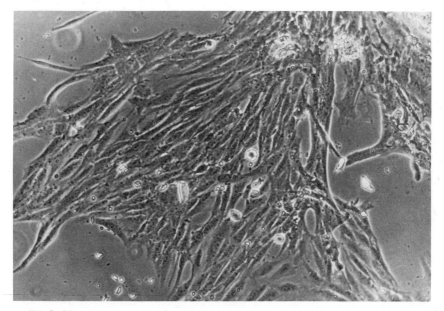

Fig. 3. Most common type of cell in outgrowth from a retinoblastoma in a plasma clot. Cell type is intermediate between epithelial and fibroblastic. This picture also shows good contact inhibition (phase contrast 100X).

blastic (Fig. 2) in appearance but most cells were something in between the two (Fig. 3). After some time we had well over a thousand pictures taken from about 20 cases and the enormous task began of trying to find some common denominator relevant to our problem. Careful examination suggested a systematic difference and since that time we have had over 90 cases and what was at first only a hint has come true! There is a difference of growth pattern in culture between all retinoblastomas that are known to be hereditary and the majority of the cases in which one eye was affected in a family that until then was free from retinoblastoma. A minority of the latter group show the same growth pattern as the hereditary group. This difference in growth pattern may be an expression of absence or presence of heredity for the tumour.

The difference in growth pattern is best seen in the classical Carrel-type of culture in a plasma clot and is probably due to a difference in contact inhibition of motion. Good contact inhibition is shown in Figs 1, 2 and 3, which all show a very regular "quiet" growth pattern. The other type of growth is probably an expression of diminished contact inhibition of motion. Figure 4 for example, shows a kind of basket-work-like interlacing of cells giving the

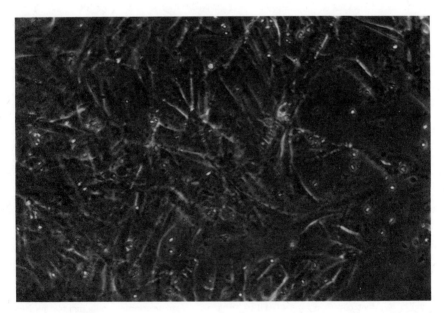

Fig. 4. Interlacing basket-work-like growth from a retinoblastoma due to impaired contact inhibition of motion. Plasma clot (phase contrast 100X).

cultures a more disorganised "wild" aspect. This "wild" aspect often occurs only in patches amidst large areas of "quiet" growth. The very regular "quiet" growth of Figs 1, 2 and 3 was observed without exception in all cultures obtained from patients with known heredity. The more "wild" type of growth occurred in a rather high percentage of the unilateral primary cases, of unknown heredity. As we might expect that in this latter group 80% should be non-hereditary, this gave us a hint that the growth pattern might be correlated with heredity.

Before we could draw even tentative conclusions we had to learn to avoid several pitfalls. First the patches of "wild" growth are sometimes rather rare and small amidst large regions of "quiet" growth. In the earlier cases, when we did not yet know what to look for, these often rather inconspicuous small patches were overlooked, and not photographed. The "score" of these patches was considerably lower in the earlier cultures—ca. 50%—than in the cultures taken when the one of us (E) who takes the pictures knew what to look for. There is of course still a small hazard that no patch of "wild" growth will develop in cultures from a tumour that would potentially show some patches if more cultures had been made.

Another pitfall arises from the use of the plasma clot culture. In such a clot cells sometimes grow in two or even more parallel layers, each layer separated from the other by a thin layer of plasma. The direction of the cells in the different layers may not be the same, suggesting on superficial examination a "wild" type of growth even though each of the cell layers is quite regular (Fig. 5). Careful differential focussing will show the separate cell layers within which there may be "quiet" or "wild" growth.

Another misleading feature that can be found in the cultures is shown in Fig. 6. Here we have not the embryonic-type retinoblastic tumour cells, but fully developed retinal neurons or glial cells with numerous pseudopods or dendrites. These cells, if numerous, will also form a basket-work-like aspect that may mislead the inexperienced investigator to report "wild", i.e. badly contact inhibited growth.

Figure 7 summarises all results for successful cultures from the beginning. *All* tumours from patients with known heredity showed the "quiet" type of growth. The "typing" of the pictures was always done blind, i.e. without knowing from which patient the culture was derived. In the group of cultures from patients with unknown heredity the majority show the impaired contact inhibition "wild" type of growth. If this growth pattern were an expression of

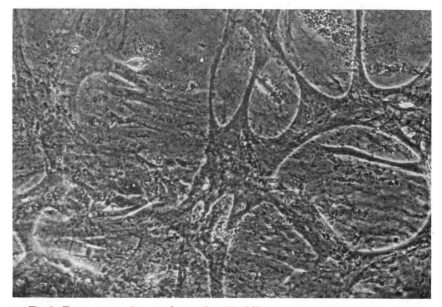

Fig. 5. Two separate layers of growth with different preferential directions. Though each layer is well contact inhibited, the crossing of the two layers simulates a "wild" type of growth; note however, the difference in levels of focus. Plasma clot (phase contrast 100X).

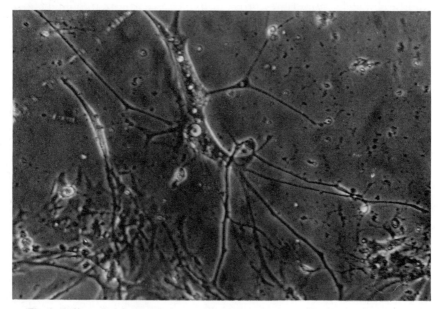

Fig. 6. Differentiated neurons from retinoblastoma culture. Plasma clot (phase contrast 100X).

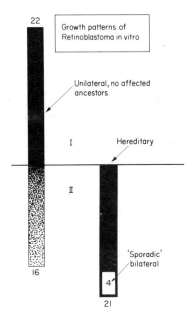

Fig. 7. Histogram showing the distribution of the two types of growth pattern over the two groups of patients. Below the horizontal line the cases with good contact inhibition are compiled (I). Above the line the cases with patches of impaired contact inhibition are shown (II). The left-hand column represents cases of unknown heredity. The right-hand column shows all cases with known heredity, including those with affected parents and first cases in a family which are known to be hereditary because they are bilateral.

non-heredity, it should occur in 80% of the cases. The main reason why the figure is lower here stems from the fact that earlier cultures are included. If we look only at those cases photographed after we had learnt what to look for, the ratio begins to approach the 80/20 figure. The number of cases, however, is for the moment still too small to be sure.

To summarise, the growth pattern in cell culture of retinoblastomas known to be hereditary always shows very good contact inhibition of motion, whereas the majority of cultures from sporadic unilateral tumours of unknown heredity show patches with defective contact inhibition. In this latter group only a minority has good contact inhibition all over.

The question arises: "Are these cultures with defective contact-inhibition the non-hereditary tumours?" Proof of this will only be obtained when our patients grow up and have children. For the moment our best evidence is that this growth pattern has never been observed in hereditary tumours and the percentage for tumours of unknown heredity is approximately the same as that observed clinically. One additional pointer, not previously mentioned in this paper, is that if we culture normal enbryonic retinoblastic cells they show the same "wild" type of growth as the tumours that we consider to be non-hereditary.

Ultimately, the only way to know whether this test discriminates between hereditary and non-hereditary retinoblastoma, will be to wait till our patients get children. Let us hope that by that time—in the years around 1990—contact will not have been lost. In Holland we have a good registration system for these patients to ensure that progeny will be examined in time, so we hope this goal can be reached.

On the other hand a lot of work has to be done to explain the mechanisms of the features described here.

REFERENCE

Schappert-Kimmijser, J., Hemmes, G. D. and Nijland, R. (1966). *Opthalmologia,* *151*, 197.

DISCUSSION

Dickson said that since this tumour is so very malignant, a biochemical back-up or a back-up of the type described by D. Easty (see page 45) would provide a much stronger case for differentiating between the two types and for saving ophthalmological examination. Although there are problems of general anaesthesia in children, the tumour is so malignant and the number of cases is so small, that an ophthalmologist would need very strong evidence to avoid carrying out such examinations on children with this tumour. An alternative extension was perhaps scanning electron microscopy.

Prop said all their histochemical and cytochemical studies had led to nothing. There are all kinds of enzymes present in this type of tumour and the patterns for different tumours are not the same but these differences have nothing to do with the decision between hereditary and non-hereditary.

Because of the limited amount of material, new ideas have to be investigated sequentially. It is hoped some time in the future to be able to freeze cells in liquid nitrogen and serially passage them but only a very small part of the tumour is available, the rest going to pathologists for checking invasiveness and diagnosis.

Boss asked why, although the retinoblastoma is very malignant, the people who suffer from this disease come to be able to have children. Prop replied that the very favourable factor is that the tumour occurs in the eye and if not treated too late can be removed completely with the eye. Furthermore, it is radio-sensitive, so if possible in most bilateral cases one eye is removed and the other eye, assuming it contains only a small tumour, is treated with radiation and even with cytostatics. In this way survival rate is not bad, though of course there are fatalities.

Chapter 3

EVALUATION OF SHORT TERM
CULTURES: CHEMOSENSITIVITY

(Moderator:L. F. Lamerton)

1. *In vitro* Sensitivity Testing of Human Tumour Slices to Chemotherapeutic Agents—Its Place in Cancer Therapy

John A. Dickson and Mohammad Suzangar

INTRODUCTION

In vitro methods for assessing the response of human cancers to cytotoxic drugs have been described by numerous authors, and some workers have found a correlation between *in vitro* effects of a drug and the response of the tumour in the patient to that agent (*see* Byfield and Stein, 1968; *Natl. Cancer Inst. Monogr. 34*, 1971). However, with a few notable exceptions, the long-term clinical response of human solid tumours to drugs has not been encouraging and recurrence of the disease is usual. Consequently, no assay techniques have been acclaimed as warranting general acceptance for predictive testing, and there is considerable scepticism amongst practising oncologists towards such *in vitro* systems. It is our belief that much of the circumspection regarding *in vitro* testing of tumours derives from over-optimistic attitudes generated by the success of bacterial chemotherapy. Our knowledge of neoplasia has now reached a stage when we can appreciate more clearly the factors involved in the response of a tumour to cytotoxic drugs; at the same time, the meaning and limitations of results which can be obtained with *in vitro* tumour assay systems are becoming more defined.

1. APPROACHES TO TUMOUR CULTURE

Figure 1 shows the commonly used methods for testing the sensitivity of solid tumours to cytotoxic drugs *in vitro*. The tumour is disaggregated into its component *cells*, enzymes (such as trypsin or collagenase) being the usual means of doing this. The cells are then cultured in the presence of the drugs to be tested and the cells examined for inhibition of proliferation or other evidence of damage. On the other hand, the tumour sample can be cut into *slices* which are cultured in the presence of the chemotherapeutic agents. In this case, drug efficacy is not assessed by direct inspection of the cells but by the effect upon tumour cell metabolism as measured by

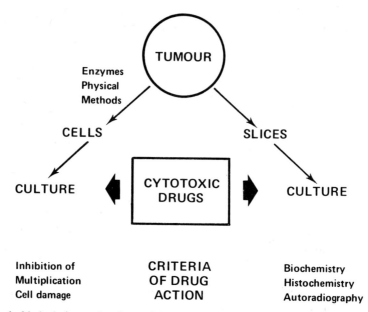

Fig. 1. Methods for testing the sensitivity of solid tumours to cytotoxic drugs *in vitro*

biochemical, histochemical or autoradiographic examination. The two methods represent alternatives only in that the limited amount of tumour material usually available precludes the use of more than one procedure routinely.

The preference for cells or slices of tumour material, involve different philosophies of tumour growth and should be regarded as different approaches to chemotherapy testing. Figure 2 lists the relative advantages of, and factors to be considered in using, the two methods. Because of the tough consistency of some tumours (e.g. breast cancers), it may be possible to obtain adequate numbers of cells from them only with difficulty, or after prolonged disaggregation, when the viability of the cells may be poor. If the cell yield is adequate, and the cells proliferate in the culture dishes, the problem of cell identity arises. Are the multiplying cells malignant cells or are they fibroblasts from the tumour stroma? If the cells *are* malignant, are they simply cancer cells that find the *in vitro* conditions to their liking—that is, are they selected or are they representative of the tumour population as a whole? Such cells are in fact selected, because at best, it is only possible to examine multiplying cells in this system. It is now well recognized that a tumour is not simply a mass of replicating cells, but is a heterogeneous system composed of

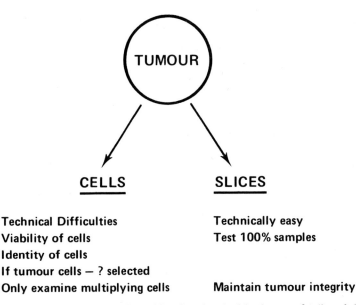

TUMOUR

CELLS

SLICES

Technical Difficulties
Viability of cells
Identity of cells
If tumour cells — ? selected
Only examine multiplying cells

Technically easy
Test 100% samples

Maintain tumour integrity

Fig. 2. Relative advantages and considerations involved in the use of cells and slices for *in vitro* assay systems.

several compartments (DeVita, 1971; Gavosto and Pileri, 1971; Lala, 1972)—a population of multiplying cells (the Growth Fraction) and, at any given time, cells that are not multiplying and are out of cycle for an indefinite period. Cells that have no further replicative potential but are proceeding towards cell death constitute the major part of the "cell loss factor" of tumours, but do not represent a threat to the life of the host (DeVita, 1971; Gavosto and Pileri, 1971; Lala, 1972). Tumour growth rate depends upon the numerical balance obtaining between replicating cells and cells leaving the neoplasm by death or migration (Johnson and Wolberg, 1971). As a tumour enlarges, there is an increase in the percentage of cells that leave the cycling compartment and enter a non-proliferating state (Skipper, 1971a). This shift alters the tumour response to drugs, and is presently considered to represent one of the major limiting factors in the effectiveness of solid tumour chemotherapy, since cells in the non-proliferating compartment are refractory to most currently available anti-cancer drugs, and represent a focus for tumour regrowth and the emergence of resistant cells (Skipper, 1971a).

The rapid repopulation of tumours following treatment by effective cycle-specific drugs and the "uncrowding phenomenon" whereby tumour cells removed from their environment again start dividing (Johnson and Wolberg, 1971; Skipper, 1971a) imply a dynamic relationship between the proliferating and non-proliferating cell pools of a tumour. In 1954, Greenstein stated "... the host-tumour relationship is the key to the cancer problem", and the importance of the stroma of tumours as a manifestation of host-tumour interaction has been known since 1905, when Bashford et al. showed that the stroma reaction was essential for the "take" of a tumour graft. Since that time, considerable evidence has accumulated to emphasise the dependence of the cancer cell on a stromal element for survival and proliferation (see Ambrose and Roe, 1966; Dickson, 1966). It is now clear that each tumour controls the amount and composition of its stroma (Bashford et al. 1905; Gullino, 1973) upon which it depends for nutrition, and mutual influences between neighbouring fragments of normal tissues and tumours grown in vitro have been demonstrated (Grossfield, 1932).

From these considerations of tumour population kinetics and the specificity and influence of the stroma on tumour cell behaviour, it is evident that there are compelling reasons favouring the use of tumour slices, in which structural (and hopefully functional) integrity of the tumour material is maintained, for drug sensitivity studies. Our own experience with several hundred tumours indicates that the use of slices is a convenient and rapid method applicable to testing practically 100% of human tumours in vitro.

2. PROBLEMS OF TUMOUR RESPONSE

The in vitro Drug Concentration

A major problem intrinsic to in vitro drug assay systems concerns the concentration of drug to be used in the cultures. There is no readily applicable means for determining the in vitro drug concentration which would be equivalent to the concentration achieved in vivo. Consequently, the in vitro drug levels used by different workers have varied from arbitrary concentrations (Bickis et al. 1966) and empirical levels found to inhibit the growth of HeLa cells (Wright et al. 1962), to concentrations which attempt to relate to the amount of agent given to the patient (Limburg and Heckmann, 1962; Dendy et al. 1971). We are in agreement with the latter approach and feel that the in vitro drug concentration should, if possible, bear some resemblance to the level of agent to which the tumour cells would be exposed in vivo. In the present work, the in vitro concentration for each drug was correlated with the daily patient dosage on the basis of a median body weight of 60 kg and blood volume of 5 litres, as

TABLE 1

In vitro *Drug Concentration*

Standard human being	
Wt.	60 kg
Blood volume	5 litres
Maximum concentration attained if total daily drug dose uniformly distributed in the plasma	
MTX	10 mg/day

$$\frac{10}{5000} \times 2 \times 10^3 = 4 \ \mu g/ml \ \text{plasma}$$

In vitro concentration = 4 μg/ml medium

recommended by Limburg and Heckmann (1962). The level of drug in the medium was equated with the maximum concentration attained in the blood assuming the total daily dose was distributed in the plasma only. Table 1 illustrates the calculation for methotrexate (MTX).

Table 2 gives the *in vitro* concentrations of the drugs used in the present work with the corresponding clinical dosages. In the case of fluorouracil FU, which rapidly equilibrates with total body water after administration (Chaudhuri *et al.* 1958), the *in vitro* dose has been computed as equivalent to the concentration of the clinical dose per ml in this compartment (35 litres). The range and duration of application of drug levels used in culture by several other investigators is also illustrated, with available data on peak plasma levels and half-life of the agents in man. After i.v. injection, most of the drugs are rapidly cleared from the blood and excreted. However, in the mouse L1210 solid leukaemia tumour, significant levels of the active metabolite of FU have been reported to persist for up to 72 hr after a single i.v. injection (Chadwick and Rogers, 1970), and MTX may persist for months in tissues with a high folic acid content (Delmonte and Jukes, 1962). Cyclophosphamide (CP) presents several special problems from the point of view of *in vitro* studies. The drug requires activation by the liver for production of its active derivative, and there are at least three alkylating metabolites with cytotoxic activity (Torkelson *et al.* 1974). In the rat, 60 min after CP injection, derivatives with alkylating activity represent only 10-15% of the serum level of CP and its metabolites (Brock and Hohorst, 1962). Although there is an initial rapid distribution of administered CP throughout the body tissues, reflux recruitment of this tissue-stored drug to the liver occurs (Brock *et al.* 1971). Consequently,

TABLE 2

In vitro Concentrations (μg/ml culture medium) of Cytotoxic Drugs Used by Various Investigators

	Peak plasma level (μg/ml)	Plasma half-life	Wright Cells 4 days (1962)	Wolberg Slices 24 hr (1964)	Bickis Slices 2½ hr (1966)	Tchao Slices 3-5 days (1968)	Byfield Cells 2 hr (1968)	Dendy Cells 2 days (1971)	This paper Slices 24 hr
MTX	$3{\cdot}0^1$ (A)	1-3 hr (A,B)	50	—	50	1-10	1·4	—	4 (165)*
FU	$28{-}52^2$ (C,D)	30 mins (C,D)	5	23	500	—	430	—	26^5 (15 × 10³)
CP	$4{\cdot}0^3$ (E)	>8 hr (E)	—	—	—	—	—	20	70^6 (3 × 10³)
TT	$0{\cdot}3^4$ (F)	40 mins (F)	19	—	50	1-10	4	—	6 (250)
PAM	(F)	3 hr (G)	—	—	—	1-10	—	—	2·5 (100)
VB		1 hr (H)	—	—	50	—	300	0·1	2·5 (100)
ACT D	1-5 × 10⁻⁴ (G)	few mins	—	—	1	—	0·4	—	0·2 (8)

* The figures in brackets are the corresponding in vivo drug dosages (μg/kg/day) used to calculate the in vitro concentrations in the last column.

[1] Following 50 mg by single i.v. injection.
[2] Following 15 mg/kg by single i.v. injection.
[3] Values refer to active metabolites following CP 10 mg/kg by single i.v. injection.
[4] Following 0·3 mg/kg by single i.v. injection.
[5] This value is $\frac{1}{14}$ the concentration calculated from the formula in Table 1.
[6] Concentration in the activating mixture (1 g fresh rat liver slices in 9 ml CP solution, incubated 20 min at 37° C. The solution was then filter-sterilised and added to the culture dishes at 70 μg/ml). The percentage activation of the drug and the concentration in the culture medium of the active metabolites were not known.

References: A. Liguori et al. (1962); B. Berlin et al. (1963); C. Chaudhuri et al. (1958); D. Clarkson et al. (1964); E. Torkelson et al. (1974); F. Mellett et al. (1962); G. Calabresi and Parks (1970); H. Morasca et al. (1969).

plasma alkylating metabolite levels which peak 2-3 hr after i.v. injection remain at over 70% of the peak value 8 hr after therapy in man and these levels are not correlated with plasma half-life of the inactive drug (Bagley *et al.* 1973). It has been suggested that the cytotoxic activity of CP depends upon conversion of the primary active metabolite(s) into further active products at the site of action with the cellular receptor (Brock and Hohorst, 1962). These considerations indicate the many difficulties involved in trying to compute a tissue-culture level for CP.

Clinically, drug absorption and distribution are affected by dosage schedules and route of administration, as well as the type and stage of the disease and the state of metabolism and nutrition of the patient (Delmonte and Jukes, 1962; Brock *et al.* 1971). There is also the possibility that the metabolic fate of a drug, e.g. FU, may be altered by the route of administration (Miller, 1964). This, in turn, would affect its blood level and biological activity. Following administration by the same route, variability in drug blood levels between individual patients is considerable (Chaudhuri *et al.* 1958; Liguori *et al.* 1962; Mellett *et al.* 1962; Clarkson *et al.* 1964). In the clinic, many different dosage regimens have been used with these cytotoxic drugs, and even with such a well-tried agent as CP there is no general agreement as to dosage schedule (Greenwald, 1973). Dosage programmes are continually being modified and the current trend is towards more intensive high dosage regimens in suitably selected patients (Ansfield, 1973; Greenwald, 1973)—with MTX, for example, the dosage schedule is now tentative and depends upon the type of disease being treated and the condition of the patient. For the current work, the most popular clinical dosages (usually involving i.v. administration (Greenwald, 1973)) have been selected as the basis for calculating *in vitro* dose levels.

It has been stated that "the effectiveness of an anti-tumour agent is directly related to its concentration in the blood and the duration of time that an effective level is maintained—the concentration by time $(C \times T)$" (DeVita, 1971). Definition of an "effective" drug level for an individual bearing a tumour is not possible at the present time, and the complexities inherent in such a measurement must not be underestimated. The final effect of a drug is related to its concentration in the immediate neighbourhood of receptors in the cell, and this in turn is related to the absorption, penetration, distribution and metabolism of the drug (Wenke, 1971). Because of these factors, measurement of the drug concentration in the plasma is not of itself very helpful. Nor can the tissue level of the drug (if it

HTSTC–5

can be measured) be readily equated with the concentration at the active sites, since this is governed by the volume of drug-containing tissue fluid to which the cells are exposed and the tissue to volume ratio (Gillette, 1968). A formula, taking many of these factors into consideration, has been devised by Gillette for computing the amount of drug to be added to the medium for *in vitro* experiments. However, the formula requires measurement of the drug concentration in the extracellular fluid and in the tissue cells under equilibrium conditions, and is not readily applicable to the human situation.

From these considerations, it would seem unprofitable at the present time to place too much emphasis on *in vitro—in vivo* drug dosage relationships. The response of a tumour in the host depends greatly on the dosage regimen, and optimal scheduling can make the difference between therapeutic success and failure (Skipper, 1971*b*). Factors such as scheduling and the effects of different routes of drug administration cannot be mimicked *in vitro*. Our brief, therefore, is to use a dosage level which will be a measure of the *in vitro* potential of each drug, and at the same time is realistic in terms of the amount of the agent that can be given to the patient.

Definition of in vitro Response

When tumour slices are exposed to the action of a cytotoxic drug, the response is not "all-or-none". If the drug is effective, it depresses metabolism to some degree, and difficulty then arises regarding what degree of metabolic inhibition correlates with inhibition of tumour growth. We have examined this question in an animal (rat) model system and correlated the minimal drug dose that cures the tumour *in vivo* with the degree of metabolic inhibition produced in culture by the equivalent *in vitro* dosage calculated as described earlier.

The solid Yoshida sarcoma in the rat is sensitive to alkylating agents (Fox, 1969), and a single dose of 2·5 mg MDMS i.p. leads to a cure rate of 100% in rats bearing 1·5 ml foot tumours (Dickson and Suzangar, 1974). *In vitro*, MDMS caused a concentration-dependent inhibition of respiration, glycolysis and radioactive thymidine, uridine and leucine uptake into Yoshida slices over 24 hr (Fig. 3). At a medium level of 100 μg/ml ($\equiv$ 2·5 mg/kg on a body wt, blood volume basis), there was 25% inhibition of O_2 uptake and 45-50% inhibition of CO_2 production (glycolysis) and isotope uptake; after culture, the treated tumour did not grow when inoculated into host rats. Table 3 depicts the *in vitro/in vivo* response of the Yoshida tumour to a series of other cytotoxic drugs. Only phenylalanine mustard (PAM) and thiotepa (TT) caused tumour cure and metabolic

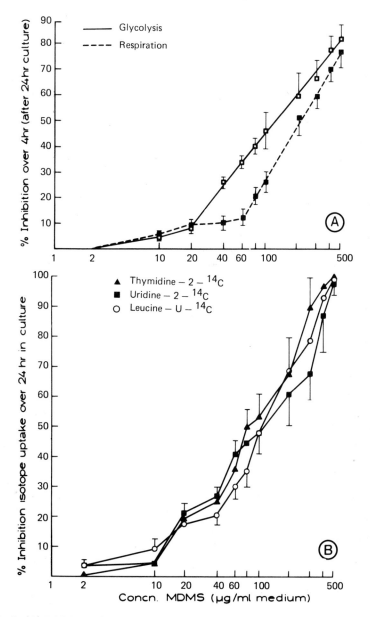

Fig. 3. (A) Inhibition of respiration and anaerobic glycolysis in Yoshida tumour slices at 38° C following 24 hr culture in the presence of different concentrations of MDMS. (B) Inhibition of radioactive thymidine, uridine and leucine uptake into Yoshida slices over 24 hr in culture with different concentrations of MDMS. The isotopes were present at an initial activity of 0·2 μCi/ml medium.

TABLE 3

Response of the Solid Yoshida Tumour to Cytotoxic Agents

Drug	In vivo	In vitro (% inhibition)		Transplant after in vitro treatment
PAM	+	Respn	42	−
0·5 mg/kg		Gly	54	
TT	+	Respn	30	−
1·0 mg/kg		Gly	25	
CP	−	−		+
7 mg/kg				
FU	−	−		+
25 mg/kg				
VB		−		+
1·0 mg/kg				
ACT D	−	−		+
0·1 mg/kg				

inhibition *in vitro*. The minimal curative dose of the drugs was associated with as little as 25-30% inhibition of tumour biochemistry in culture and failure of the tumour to take on transplantation. The other drugs were ineffective *in vivo* and *in vitro*.

Tumour regression, therefore, correlated with as little as 25-30% inhibition of metabolism *in vitro* by effective drugs over 24 hr in culture, while lesser degrees of inhibition were not associated with tumour cure when the appropriate drug dosage was given to the animal (Dickson and Suzangar, 1974). Black and Speer (1954) reported a positive correlation between the *in vitro* effects of cancer chemotherapeutic agents and their clinical effectiveness when the agent caused a 30% or more inhibition of dehydrogenase activity after 1 hr *in vitro*. Bickis *et al.* (1966) examined the effect of drugs on the respiration, glycolysis and isotope precursor uptake into slices of human tumours over $2\frac{1}{2}$ hr in Warburg flasks. From clinical correlation studies on a limited number (eight) of tumours, these workers found that at least 50% inhibition of isotope uptake into DNA, RNA or protein over this period was necessary for reasonable expectation of a favourable clinical response to a given drug.

It is now established that currently available anti-cancer drugs exert their effects chiefly on multiplying cells, their biochemical targets being DNA synthesis (MTX, FU), DNA replication (alkylating agents) RNA synthesis (actinomycin D, ACT D) or synthesis of both DNA and RNA (vinca alkaloids, which also have a direct damaging effect on the mitotic spindle) (*see* Greenwald, 1973 for refs). The effects of the drugs on the synthesis of DNA, RNA and also protein by organ cultures of tumour can be expressed quantitatively by measuring the uptake of radioactive precursors into these macromolecules (Bickis *et al.* 1966; Tchao *et al.* 1967, 1968; Wolberg, 1971*a*). It has been known since the 1930s that alkylating agents that are active against tumours also inhibit their glycolysis (Holzer, 1964), and in regressing animal tumours there is a depression of both respiration and glycolysis, the degree of inhibition corresponding to the sensitivity of the tumour to the drug (Larionov, 1965). Vinblastine (VB) has been reported to cause a similar NAD-mediated inhibition of anaerobic glycolysis in the Jensen sarcoma in rats, the decrease reaching its maximum (20%) after 24 hr (Obrecht, 1964). This was accompanied by an increase in respiration of 50%, but it is of note that these metabolic changes were not associated with a cytostatic effect on the tumour (*see later* "Comment"). In the small series of human tumours studied *in vitro* over $2\frac{1}{2}$ hr by Bickis *et al.* (1966), significant inhibition (>50%) of isotope uptake by cytotoxic drugs was accompanied by inconsistent and smaller (<30%) inhibition of respiration or glycolysis.

In recent years, evidence has accumulated in favour of the biochemical uniqueness of individual human cancers (Busch, 1965; Lemon and Foley, 1966; Bickis and Henderson, 1966; Bickis *et al.* 1966), and the work of Wolberg (1964, 1971*a*) has indicated clearly the problems posed in drug assay systems by the availability to tumours of alternative metabolic pathways (*see also later* "Comment"). In view of these considerations and the various findings discussed above, we have employed multiple biochemical parameters in the assessment of tumour sensitivity to cytotoxic agents. Tumour slices were cultured for 24 hr in the presence of the drug(s); the effect on energy processes of the cells was assayed by measurement of respiration and glycolysis, and precursor isotope uptake into nucleic acids and protein was used to indicate the effect on cell replicative potential. Tumour response to a cytotoxic drug is defined as a minimum 30% depression of respiration and/or glycolysis accompanied by 50% or more inhibition of precursor uptake into DNA, RNA or protein, measured over 6 hr after 24 hr in culture in the presence of the drug.

3. METHODOLOGY

Upon removal from the patient, a piece of the tumour was taken for routine pathological examination and the remainder of the specimen was placed in a sterile ice-cooled container for transport to the laboratory. As the tumours were obtained from four hospitals within a 100-mile radius of Newcastle, a delay of 1-3 hr was sometimes incurred between operating theatre and culture room.

In the laboratory, a frozen section was performed to confirm the diagnosis of malignancy and assess the degree of cellularity of the specimen. The tumour was placed on ice, in a sterile Petri dish, washed with cold Rinaldini saline (Rinaldini, 1959) containing penicillin (100 units/ml), streptomycin (100 μg/ml), and Mycostatin (100 units/ml), and carefully dissected free of necrotic material and surrounding normal tissue. Using cataract knives, the tumour was cut into thin sections (less than 1 cu mm); these were then allocated at random into aliquots of approximately 100 mg to minimise the effects of tumour heterogeneity.

For *culture*, approximately 100 mg tissue was placed in 3 ml Waymouth medium MB 752/1, supplemented with 10% pooled human AB serum, in 5 cm diameter plastic Petri dishes (Esco Grade A; Esco Rubber Ltd., London), and placed in a CO_2 incubator (5% CO_2 in air) at 37·5°C. Cytotoxic drugs were prepared as the pure compound fresh in aqueous solution just before use and added to the medium of the test cultures in 0·1 ml. At the same time as the cultures were being set up, respiration and anaerobic glycolysis of tumour aliquots were measured over 2 hr. By this means, tumours with a very low O_2 uptake or CO_2 production were identified rapidly and unproductive biochemical studies on the cultured material avoided. The great individual variation in respiration and glycolysis values between tumours of the same organ, e.g. breast, is illustrated in Table 4. In many cases, detailed Warburg manometry

TABLE 4

Respiration and Anaerobic Glycolysis of Human Tumour Slices

	* Respiration	† Anaerobic Glycolysis
Breast (60)	4-48	11-75
Lung (71)	4-40	7-76
Stomach (26)	6-56	8-83
Colon (32)	10-61	11-120
Melanoma (22)	11-40	23-93

* μl O_2 uptake/10 mg tissue dry wt/hr in air.

† μl CO_2 produced/10 mg tissue dry wt/hr in 5% CO_2/95% N_2.

In these values no account has been taken of the percentage tumour in the slices. Figures in brackets are the numbers of tumours examined.

was performed on the fresh tumours for comparison with the values after culture.

Further details of the culture technique are given in the "Methods" section of Chapter 1 (page 31).

Warburg Manometry

Classic Warburg manometry using 50-100 mg tumour slices was used in the metabolic studies. Respiration was studied in a Krebs-Ringer phosphate buffer, pH 7·4, containing sodium succinate (0·013M), with 0·2 ml 10% KOH in the centre well and air as the gas phase. Anaerobic glycolysis was measured in a KRBP solution (Mondovi *et al.* 1969), pH 7·4, containing glucose (2 g/l) and a gas phase of 95% N_2 : 5% CO_2 (initial O_2 content of mixture less than 20 ppm, Air Products Ltd., Gateshead). The KRBP maintained a more stable pH over the incubation period than did the traditional Krebs-Ringer bicarbonate buffer. Results were expressed as μl O_2 consumed (respiration), or μl CO_2 produced (anaerobic glycolysis), per 10 mg tumour dry wt, per hr.

Radioactivity Measurements

Thymidine-2-[14]C ($>$50 mCi/mmole), uridine-2-[14]C ($>$50 mCi/mmole), and uniformly labelled L-leucine-[14]C (344 mCi/mmole) were obtained from the Radiochemical Centre, Amersham, and were added to the culture medium at an initial concentration of 0·5 μCi/ml. At the end of the culture period, the tissue was treated by a modified Schneider procedure (Hutchison and Munro, 1961). After preliminary removal of the acid-soluble fraction and lipids, the nucleic acids were extracted with 1·0 N perchloric acid at 70° C, and incorporation of thymidine-^{14}C or uridine-^{14}C was measured by counting this extract. The protein pellet was dissolved in 1·0 N NaOH and counted for leucine-^{14}C activity. For radioactive counting, the toluene : Triton X-100 scintillation mixture of Patterson and Greene (1965) was used. The tissue extracts were neutralised with 5 N NaOH or 5 N trichloroacetic acid before addition to the counting fluid, and an internal standard of methanol-^{14}C was used to correct for quenching. Activity in the samples was expressed as cpm/mg DNAP, which was determined by the method of Burton (1956).

Measurements for manometry and radioactivity were each performed on duplicate samples of tumour, reducing the amount of material examined to 50 mg as required.

4. RESULTS

Over a 6-year period, more than 200 solid human tumours have been tested for sensitivity to cytotoxic drugs. All material came from primary tumours (2-12 g but occasionally larger), except for the melanoma group, some of which were recurrent lesions or involved regional lymph nodes. None of the patients had received drug or X-ray therapy prior to removal of the specimen.

Table 5 illustrates the experimental protocol and calculation of the sensitivity to drugs for a scirrhous carcinoma of the breast. Slices

TABLE 5

Response of Breast Cancer (Scirrhous Carcinoma) to Cytotoxic Drugs

Drug	μl gas exchanged/ 10 mg tissue/hr		Isotope uptake (cpm/mg DNAP)		
	Respn	Gly	Thymidine	Uridine	Leucine
No drug (Control)	11	45	5933	3179	4670
FU	7 (36)	17 (62)	1060 (82)	640 (80)	3390 (28)
CP	7 (36)	47 (nil)	1310 (78)	680 (79)	3000 (35)
MTX	12 (nil)	42 (nil)	6410 (nil)	3706 (nil)	4500 (nil)
VB	12 (nil)	41 (nil)	5610 (nil)	3400 (nil)	4460 (nil)
FU, CP, MTX, VB	5 (55)	12 (73)	405 (93)	250 (92)	2700 (43)

Figures in brackets are percentage inhibition in relation to the control values.

of the tumour were cultured for 24 hr in the presence of 4 individual drugs, and also with all 4 drugs present in the medium. Following culture, the respiratory and glycolytic capacity, as well as the uptake of labelled thymidine, uridine and leucine into the cultures was measured over a 6 hr period; the results were expressed as a percentage inhibition of each parameter in the presence of the drug(s) compared to the control untreated tissue. In this tumour, FU caused an inhibition of both respiration (36%) and anaerobic glycolysis (62%); this was associated with a significant decrease in thymidine (82%) and uridine (80%) uptake into the tumour slices. The response to CP illustrates that a significant inhibition of thymidine and uridine uptake may accompany a decrease in O_2 uptake (36%) with no change in glycolysis. The mixture of 4 drugs had a greater inhibitory effect on all parameters examined than any individual agent.

Tables 6-10 record the response of tumours of the breast, lung, stomach and colon and also malignant melanoma to cytotoxic agents. The specific drugs and drug combinations tested against each tumour type were those found to be most useful clinically against such cancers. No correlation has been found between histological classification of any of the tumour types examined and the rate of metabolism (respiration, glycolysis, nucleic acid and protein pre-cursor uptake) or response to specific cytotoxic drugs. Nor has any evidence emerged that the age of the patient influences drug sensitivity of tumours. In the case of breast cancer, it has been reported that the clinical predictive factors (e.g. the patient's menstrual status) which have been described for endocrine therapy do not operate in the response to drug therapy (Ansfield, 1973; Greenwald, 1973; Edelstyn, 1974). The tumours in Tables 6-10, therefore, have not been categorised according to the age or sex of the patients in whom they originated; the breast cancers were all from female patients.

There were large variations in the response to drugs of individual tumours of all types examined. Specific patterns of response did not emerge in relation to individual drugs or tumour types, e.g. FU did not always exert its main effect on glycolysis or on thymidine or uridine uptake. The pattern of response was an individual one for each tumour. Either respiration or glycolysis was inhibited >30% leaving the other parameter unaffected; respiration and glycolysis could both be depressed to equal or unequal degrees. In general, these changes were accompanied by a 50% or more decrease in at least two of the isotope uptake measurements. Total inhibition of all parameters by a drug(s) was uncommon. This occurred in 4 cases of breast cancer and 2 of lung cancer; in 2 of the breast tumours, FU was the drug responsible, and in the other 4 cases the tumour was cultured in the presence of the 4 drug mixture. A more common response to a single drug (e.g. FU in breast tumours) or drug combination was a high degree of inhibition of thymidine and uridine uptake accompanied by a 50% or greater decrease in respiration or glycolysis. In the tumours not included in Tables 6-10 (and regarded as "non-responders"), a further variety of drug effects was observed: the drug(s) had no significant effect on any of the 5 parameters measured; respiration was decreased and glycolysis increased or *vice versa*; both respiration and glycolysis were increased. In some tumours, an increase in respiration and/or glycolysis was accompanied by an increased isotope uptake into the slices in the presence of the drug. There was no marked overlap of tumour response to individual agents, and in combination the drugs seemed to have additive effects. Tumours that responded to a mixture of drugs comprised the tumours that were sensitive to one or more components of the mixture; there were few tumours that responded to multiple agents but were not susceptible to single drug exposure. In general, drug combinations (especially the 4 drug combination of FU, CP, MTX and VB) were more effective in inhibiting metabolism than single agents.

Breast Cancer

Table 6 shows that the 4 drugs tested each had an inhibitory effect on some of the breast tumours examined. The number of tumours responding to the agents increased as the combinations became more complex, 4 drugs being better than 3, and 3 drugs being better than 2. The results were more uniform with combination treatment, there being a larger percentage of tumours in which both respiration and glycolysis were inhibited, and there was a concomitant significant inhibition of uptake with 2 or more of the isotopes.

Clinically, each of the 4 drugs used in culture has been shown to have significant activity against breast cancer, with an overall response rate in the region of 30% in various clinical trials (*see* the review of Carter, 1972). In recent years, the use of multiple drugs in combination chemotherapy has become popular. Of the major solid tumours, breast cancer has attracted most attention in this respect. The tumour would seem to offer the greatest potential for success with a combination approach because of its clinical response to a variety of agents with different mechanisms of action. Several drug combinations have been tried over the past 10 years in the treatment of breast cancer. The most popular of these is that of FU, CP, MTX and vinblastine or vincristine, advocated in 1969 by Costanzi and Coltman. With this combination (or these drugs plus prednisone, given to protect the marrow—so-called "5 drug therapy") short-term remissions have been reported in as many as 90-100% of patients with advanced breast cancer (*see* Hanham *et al.* 1971; Carter, 1972; and the Symposium Proceedings edited by Shedden, 1974).

Lung Cancer

The 6% five-year survival rate in this disease attests to the ineffectiveness of cytotoxic drugs in unresectable bronchogenic carcinoma as well as in disseminated disease. Of the various agents found to produce a short-term improvement in patients with this tumour, the vinca alkaloids in combination with other drugs are worthy of note. Although ACT D has proved generally disappointing in its clinical usefulness, Chanes and Condit (1971) reported a 60%

TABLE 6

Response of Tumour Slices to Cytotoxic Drugs—Breast Cancer

Drug(s)	Number of tumours showing > 30% inhibition				Percentage inhibition isotope uptake		
	Responders	Respn	Gly	Respn + Gly	TdR	UdR	Leu
FU	6/16		4	2	75-91	60-100	40-62
CP	5/16	1	3	1	62-88	41-73	51-67
FU, CP	10/16	1	1	8	81-100	57-100	36-67

Two of the 5 CP responders also responded to FU, and are included in the 6 FU responders. One of the 10 FU + CP responders did not respond to either drug alone.

FU	4/10	1	3		90-100	72-86	30-47
MTX	3/10		1	2	58-85	46-70	25-46
VB	3/10	1	2		43-60	60-70	48-66
FU, MTX, VB	7/10		1	6	90-96	71-98	55-77

One tumour responded to all 3 drugs individually; otherwise there was no overlap in the response to individual drugs.

FU	8/16	1	6	1	60-94	40-73	30-52
FU, CP, MTX, VB	15/16		3	12	79-100	78-100	50-81

Seven of the 8 FU responders had an increased response to the mixture.

In Tables 6-10, each tumour type was tested against single drugs and also against the drugs in combination, as indicated by the results separated by horizontal lines.

The numerator in the "Responders" column gives the number of tumours showing significant inhibition of metabolism in the presence of cytotoxic drug(s), and the denominator represents the number of tumours tested in each series.

For drug combinations, the concentration of each agent was reduced by a factor proportional to the number of components—e.g. for 4 drug mixtures each agent was included at $\frac{1}{4}$ of the usual single drug concentration in Table 2. This scheme is in keeping with the protocol used clinically in the administration of multiple cytotoxic drugs (Nathanson *et al.* 1969).

TABLE 7

Response of Tumour Slices to Cytotoxic Drugs—Lung Cancer

Drug(s)	Number of tumours showing > 30% inhibition				Percentage inhibition isotope uptake		
	Responders	Respn	Gly	Respn + Gly	TdR	UdR	Leu
FU	3/14	1	1	1	56-71	50-81	39-53
TT	5/14	3	2		50-73	41-71	40-48
CP	5/14	4		1	70-100	45-83	36-74

Two of the CP responders also responded to both FU and TT, and are included in the FU and TT responders; one other TT responder also responded to FU. Six tumours did not respond to any of the 3 drugs.

Drug(s)	Responders	Respn	Gly	Respn + Gly	TdR	UdR	Leu
VB	2/8	1		1	54, 51	66, 78	42, 82
ACT D	2/8			2	41, 62	52, 70	65, 75
VB, ACT D	6/8	1		5	51-70	82-95	53-77

There was no overlap between tumours in their response to VB and ACT D.

Drug(s)	Responders	Respn	Gly	Respn + Gly	TdR	UdR	Leu
FU	5/15	1	3	1	70-95	46-100	36-50
MTX	2/15			2	61, 51	44, 59	30, 62
VB	3/15	2		1	41-54	50-82	33-40
FU, MTX, VB	9/15	1	1	7	80-96	70-100	50-73

One of the 3 VB responders also responded to FU, and is included in the FU responders.

Drug(s)	Responders	Respn	Gly	Respn + Gly	TdR	UdR	Leu
FU	8/23		6	2	41-83	53-77	32-61
FU, CP, MTX, VB	16/23		3	13	87-100	72-100	63-84

Seven of the 8 FU responders had an increased response to the mixture.

initial response rate in patients with lung cancer treated with ACT D and vincristine. Hanham *et al.* (1971) obtained a partial, short-lived response in 57% of a series of lung cancer patients treated by the 4 drug Costanzi and Coltman combination.

Table 7 indicates that synergism of effect was obtained between VB and ACT D in their effect on lung tumour slices. Other combinations, containing VB with 2 or 3 other drugs, were not strikingly more effective in depressing metabolism than VB plus ACT D. The percentage of tumours responding to the mixtures was higher than that responding to single drugs, as with breast tumours (Table 6). With multiple drug combinations, a large number of the responding tumours exhibited a decrease in both respiration and glycolysis, in association with a high degree of inhibition of isotope uptake.

Gastrointestinal Cancer

FU is the only drug considered to be of value in this type of cancer, and short-term objective remissions have been obtained in 15-20% of patients with gastric or colorectal cancer (Ansfield, 1973; Greenwald, 1973). Using the Costanzi/Coltman combination, Priestman (*see* Shedden, 1974) obtained short-term objective response to treatment in 11 of 16 cases (70%) of colorectal cancer that had metastasised to the liver; the response was reflected in improved liver function tests and gamma scanning of the liver. Hanham *et al.* (1971) reported remissions in all of 4 patients with cancer of the stomach or colon treated by the Costanzi/Coltman regimen.

In the 23 gastric cancers detailed in Table 8, FU was the only single drug that produced metabolic inhibition in a significant number of tumours. In combination with CP, MTX and VB, the percentage of cancers responding was significantly increased compared to FU alone (7/10 versus 8/23). Five of the 7 responders to the mixture had inhibition of both respiration and glycolysis as well as very significant inhibition of isotope uptake values.

With the colon cancers investigated (Table 9), the results were similar to those for gastric cancer. FU was the only effective single drug of those tested, and its combination in the Costanzi/Coltman mixture increased the number of cancers showing biochemical inhibition.

Malignant Melanoma

Table 10 shows the biochemical response of this type of tumour to PAM and ACT D. Clinically, objective responses have been obtained

TABLE 8

Response of Tumour Slices to Cytotoxic Drugs—Stomach Cancer

Drug(s)	Responders	Number of tumours showing > 30% inhibition			Percentage inhibition isotope uptake		
		Respn	Gly	Respn + Gly	TdR	UdR	Leu
FU	3/9	2		1	66-81	49-97	35-53
CP	2/9	1	1		60, 81	73, 51	33, 46
FU	2/4	1		1	90, 52	80, 44	40, 23
ACT D	1/4	1			52	70	36
FU, ACT D	2/4	1		1	45, 72	76, 80	44, 51

One of the 2 FU, ACT D responders reacted to FU alone, and is included in the 2 FU responders.

Drug(s)	Responders	Respn	Gly	Respn + Gly	TdR	UdR	Leu
FU	3/10	2		1	51-84	54-70	23-53
VB	1/10	1			52	72	71
FU, CP, MTX, VB	7/10	2		5	80-100	64-100	42-76

The VB responder and 2 of the 3 FU responders had an increased response to the mixture.

TABLE 9

Response of Tumour Slices to Cytotoxic Drugs—Colon Cancer

Drug(s)	Number of tumours showing > 30% inhibition				Percentage inhibition isotope uptake		
	Responders	Respn	Gly	Respn + Gly	TdR	UdR	Leu
FU	4/10		4		61-91	51-62	30-46
TT	0/10				0-55	0-33	0-28
CP	0/10				0-22	0-15	0-12
VB	1/6	1			43	61	26
ACT D	0/6				0	0	0
VB, ACT D	1/6	1			60	56	40

The VB responder and VB, ACT D responder were the same tumour.

FU	4/12		3	1	52-90	46-91	34-55
FU, CP, MTX, VB	9/12		2	7	77-100	72-100	57-82

All 4 FU responders had an increased response to the mixture.

TABLE 10

Response of Tumour Slices to Cytotoxic Drugs—Malignant Melanoma

Drug(s)	*Number of tumours showing > 30% inhibition*				*Percentage inhibition isotope uptake*		
	Responders	*Respn*	*Gly*	*Respn + Gly*	*TdR*	*UdR*	*Leu*
PAM	6/18	2	3	1	52-92	44-62	38-58
ACT D	5/18	4	1		31-59	67-93	50-81
PAM, ACT D	10/18	4	4	6	66-92	60-82	40-73

One of the ACT D responders also responded to PAM and is included in the 6 PAM responders.

in 30%-70% (depending on the stage of the disease) of patients with this cancer treated by regional perfusion with PAM (Greenwald, 1973). ACT D has also been used in combination with PAM and nitrogen mustard, again by regional perfusion. With these 3 agents, a 50% regression rate was obtained in advanced melanoma of the extremities (McBride, 1970). In Table 10, only 2 of the responders (both to PAM) were primary tumours; the other responders to both PAM and ACT D were recurrent tumours or slices obtained from involved regional lymph nodes. The response to both drugs in combination was an additive one, just over 50% of the tumours tested exhibiting a significant inhibition of metabolism.

5. COMMENT

The present results indicate that it is possible to select *in vitro* cytotoxic drugs that inhibit the metabolism of the common types of solid human cancer. Numerous papers dealing with the feasibility of estimating human tumour sensitivity to drugs by *in vitro* methods have appeared in the literature over the past 20 years (*see* the *Natl. Cancer Inst. Monogr.* (1971) for refs). Several of these publications have reported a generally good correlation between *in vitro* and *in vivo* tumour sensitivities. In spite of this, no method(s) of predictive testing have gained general acceptance. We believe this reflects the complexities inherent in such testing rather than the perversity of investigators to persevere with their own approach. It behoves us, therefore, to define clearly our objectives in relation to *in vitro* drug testing of human tumours, and to interpret the present results in terms of the limitations of such systems. It is clear that *in vitro* systems cannot predict drugs that will cure patients of cancer, because drugs with such lethal potential towards the common solid cancers of man are not available. The most that can be expected from *in vitro* assay systems is the ability to select drugs that have a high chance of producing a short-term remission in the patient. Such drugs would not only achieve clinical palliation of the disease and improve the quality of the patient's remaining life, but would prevent the needless exposure of patients to the toxicity of ineffective agents.

Tumours are heterogeneous populations, not only from the kinetic point of view (DeVita, 1971; Gavosto and Pileri, 1971; Lala, 1972), but are composed of a mixture of biochemically sensitive and resistant cells in relation to drug therapy (Johnson and Wolberg, 1971). From growth curve studies, Israel *et al.* (1971) have calculated that in human solid tumours 15-30% of the cells may be initially resistant to a single agent such as CP, and between 1% and 10% of cells in the untreated tumour may be resistant to a 5-drug combination. The *in vitro* responses obtained in the present work are therefore interpreted as indicating that there exists in the tumour examined a population of cancer cells that is sensitive to a particular drug, or drug combination, under the experimental conditions described.

The significance of this interpretation in terms of tumour response in the patient requires consideration. It must be remembered that the tumour usually tested *in vitro* has (it is hoped) been radically removed from the host. Tumour subsequently confronting the therapist will represent recurrent or metastatic disease, and the metabolism and response to drugs of such secondary cancer cells may differ considerably from that of the primary cells (Bickis *et al.* 1966; Wolberg, 1971a). Evolution by selection occurs throughout the life of a neoplastic cell population, and from its inception the characteristics of a cancer are continually changing. The biological basis for this Tumour Progression was proposed by Foulds over 20 years ago (*see* the review by Foulds, 1954), and the biochemical basis for such progression has since been firmly established by the work of Potter (1963). As a tumour enlarges, alterations in the cell kinetics of the population also occur, there being a reduction in the number of proliferating cells or growth fraction (Gavosto and Pileri, 1971; DeVita, 1971; Johnson and Wolberg, 1971; Skipper, 1971b). The importance of these considerations has been verified both in animal systems and in the clinic by work indicating that as a tumour enlarges and/or metastasizes, its response to drugs alters; as the total host burden of cancer cells increases, it becomes more difficult to influence the disease, and even initially sensitive tumours in animals can no longer be cured (DeVita, 1971; Johnson and Wolberg, 1971; Skipper, 1971b and c).

From the point of view of therapy, therefore, a tumour represents a moving target. As pointed out by Di Paolo (1971), this means that *in vitro* screening must be viewed as selecting the best anti-tumour agent for a particular patient at a specific time in the course of his disease. The good correlation obtained by various workers between the response of primary tumours to drugs and the subsequent response of the host to those drugs in no way contradicts this statement, when it is remembered that by response we are referring to a cell *population* in the tumour. The size of the sensitive population will determine the extent of the remission in the patient, but it is the population of *resistant* cells that brings about the almost inevitable escape of most common solid cancers from therapeutic control. The results in Tables 6-10 indicate that reasonable agreement exists between the assessment of sensitive cell populations in solid tumours by the present method, and the clinical response rate for various cancers reported in the literature. A higher percentage of the cancers examined responded *in vitro* than have been reported to respond *in vivo* (*see* "Results" section): this may be ascribed to the problems involved in detecting drug effects on tumours in the host (*see later*), and because of these difficulties, *in vitro* assessment of tumour sensitivity to drugs may be more precise than is the evaluation of tumour response in the patient (Wolberg, 1971b).

It is often assumed that the use of drug combinations increases the likelihood of destroying resistant cells. Our experience has been that the metabolic inhibition produced in tumours by a single drug can usually be markedly increased by drug combinations. Clinical data to date supports the soundness of the rationale that a combination of drugs, each of which produces a different biochemical lesion so as to attack multiple sites in biosynthetic pathways (Schein, 1973), should be more effective against tumours than single agents. The use of multiple drug combinations such as the Costanzi/Coltman regimen has led to a dramatic increase in the percentage of objective remissions in solid tumours (*see* "Results" section). However, such remissions have been of limited duration, and overall long-term survival rates have not shown a significant improvement to date. Because anti-cancer drugs kill cells according to first order kinetics, a high degree of selectivity is required to eradicate even small tumours and Johnson and Wolberg (1971) state that, in relation to clinical practice, we are seeking specificity which is not likely to be obtained from any single drug. Israel *et al.* (1971) have also emphasised that a single drug has only a poor chance of controlling 100% of the cells in large multiclonal populations; these workers believe it is unlikely that any of the available drug combinations could prevent the selection of resistant cells in tumours containing more than 10^9 cells (1 g of tumour—a small host burden of cancer cells).

The problem of resistant cells looms large, therefore, in both the *in vitro* and *in vivo* response to drugs.

The increased ability of drug combinations to produce inhibition of metabolism in the different types of tumour in the present work (Tables 6-10) inevitably calls to mind Toman's famous law that "enough of anything will inhibit anything". Birnie and Heidelberger (1963) originally recognised this type of problem in relation to *in vitro* drug assay systems. These workers pointed out that due to competition between metabolites (thymidine and uridine) and antimetabolites (FU or FUDR) for the same anabolic enzymes, and because the antimetabolites are usually added at much higher concentrations than that of metabolites, there can result a decrease in thymidine or uridine incorporation, even though no metabolic block is produced by the drug. Nevertheless, in discussing this metabolite pool effect, Wolberg (1964) concluded that tumours were generally clinically sensitive to the fluorinated pyrimidines when there was a decreased incorporation of thymidine and uridine *in vitro* in the presence of the drug (concn. 23 µg/ml). It is also of note that in a large series of different types of cancer, Israel *et al.* (1971) found that clinically 5-drug combination therapy was superior to single drugs, and commented that with multiple drugs the results were very similar regardless of the site of the tumour. These workers felt that a possible explanation of this similarity was that "specific" sensitivities were obliterated under a large spectrum of different drugs, due to the smaller percentages of cancer cells resistant to the combination drugs than to any single drug. In the current results, tumours that responded to drug mixtures were usually sensitive to one or more individual components of the cocktail; there were also tumours of different types that showed no response to multiple drug combinations. In view of these various considerations, it is believed that the tumour responses obtained to multiple drugs (Tables 6-10) reflect pharmacological effects and are not merely non-specific blunderbuss toxic manifestations.

It may be argued that the drug concentrations employed in the present work are too high, especially on a C x T basis, since the plasma half-life of the drugs is so short. It is usually assumed that the pharmacological response is determined by the quantity of agent that is fixed to the drug receptors. Although the therapeutic effects of some drugs are related to their plasma level, this does not apply to drugs that act non-reversibly (so-called "hit-and-run" drugs) such as alkylating agents (Brodie and Reid, 1971); nor does the activity of drugs such as CP that require activation and have a biphasic activity peak in the plasma, or MTX that has a cumulative effect in tissues, have a well-defined relationship with the plasma level. It is of note that Wolberg (1971*b*) obtained clinical regression in tumours treated by FU when the drug (23 µg/ml) caused over 50% inhibition of formate incorporation into slices of the tumour *in vitro*. Bickis *et al.* (1966) contended that suppression of neoplastic cells in the host may be attainable by sufficient inhibition of any one of the three syntheses DNA, RNA or protein measured *in vitro*. These workers found that, under their experimental conditions, at least 50% *in vitro* inhibition of one of these parameters was necessary for reasonable expectation of a favourable clinical response. In the present work, results with the Yoshida tumour indicated that tumour regression *in vivo* can be associated with less than 50% inhibition of metabolism *in vitro*. Animal tumour systems exhibit important differences to human tumours from the point of view of chemotherapy. There are several animal tumours that are susceptible to cytotoxic drugs (*see* Larionov, 1965; Skipper, 1971*b* and *c*; Dickson and Suzangar, 1974) and with these neoplasms drug-induced tumour regression is usually synonymous with host cure. Such a degree of susceptibility to drugs is only rarely observed in human tumours, and may reflect a greater degree of homogeneity, with less importance of resistant cell populations, in the transplantable tumours. Nevertheless, results with animal tumours can provide valuable guidelines for work with human tumours, and it was found that a 30% or more inhibition of respiration and/or glycolysis in human tumour slices was usually associated with an inhibition of isotope uptake into DNA and/or RNA in excess of 50% and an inhibition of leucine uptake into protein of 30% or more. It was also found that in such "responsive" tumours, the effective drug(s) caused inhibition of respiration and/or glycolysis in fresh uncultured slices over 4-6 hr, when the drug was added to the Warburg flasks (drug concentrations as in Table 2). This approach, which correlates with the more detailed results given in Tables 6-10, is an extension of the shorter incubation technique of Bickis *et al.* (1966) and represents a rapid method of testing the susceptibility of solid human tumours to drugs.

Wolberg's extensive studies over the past 10 years on the mechanism of action of the fluorinated pyrimidines have emphasised the complex nature of the mode of action of these drugs on human tumours (*see* Wolberg, 1971*a*). Because of metabolite-anti-metabolite competition and the availability of alternative pathways for DNA synthesis, accurate assessment of the effect of FU requires simultaneous evaluation of more than one pathway of DNA synthesis, using labelled deoxycytidine, serine or formate in addition to thymidine. Only by this means can the significance of an increase in thymidine uptake by tumour *in vitro* in the presence of FU be assessed, for example; such an increase may indicate sensitivity to FU. However, tumours exhibiting an increase in thymidine uptake *in vitro* in the presence of FU are not uniform in their clinical response to FU (Wolberg, 1964). A stimulation of biochemical parameters (nucleic acid and protein precursor uptake, respiration, glycolysis) in tumour tissue *in vitro* as a response to cytotoxic drugs has been reported by other workers also, and has usually been interpreted as indicating non-sensitivity of the tumour to the particular drug tested (Bickis *et al.* 1966; Tchao *et al.* 1968). There is, however, the distinct possibility that such an increased metabolism occasioned by a drug could be accompanied *in vivo* by an increased biological malignancy of a tumour. It has been shown by several workers that respiration and glycolysis in tumours are coupled in such a way that any failure to produce adequate energy by one mechanism is compensated by an increased production by the other (*see* Bickis and Henderson, 1966 for refs). In the current work, only *inhibition* of biochemical parameters has been considered as indicating response to a drug. From the point of view of predictive testing, the availability of alternative metabolic pathways render extrapolation of *in vitro* results to the *in vivo* situation hazardous. Even a considerable (>50%) inhibition of all parameters measured in these experiments must be interpreted with caution. The heterogeneous nature of human tumours, and the inherent problems of tumour sampling, militate against even a high degree of metabolic inhibition *in vitro* being equated with more than temporary suppression of the biological malignancy of the tumour in the patient. Even xenogeneic transplantation of human cancers into laboratory animals is of little help in this situation, since the ability of a human tumour, before or after drug treatment, to grow in a rodent may have little relevance to its growth potential in the human host.

Nor is it especially helpful at present to attempt to vindicate the results of *in vitro* drug assay by using the drugs in clinical trial on patients whose tumours have been screened. This is because problems of assessing the sensitivity of tumours to cytotoxic drugs are not the monopoly of the experimentalist. The usual means of appraising a response to chemotherapy in man, is by estimating reduction in tumour size, and it is well recognised that tumour volume measurements can underestimate tumour cell kill by several orders of magnitude (Israel *et al.* 1971; Wolberg, 1971a and b; Greenwald, 1973). This serious underestimation of tumour cell kill based solely on tumour mass behaviour was first described by Wilcox and his group (the "Wilcox phenomenon"—see Skipper, 1971c), and represents a major problem currently facing medical oncologists. In addition to the effect of variables, such as the slow rate of dead tumour cell lysis and absorption following effective therapy, exponential multiplication of resistant cells can rapidly repopulate the tumour and mask effective cell kill by the drug. As many as 99% cells may require to be killed for a tumour to regress in size (*see* Johnson and Wolberg, 1971 for refs). In the absence of a biopsy, therefore, the effectiveness of a drug may pass undetected. Nor is there general agreement as to the clinical criteria that constitute response to therapy (*see* Ansfield, 1973; Greenwald, 1973). Also, as mentioned earlier, response of a tumour in the host to a drug is influenced by the route and schedule of administration. So again, a clinical response may be missed, because of inadequate therapy.

6. SUMMARY

It is possible to select *in vitro* cytotoxic drugs that inhibit to a considerable degree the metabolism of human tumours. A short-term culture system employing tumour slices is described; tumour sensitivity to a drug is defined as a minimum 30% inhibition of major energy-yielding processes of the cancer cell (respiration, anaerobic glycolysis), associated with a minimum 50% reduction of isotope precursor uptake into DNA, RNA or protein. These results correlate well with reduction of respiration and anaerobic glycolysis produced by the drugs over 4-6 hr in fresh tumour slices. Such inhibition of metabolism in this *in vitro* system is interpreted as implying the presence in the tumour of a drug-sensitive cancer cell population; this should not be equated with potential cure of the host given the drug, and even extensive tumour cell kill *in vivo* by the selected drug may pass undetected because of the presence and/or emergence of resistant cells. By using a multi-parameter assessment for the assay system, the hazards involved in extrapolating the results to predicting tumour response in the host may be reduced, but they cannot be eliminated. The nature of tumours and of the neoplastic process, as well as the pharmacodynamics of cytotoxic drugs and the rapidly changing concepts of drug administration, pose problems that at present seem unreceptive to experimental attack *in vitro*. We are also greatly hampered by the lack of drugs with a specific action against cancer cells, and it could be argued that the methods of *in vitro* tumour sensitivity testing to hand are as good as the available drugs permit them to be. The demonstration that there is no differential sensitivity to FU *in vitro* between human cancers and their normal tissues of origin (Wolberg, 1972) is a sobering reminder of the importance in chemotherapy of drug scheduling and other factors that cannot be assessed in *in vitro* systems. *In vitro* drug testing of human cancers must not be regarded solely as the domain of the experimentalist. Maximum benefit to the individual patient from the use of currently available cytotoxic drugs requires close cooperation between research scientists and clinicians versed in the problems posed by the use of these agents both *in vitro* and *in vivo*.

ACKNOWLEDGMENTS

We thank Mr. R. McCoy, Miss I. Beldon and Mr. S. Cohen for skilled technical assistance; the surgeons of the Royal Victoria and Newcastle General Hospitals, Shotley Bridge Hospital, and Dumfries and Galloway Royal Infirmary, for their enthusiastic co-operation in obtaining tumour material; the various drug firms for the kind gift of cytotoxic agents. M. S. gratefully acknowledges the financial assistance of the W.H.O. during the tenure of a W.H.O. Fellowship (1968-72). The work was also supported by the North of England Council of the Cancer Research Campaign.

Abbreviations used.

MTX, methotrexate (Lederle); FU, 5-fluorouracil (Roche); CP, cyclophosphamide (Ward Blenkinsop); TT, triethylene thiophosphoramide (Thiotepa; Lederle); PAM, L-phenylalanine mustard (melphalan; Burroughs Wellcome); VB, vinblastine (Lilly); ACT D, actinomycin D (Dactinomycin: Merck, Sharp and Dohme); MDMS, methylene dimethane sulphonate (Ward Blenkinsop); DNAP, DNA phosphorus.

REFERENCES

Ambrose, E. J. and Roe, F. J. C. (1966). "The Biology of Cancer". Van Nostrand Company, London.

Ansfield, F. J. (1973). "Chemotherapy of Malignant Neoplasms". Charles C. Thomas, Springfield, Illinois.

Bagley, C. M., Bostick, F. W. and DeVita, T. V. (1973). *Cancer Res. 33,* 226.

Bashford, E. F., Murray, J. A. and Cramer, W. (1905). *Scient. Rep. Invest. Imp. Cancer Res. Fund,* 2, 1.

Berlin, N. I., Rall, D., Mead, J. A. R., Freireich, E. J., Van Scott, E., Hertz, R. and Lipsett, M. B. (1963). *Ann. Intern. Med. 59,* 931.

Bickis, I. J. and Henderson, I. W. D. (1966). *Cancer, 19,* 89.

Bickis, I. J., Henderson, I. W. D. and Quastel, J. H. (1966). *Cancer, 19,* 103.

Birnie, G. D. and Heidelberger, C. (1963). *Cancer Res. 23,* 420.

Black, M. M. and Speer, F. D. (1954). *J. Natl. Cancer Inst. 14,* 1147.

Brock, N., Gross, R., Hohorst, H. J., Klein, H. O. and Schneider, B. (1971). *Cancer, 27,* 1512.

Brock, N. and Hohorst, H. J. (1967). *Cancer, 20,* 900.

Brodie, B. B. and Reid, W. D. (1971). *In* "Fundamentals of Drug Metabolism and Drug Disposition" (B. N. LaDu, H. G. Mandel and E. L. Way, eds.), p. 328. Williams & Wilkins Co., Baltimore.

Burton, K. (1956). *Biochem. J. 62,* 315.

Busch, H. (1965). *In* "The Scientific Basis of Surgery" (W. T. Irvine, ed.), p. 496. Churchill, London.

Byfield, J. E. and Stein, J. J. (1968). *Cancer Res. 28,* 2228.

Calabresi, P. and Parks, R. E. (1970). *In* "The Pharmacological Basis of Therapeutics" (L. S. Goodman and A. Gilman, eds.), p. 1348. MacMillan Co., New York.

Carter, S. K. (1972). *In* "The Design of Clinical Trials in Cancer Therapy" (M. Staquet, ed.), p. 336. Editions Scientifiques Européennes, Brussels.

Chadwick, M. and Rogers, W. I. (1970). *Proc. Amer. Assoc. Cancer Res. 11*, 15.

Chanes, R. E. and Condit, P. T. (1971). *Cancer, 27*, 613.

Chaudhuri, N. K., Montag, B. J. and Heidelberger, C. (1958). *Cancer Res. 18*, 318.

Clarkson, B., O'Connor, A., Winston, L. and Hutchison, D. (1964). *Clin. Pharm. Therap. 5*, 581.

Costanzi, J. J. and Coltman, C. A. (1969). *Cancer, 23*, 589.

Delmonte, L. and Jukes, T. H. (1962). *Pharm. Rev. 14*, 91.

Dendy, P. P., Bozman, V. G., Wheeler, T. K. and Dawson, M. P. (1971). *In* "Some Implications of Steroid Hormones in Cancer" (D. C. Williams and M. H. Briggs, eds.), p. 107. Wm. Heinemann Ltd., London.

DeVita, V. T. (1971). *Cancer Chemotherap. Reports, 2*, 23.

Dickson, J. A. (1966). *Brit. Med. J. 1*, 817.

Dickson, J. A. and Suzangar, M. (1974). *Cancer Res. 34*, 1263.

DiPaolo, J. A. (1971). *Natl. Cancer Inst. Monogr. 34*, 240.

Edelstyn, G. J. A. (1974). *In* "The Vinca Alkaloids in the Chemotherapy of Malignant Disease" Vol. 2, (W. I. H. Shedden, ed.), p. 80. Sherratt and Son Ltd., Altrincham, Cheshire.

Foulds, L. (1954). *Cancer Res. 14*, 327.

Fox, B. W. (1969). *Intern. J. Cancer, 4*, 54.

Gavosto, F. and Pileri, A. (1971). *In* "The Cell Cycle and Cancer" (R. Baserga, ed.), p. 99. Marcel Dekker Inc., New York.

Gillette, J. R. (1968). *In* "Importance of Fundamental Principles in Drug Evaluation" (D. H. Tedeschi and R. E. Tedeschi, eds.), p. 69. Raven Press, New York.

Greenstein, J. P. (1954). "Biochemistry of Cancer". 2nd edn. Academic Press, New York and London.

Greenwald, E. S. (1973). "Cancer Chemotherapy". 2nd edn. Henry Kimpton, London.

Grossfield, H. (1932). *Z. Krebsforsch. 37*, 49.

Gullino, P. M. (1973). *In* "Chemotherapy of Cancer Dissemination and Metastasis" (S. Garattini and G. Franchi, eds.), p. 89. Raven Press, New York.

Hanham, I. W. F., Newton, K. A. and Westbury, G. (1971). *Brit. J. Cancer, 25*, 462.

Holzer, H. (1964). *In* "Chemotherapy of Cancer" (P. A. Plattner, ed.), p. 44. Elsevier, Amsterdam.

Hutchison, W. C. and Munro, H. N. (1961). *Analyst, 86*, 768.

Israel, L., Depierre, A. and Chahinian, P. (1971). *Cancer, 27*, 1089.

Johnson, R. O. and Wolberg, W. H. (1971). *Cancer, 28*, 208.

Lala, P. K. (1972). *In* "Methods in Cancer Research" (H. Busch, ed.), Vol. 6, p. 3. Academic Press, New York and London.

Larionov, L. F. (1965). "Cancer Chemotherapy". Pergamon Press, London.

Lemon, A. M. and Foley, J. F. (1966). *In* "Controversy in Internal Medicine" (F. J. Ingelfinger, A. S. Relman and M. Finland, eds.), p. 575. Saunders, Philadelphia.

Liguori, V. R., Giglio, J. J., Miller, E. and Sullivan, R.D. (1962). *Clin. Pharm. Therap. 3,* 34.

Limburg, H. and Heckmann, U. (1968). *J. Obstet. Gynecol. Brit. Commonwealth, 75,* 1246.

McBride, C. M. (1970). *Arch. Surg. 101,* 122.

Mellett, L. B., Hodgson, P. E. and Woods, L. A. (1962). *J. Lab. Clin. Med. 60,* 818.

Miller, E. (1964). *In* "Chemotherapy of Cancer" (P. A. Plattner, ed.), p. 251. Elsevier, Amsterdam.

Mondovi, B., Strom, R., Rotilio, G., Agro, A. F., Cavaliere, R. and Fanelli, A. R. (1969). *Europ. J. Cancer, 5,* 129.

Morasca, L., Rainisio, C. and Masera, G. (1969). *Europ. J. Cancer, 5,* 79.

Nathanson, L., Hall, T. C., Schilling, A. and Miller, S. (1969). *Cancer Res. 29,* 419.

Natl. Cancer Inst. Monogr. 34, (1971). "Prediction of Response in Cancer Therapy" (T. C. Hall, ed.) U.S. Govt. Printing Office, Washington, D.C.

Obrecht, P. (1964). *In* "Chemotherapy of Cancer" (P. A. Plattner, ed.), p. 165. Elsevier, Amsterdam.

Patterson, M. S. and Greene, R. C. (1965). *Anal. Chem. 37,* 854.

Potter, V. R. (1963). *Adv. Enzyme Regln. 1,* 279.

Rinaldini, L. M. J. (1959). *Exptl. Cell Res. 16,* 477.

Schein, P. S. (1973). *In* "Current Research in Oncology" (C. B. Anfinsen, M. Potter and A. N. Schechter, eds.). Academic Press, London and New York.

Shedden, W. I. H. (ed.) (1974). "The Vinca Alkaloids in the Chemotherapy of Malignant Disease". Proceedings Third Lilly Symposium, Sherratt and Son, Altrincham, Cheshire.

Skipper, H. E. (1971*a*). *Cancer, 28,* 1479.

Skipper, H. E. (1971*b*). *In* "The Cell Cycle and Cancer" (R. Baserga, ed.), p. 358. Marcel Dekker Inc., New York.

Skipper, H. E. (1971*c*). *Natl. Cancer Inst. Monogr. 34,* 2.

Tchao, R., Easty, G. C. and Ambrose, E. J. (1967). *Brit. J. Cancer, 21,* 821.

Tchao, R., Easty, G. C., Ambrose, E. J., Raven, R. W. and Bloom, H. J. G. (1968). *Europ. J. Cancer, 4,* 39.

Torkelson, A. R., LaBuddhe, J. A. and Weikel, J. H. (1974). *Drug Metab. Rev. 3,* 131.

Wenke, M. (1971). *In* "Fundamentals of Biochemical Pharmacology" (Z. M. Bacq, ed.), p. 367. Pergamon Press.

Wolberg, W. (1964). *Cancer Res. 24,* 1437.

Wolberg, W. (1967). *Ann. Surg. 166,* 609.

Wolberg, W. (1971*a*). *Natl. Cancer Inst. Monogr. 34,* 189.

Wolberg, W. (1971*b*). *Arch. Surg. 102,* 344.

Wolberg, W. (1972). *Cancer Res. 32,* 130.

Wright, J. C., Cobb, J. L., Gumport, S. L., Safadi, D., Wacker, D. G. and Golomb, F. M. (1962). *Cancer, 15,* 284.

2. Quantitative Assays of *in vitro* Drug Damage

P. P. Dendy, M. P. A. Dawson, D. M. A. Warner and D. J. Honess

INTRODUCTION

The main object of this work is to establish a simple predictive test, the results of which can be used in the management of patients with malignant disease. If the sensitivity of tumour cells from each patient to various cytotoxic drugs can be determined ("Oncobiogram"– Tanneberger and Bacigalupo, 1970), chemotherapy can be planned to give the best chance of success. Percival (1974) has recently emphasised the need for such tests because there is good evidence that for carcinoma of the ovary at least the most successful course of drug treatment is the first, which should be as radical as possible. Attempts to demonstrate that *in vitro* tests of this type are of benefit to patients (Limburg *et al.* 1971; Wheeler *et al.* 1974) are extremely difficult for a variety of clinical and ethical reasons. However, a valuable step forward is to show that the *in vivo* biochemical properties of tumour cells are retained *in vitro* and can be studied in short term culture.

Using the monolayer technique described on page 24 we can establish within 24 hr to 7 days a number of comparable replicate tubes. Monolayer cultures are particularly satisfactory for biopsy specimens of advanced carcinoma of the ovary and for tumour cells from ascites fluid and pleural effusions. We have also cultured successfully smaller numbers of several other types of tumour including melanomas, especially of the eye, and brain tumours. These replicate tubes are subjected to a spectrum of cytotoxic drugs (Table 1) chosen to represent the widest possible range of biochemical actions and including alkylating agents, steroids, antimetabolites and plant alkaloids. Supply of material and laboratory facilities limit the number of drugs that can be tested against any one specimen.

An important cytotoxic which does not appear in Table 1 but is used frequently in the management of advanced carcinoma of the ovary, is cyclophosphamide. This drug is quite inactive against cells

TABLE 1

Drug Concentrations which Provide Useful Information in the in vitro *test*

Drug	Range of concentrations $\mu\,gm/ml$
Triaziquone (Trenimon-Bayer)	$10^{-2}\text{-}10^{-4}$
Chlorambucil (Burroughs-Wellcome)	0·1-0·3
Mustine hydrochloride (Boots)	0·1-0·4
5-fluorouracil (Roche Products)	1·5-15
Vinblastine sulphate (Velbe-Eli Lilly)	0·01-0·1
Vincristine sulphate (Oncovin-Eli Lilley)	0·01-0·1
Prednisolone 21 phosphate (Merck Sharpe and Dohme)	16
Oxymetholone (Anapolon-Syntex)	3-12

in culture but can be metabolised to extremely cytotoxic products in the body. Connors *et al.* (1970) have shown that toxic derivatives can be obtained *in vitro* by treating cyclophosphamide with microsomes. We have found this procedure rather too elaborate for almost daily use on fresh tumour specimens and, in any event, it is not yet clear which of the numerous derivatives isolated *in vitro* (Connors, 1974) is the active product *in vivo*. Preibach *et al.* (1974) have reported that the urine taken from a patient being treated with cyclophosphamide contains the cytotoxic metabolites, but our attempts to standardise this procedure against an established cell line *in vitro* have so far been unsuccessful.

In our early work the test was assayed by the morphological damage caused to the monolayer. The drugs were left in contact with the cells for 24 hr, after which they were removed and the cultures re-fed with normal medium. Cell damage was assessed under the microscope for the next 48 hr and signs of recovery from drug damage were also noted. Figures 1 and 2 show examples of specimens which were respectively sensitive and resistant to a 24 hr exposure to 0·1 μgm/ml vincristine sulphate.

This method had all the disadvantages of a subjective assay, and we have subsequently developed two quantitative methods (Dendy *et al.* 1973). Since it is important to remember that the ability or otherwise of a cell to replicate after treatment will determine the efficacy of a drug, both the assay methods we have chosen relate to the ability of the cell to proceed through the cell cycle after drug treatment.

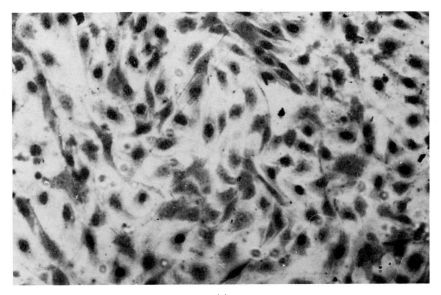

(a)

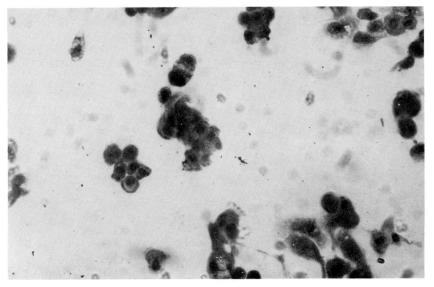

(b)

Fig. 1. Monolayer cultures prepared from a solid biopsy of an ovarian tumour (a) Control (b) After 24 hr exposure to 0·1 μgm/ml Oncovin.

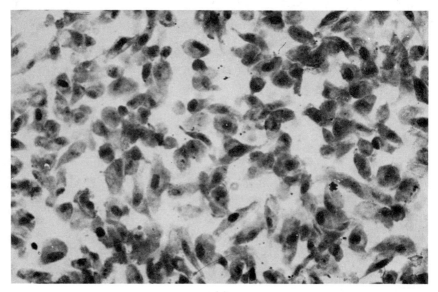

(a)

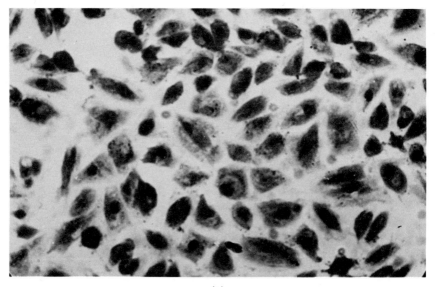

(b)

Fig. 2. Monolayer cultures prepared from malignant cells in ascites fluid taken from a different patient with an ovarian tumour (a) Control (b) After 24 hr exposure to 0·1 μgm/ml Oncovin.

1. PERCENTAGE OF CELLS PROCEEDING THROUGH S PHASE BETWEEN 24 AND 48 HR AFTER THE END OF DRUG TREATMENT

The first method uses the uptake of tritiated thymidine (^{3}HTdR) as a measure of cell survival. For this test, cells are seeded onto coverslips in petri dishes at 2×10^5 cells/coverslip and allowed to establish. Drugs are added for 24 hr, then the cells are fed with drug-free medium for 24 hr and then exposed to feeding medium containing 1 μCi/ml ^{3}HTdR for 24 hr. Cultures are washed and fixed and autoradiographs are prepared. The cells are lightly stained and the labelling index on each slide is counted and recorded. The labelled cells are those which have entered S phase of the cell cycle sometime during the 24 hr exposure to ^{3}HTdR. Labelling indices for the cultures shown in Figs 1 and 2 were as follows:

	Control (a)	0·1 μgm/ml vincristine sulphate (b)
Fig. 1	45%	11%
Fig. 2	34%	35%

These results confirm very well deductions made from the morphological appearance of the cultures. A wide variation in sensitivity as measured by the ^{3}HTdR labelling index, and good correlation with the morphological damage is shown in Table 2 for 5 different specimens following 10^{-2} μgm/ml triaziquone.

TABLE 2

Variation in ^{3}H Thymidine Labelling Index between Specimens following 10^{-2} μgm/ml Triaziquone

		Labelling index	
Tumour	Morphological damage	Control	10^{-2} μgm/ml triaziquone
Disgerminoma or endometrial carcinoma or granulosa cell carcinoma of ovary	0	35	38
Melanoma	0	12	9
Cystadenocarcinoma of ovary	+	37	2·5
Carcinoma of breast and liver secondaries	+	45	5
Ovarian carcinoma	+++	46	0

2. TOTAL DNA SYNTHESISED BY THE CULTURE BETWEEN 24 HR AND
48 HR AFTER THE END OF DRUG TREATMENT

The second assay method is the ability of drug-treated cells to take up 125 Iodine labelled Iododeoxyuridine (^{125}IUdR) from the culture medium. This precursor appears to be specifically incorporated into newly synthesised DNA and is a stable DNA label (Commerford, 1965). It was first used to label human tumour cells *in vitro* by Andrysek *et al.* (1969). Replicate monolayers are set up in test tubes as for the earlier morphological work and the cultures are subjected to 24 hr drug treatment. The drugs are given in 50% feeding medium mixed with 50% Hanks balanced salt solution to discourage excessive growth during the test period. A further 24 hr on 50% medium without drugs allows for any recovery from drug action which might take place. 0·06 μCi/ml ^{125}IUdR in full feeding medium is then given to the cultures for 24 hr. The return to full feeding medium encourages growth and uptake of ^{125}IUdR in control and undamaged cultures. The cultures are then washed three times in saline and re-fed. Not less than 6 hr later they are washed once more and the bound ^{125}I activity is counted using a sodium iodide well crystal scintillation counter system. The double washing procedure is important, both to wash away unincorporated ^{125}IUdR, and to remove label released by degenerating cells. Re-utilisation of ^{125}IUdR is very low.

The drug damage is estimated by expressing the count obtained from the drug-treated cells as a percentage of the count obtained from untreated control cultures.

Figure 3 shows the effect of 0·3 μgm/ml chlorambucil on 186 specimens. There is a wide range of sensitivities. Figure 4 shows the distribution of results for 1·5 μgm/ml fluorouracil. The spread is even greater and ^{125}IUdR incorporation is actually stimulated for a few specimens—above 100%.

To verify that this variation is not caused by an inability to standardise conditions during the test, a culture of human embryonic skin and muscle cells was tested against two different concentrations of 5-fluorouracil on seven occasions. Cell numbers were varied to cover the acceptable range (vide infra) for testing tumour specimens. The results are shown in Table 3 and indicate that the response at each dose was very consistent. The use of two drug concentrations helps to eliminate small variations in sensitivity which might seem significant if only one concentration were used, and we generally use two concentrations of each drug in the test. It may be noted that the

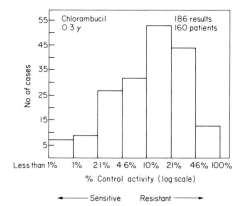

Fig. 3. Uptake of ^{125}IUdR after treatment with 0·3 μgm/ml chlorambucil for 186 specimens from different human tumours expressed as a percentage of the control activity.

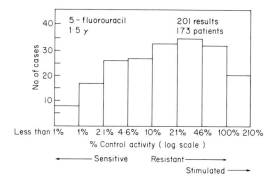

Fig. 4. Uptake of ^{125}IUdR after treatment with 1·5 μgm/ml 5 fluorouracil—expressed as a percentage of the control activity.

TABLE 3

Effect of 24 hr Exposure to 1·5 μ gm/ml 5-fluorouracil on ^{125}IUdR Uptake into Cultures of Human Embryonic Skin and Muscle

| Date | Final cell count | % of Control count | |
		1·5 γ 5 FU	0·15 γ 5 FU
18/6/74	6·7 x 10^4	2·4%	55·6%
25/6/74	14·1 x 10^4	0·2%	60·0%
2/7/74	5·8 x 10^4	1·4%	50·4%
9/7/74	16 x 10^4	1·1%	78·5%
23/7/74	6·7 x 10^4	0·9%	84·7%
30/7/74	19 x 10^4	0·2%	83·8%
6/8/74	4·3 x 10^4	1·1%	72·2%

Effect of 5-fluorouracil on cultures of human embryonic skin and muscle.

HTSTC–6

human embryonic skin and muscle cells were more sensitive than nearly all the tumour specimens.

Figure 5 shows the spread for the drug triaziquone at 10^{-3} μgm/ml for 202 specimens from 167 patients with a wide variety of tumours. Our recommendations to the clinicians are based on these histo-

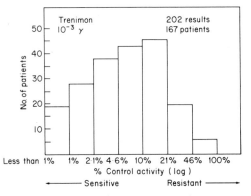

Fig. 5. Uptake of ^{125}IUdR after treatment with 10^{-3} μgm/ml triaziquone for 202 specimens from different human tumours—expressed as a percentage of the control activity.

grams. For triaziquone a response in the centre of the scale, between about 4% and 10% is reported as average sensitivity and the drug is not recommended. If residual uptake is more than 10% of the control, the cells are reported as resistant to the drug, and when uptake falls below 4% the cells are reported as sensitive to the drug and it is recommended.

Test results are related to clinical findings in Chapter 7 (p. 291), but we have some indirect evidence from the biochemical studies alone that the ^{125}IUdR assay method may measure *in vivo* drug sensitivity. In Fig. 5 the median value for all specimens is at about 7%. Figure 6 shows the spread of sensitivities for melanomas and sarcomas treated with 10^{-3} μgm/ml triaziquone. Clinically, melanomas and sarcomas are frequently resistant to chemotherapy, and relative to the median value of 7% for all specimens in Fig. 5, it can be seen that more specimens fall at the resistant end of the scale than at the sensitive end—in a ratio of 12 to 4.

Effects of Overcrowding

At the end of the ^{125}IUdR assay the number of cells in two control tubes is estimated by stripping the cells off the glass surface on which they are growing. To do this the cells are exposed to 1 ml 0·2%

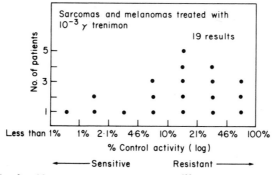

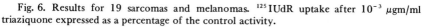

Fig. 6. Results for 19 sarcomas and melanomas. ^{125}IUdR uptake after 10^{-3} μgm/ml triaziquone expressed as a percentage of the control activity.

Versene for 1 min. 1 ml of 0·1% trypsin is then added, the pH is adjusted to 7·2 and the cells are incubated until they come off the glass (see page 26). A single cell suspension is normally obtained in this way, and is counted with a Coulter counter. This count is important because although the number of viable tumour cells seeded can be standardised, the percentage which grow is very variable for different specimens. Experiments with both mouse L cells and normal adult human ovary show that at about 2×10^5 cells per tube, ^{125}IUdR uptake per cell falls sharply (Fig. 7). If the control is inhibited in this way, an apparent, but false, drug resistance may be reported for a treated tube where the ^{125}IUdR uptake has not been cell density inhibited.

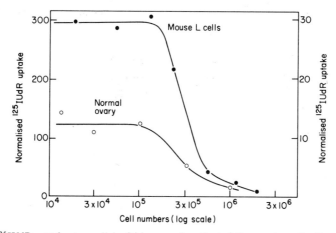

Fig. 7. ^{125}IUdR uptake per cell in 24 hr as a function of the number of cells per test tube. Mouse L cells—left hand scale. Normal adult human ovary—right hand scale. Uptake is expressed as counts/10 sec and normalised to 10^5 cells/tube.

Below 3×10^4 fresh tumour cells per tube, ^{125}IUdR uptake is generally too low to be measurable even in the controls so the useful range for drug sensitivity work is 3×10^4 to 2×10^5 cells per tube. Measurement of the number of cells in a tube also allows ^{125}IUdR uptake to be expressed on a "per cell" basis.

3. CONCLUSIONS

(1) Both assay methods measure the ability of cells to continue cycling after drug treatment. The ^{125}IUdR/scintillation method measures the total DNA synthesised during the 24 hr exposure. The ^{3}H thymidine/autoradiographic method measures the ability of cells to enter S phase, but not the rate of DNA synthesis.

(2) A minimum of 3×10^4 cells per tube is required to give reasonable counts in the ^{125}IUdR assay: this is because ^{125}IUdR is much more toxic than ^{3}HTdR and a non-toxic concentration must be used. When using ^{3}HTdR, the cells are grown on coverslips and examined microscopically, so small numbers of cells can be assayed by growing them in the wells of plastic micro-titre plates. This method could thus be useful for testing sequential needle biopsy specimens. The method is also valuable for examining mixed populations of cells.

(3) If an automatic sample changer is available, uptake of ^{125}IUdR in each test tube can be assayed quickly and with a minimum of technical manipulation. ^{3}HTdR/autoradiography requires a 3-day autoradiographic exposure and then lengthy microscope examination.

(4) ^{3}HTdR can be re-utilized by the cells after it has been degraded, but for ^{125}IUdR re-utilisation is minimal (Dethlefsen, 1970).

(5) It is impossible to say which method is "best", as they measure different parameters and are suited to different circumstances. Routinely, the ^{125}IUdR test is better as it is quicker than the thymidine test and requires less technical skill. It would therefore be more suitable for introduction as a Hospital Service.

ACKNOWLEDGEMENT

Support for this work from the Cancer Research Campaign is gratefully acknowledged.

REFERENCES

Andrysek, O., Dvorak, O and Stranska, E. (1969). *Neoplasma, 16*, 239.

Commerford, S. L. (1965). *Nature, Lond. 206*, 949.

Connors, T. A., Grover, P. L. and McLoughlin, A. M. (1970). *Bioch. Pharm. 19*, 1533.

Connors, T. A., Cox, P. J., Farmer, P. B., Foster, A. B. and Jarman, M. (1974). *Bioch. Pharm. 23*, 115.

Dendy, P. P., Dawson, M. P. A. and Honess, D. J. (1973). *In* "Aktuelle Probleme der Therapie maligner Tumoren" (G. Wüst, ed.), p. 34. Georg. Thieme Verlag, Stuttgart.

Dethlefsen, L. A. (1970). *J. Nat. Cancer Inst. 44*, 827.

Limburg, H., Tranekjer, A. S. and Heckmann, U. (1971). *In* "Gynaecological Cancer" (T. J. Deeley, ed.), p. 243. Butterworths, London.

Percival, R. (1974). *Proc. Roy. Soc. Med. 67*, 381.

Preibach, W., Krafft, W., Marzotko, F., Schröder, M. and Hofman, K. D. (1973). *Arch. Geschwulstforsch, 41*, 248.

Tanneberger, St. and Bacigalupo, G. (1970). *Arch. Geschwulstforsch, 35*, 44.

Wheeler, T. K., Dendy, P. P. and Dawson, M. P. A. (1974). *Oncology, 30*, 362.

3. Some Observations on Assay of Anticancer Drugs in Culture

R. I. Freshney

This assay of drug sensitivity employs the prolonged growth of monolayer cultures in microtitre trays (Freshney, Paul and Kane, 1975). Each tray gives 96 identical wells enabling the testing of a large number of drugs and drug combinations at a large range of concentrations. The maximum concentration of drug is added to the left-hand side of the plate and a serial dilution is made across the plate. After removing the drugs and allowing the cells to recover, the residual ability of the cultures to incorporate tritiated leucine into protein is measured. The concentration of drug causing 50% inhibition of tritiated leucine incorporation is then referred to as the ID_{50} (Fig. 1) and this value is used in subsequent plots. (See page 20 for a more complete description of this method).

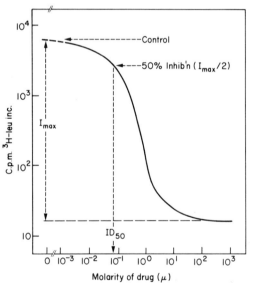

Fig. 1. Hypothetical dose response curve to show derivation of ID_{50}. "Control" counts are those from ^{3}H-leucine incorporated in wells containing no drug. The remainder of the curve is derived from gradually reduced counts with progressively higher drug concentrations. The ID_{50} is that concentration producing 50% inhibition of the control level of ^{3}H-leucine incorporation.

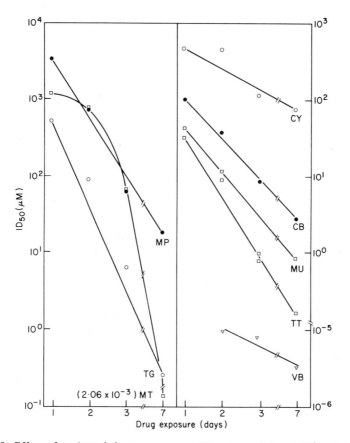

Fig. 2. Effect of prolonged drug exposure on ID_{50}. Four plates at 10^4 cells/ml (10^3 cells/well) were exposed to drugs, with daily replacement at 1, 2 and 3 days, for 1, 2, 3 and 7 days. After 22 hr recovery, 5 μCi/ml ^{3}H-leucine (10 μCi/μMole) was added to each well for 4 hr, the plates were washed, extracted and counted (see page 22). The ID_{50} was calculated and plotted against the time from the first addition of drugs.

Abbreviations: CY: cyclophosphamide
                  CB: chlorambucil
                  MP: 6-mercaptopurine

                  MT: methotrexate
                  MU: mustine
                  TG: thioguanine
                  TT: thiotepa
                  VB: vinblastine

The left-hand axis refers to MP, TG, MT, TT and CB. The right-hand axis refers to MU and CY above the break and VB below. (From: Freshney, Paul and Kane, 1975.)

We have used HeLa cells in these experiments, although many people feel that HeLa cells are not relevant to primary cultures from human tumours. However, we believe it is important to work out assay conditions using a homogeneous cell strain with predictable kinetics rather than to work with a heterogeneous culture of primary tumour cells where the proliferation rate is uncertain.

Figure 2 shows that the duration of exposure to drugs has a profound effect not only on the ID_{50} of each drug but, also on the relative ID_{50}'s of the different drugs. Although all the drugs showed an increasing effect with time of exposure, this was particularly so with mercaptopurine, methotrexate and thioguanine. While the sensitivity to these three drugs was much less than to the alkylating agents after one day, the effect was as great, and in the case of methotrexate even greater, by seven days. The drugs were replaced daily to minimise the problems of drug instability.

That all the alkylating agents show increased effectiveness with time is perhaps not too surprising but it is important to note that the relative sensitivity to different drugs changes with time. Furthermore, measurement of sensitivity to antimetabolites such as methotrexate and mercaptopurine which is very difficult unless the cells are exposed for at least two cell cycles (Hussa and Pattillo, 1970; Tidd *et al.* 1972) can be determined much more effectively with the extended regime.

Figure 3 shows that recovery after exposure to the drug can also be important. Cells were exposed to drug for 24 hr and then allowed to recover for varying periods. Tritiated leucine uptake was then measured and the ID_{50}s calculated. In the case of the antimetabolites and vinblastine, there is a reversal of the effect (an increase in the ID_{50} meaning a reduction in sensitivity). With the alkylating agents, however, the ID_{50} increases during apparent "recovery". That is to say, the cells are not in fact recovering, but are accumulating damage much as they would after radiation. The ID_{50} values for the alkylating agents plateau at a minimal value 5 days after drug removal; this is ·a much more stable region to measure drug sensitivity, rather than on the slope of the curve where small differences in time or growth rate may make a large difference in the actual measurement of ID_{50}.

An optimal procedure might be to give prolonged exposure to drugs followed by prolonged culture after removing drugs (Fig. 4); 3 days here represents 3 cell cycles for HeLa cells but longer exposure might be required for freshly cultured cells with longer cell cycle times. After this prolonged exposure the cells are allowed to recover

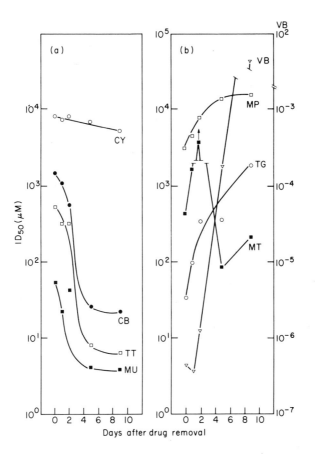

Fig. 3. Effect of prolonged "recovery". Plates were set up at 10^4/well and treated with drugs for 24 hr. One plate was labelled directly after the removal of drugs, the others after varying periods of culture in drug-free medium, and ID_{50}s derived as in Fig. 2.

(a) Cyclophosphamide, chlorambucil, thiotepa and mustine.

(b) Left-hand axis 6-mercaptopurine, thioguanine and methotrexate; right-hand axis vinblastine.

Symbols as for Fig. 2. (From: Freshney, Paul and Kane, 1975.)

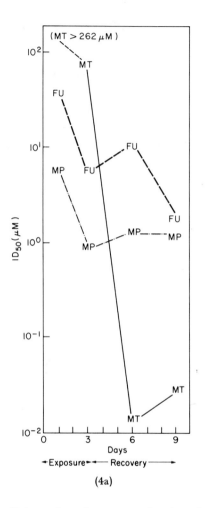

(4a)

Fig. 4. Effect of combining prolonged exposure and prolonged recovery. Plates were set up at 2×10^3 cells/well and drugs added for 3 days, with daily renewal. Plates were then incubated for a further six days in the absence of drugs. Samples were taken after 24 hr drug exposure (4 hr recovery, 3 hr label), 3 days drug exposure (4 hr recovery, 3 hr label), 3 days after drug removal (3 hr label) and six days after drug removal. ID_{50}s were determined as before.

Symbols as in Fig. 2.

(a) Methotrexate, 5-fluorouracil (FU), 6-mercaptopurine (Inhibition with methotrexate did not exceed 50% after 24 hr).

(b) Cyclophosphamide, thiotepa, chlorambucil, and mustine.

(c) Vinblastine.

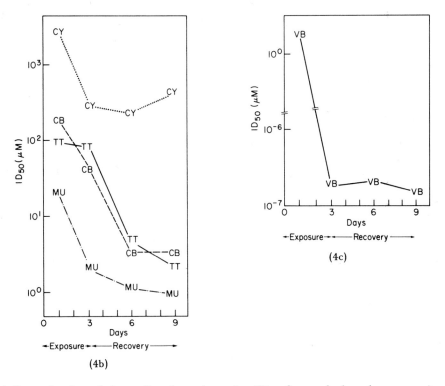

(4b)

(4c)

for a further 6 days. By that time the ID_{50} for each drug has moved into a region of stable measurement, maximal drug effect is measured, and, in addition, this applies equally well to the cycle dependent drugs.

REFERENCES

Freshney, R. I., Paul, J. and Kane, I. (1975). *Brit. J. Cancer, 31,* 89.

Hussa, R. O. and Pattillo, R. A. (1972). *Europ. J. Cancer, 8,* 523-530.

Tidd, D. M., Kim, S. C., Horakova, K., Morikaki, A. and Paterson, A. R. P. (1972). *Cancer Res. 32,* 317-322.

GENERAL DISCUSSION

Hill emphasised the need to base the use of chemotherapeutic agents for an *in vitro* test on their use clinically. First, there are quite often only certain ways in which various chemotherapeutic agents can be given to a patient. Secondly, it is important not to test an agent over a long period of time if when it is given to a patient it may only be active for a short time. It may be of no value to know what happens when a drug is in the culture for 48 hr if it remains in the patient for only 3 hr.

Freshney said an *in vitro* test should be devised in discussions with the practising chemotherapist since the duration of exposure to drug is one of the major disparities between an *in vitro* technique and *in vivo* chemotherapy. The regime he described could adjust the time of drug exposure to fit the known *in vivo* exposure by changing the exposure time per day. Then the number of days dosing could be increased to agree with clinical use. Kohorn added that since the cycling time of HeLa cells is about 18 hr, daily replacement of the drug might have something approaching a pulsing effect. The conditions with more slowly growing freshly cultured human cells might be quite different.

Dickson said a knowledge of the detailed action of cytotoxic drugs is extremely important. For example, the action of fluorouracil is not basically concerned only with thymidine metabolism (*see* Fig. 1). 5-Fluorouracil (FU) is an analogue of uracil (U) and depends for its action on conversion via the uridine (UR) or deoxyuridine (UDR) pathway to the monophosphorylated derivative (FUDRP) which then blocks the conversion of the normal substrate, deoxyuridine monophosphate (UDRP), to the thymidine derivative TDRP through the action of the enzyme thymidylate synthetase. Now if this enzyme is not present

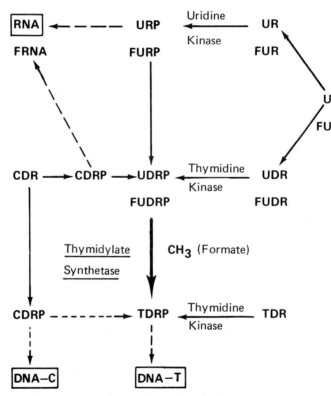

Fig. 1. Metabolic pathways for the formation of DNA-thymine and RNA uridine, and the associated anabolic pathways for FU metabolism. FU is incorporated into RNA but not into DNA.

or is insensitive to FU, there will be no action of the drug. Similarly, decreased activity or absence of either of the other two enzymes, thymidine kinase and uridine kinase, upon which FU depends for its activation to FUDRP, can be associated with drug resistance (Wolberg, 1964). Wolberg found that if the action of thymidylate synthetase is blocked by FU, the cell can synthesise its DNA thymine (DNA-T) either by uptake of thymidine (TDR), or from cytidine (CDR). To measure the action of FU upon DNA synthesis, a multiple approach with isotopically labelled substrates must be used. There must be either uracil or uridine with thymidine in the medium, cytidine must also be used and the effectiveness of FU in blocking thymidylate synthetase can also be monitored by the inclusion of formate to provide the methyl group required for the 5-methylation of the UDRP. This is a complex sequence of reactions and the use of a single labelled compound for assay of FU activity is extremely hazardous from the point of view of interpretation, because of alternative pathways. In particular, inhibition of thymidine uptake alone cannot be used as an assay of FU sensitivity. Indeed the opposite may be the case, and once the normal (de novo) pathway via thymidylate synthetase is blocked, there is increased uptake of thymidine by the cultures via the thymidine kinase (salvage) pathway (Wolberg, 1967).

Warenius said that although these considerations were certainly important if isotope uptake were assayed during exposure to FU, they might not apply to an assay made many hours after the end of FU treatment. So the relative timings of the administration of drug and ^{3}H thymidine assay are important.

Lamerton suggested this introduced another problem. When the percentage of labelled cells is scored after ^{3}H thymidine labelling, the radioactive precursor is being used to measure the rate of cell proliferation, and there can be considerable uncertainty in interpretation. Either the effect of cell loss, or a hold up in cell proliferation, or in some cases even a subsequent speed up in cell proliferation may be being measured.

Dendy said that measurements of the change in total cell number in the culture over a period of several days or even weeks after drug treatment, might be the best criterion of sensitivity. However, the importance of expediency in any test which is to be clinically applicable has already been emphasised, and it is unlikely that colony-forming ability will be a practicable method for a routine test. The methods described on pages 139-149 are a compromise which does not go as far as measuring colony formation but does allow the cell time to recover from the immediate action of a drug on the biochemical pathways. Only further experiments of the type discussed in the foregoing papers can decide if a 24 hr delay between the end of drug treatment and addition of isotope precursor, is a good time interval for the subsequent assay to reflect accurately cell killing.

REFERENCES

Wolberg, W. (1964). *Cancer Res.* 24, 1437.
Wolberg, W. (1967). *Ann. Surg. 166*, 609.

4. The Chemosensitivity of Freshly Explanted Tumour Cells of Various Origins as Determined by Clonal Assay and Six-day Growth *in vitro* and Variation in Chemosensitivity with Subsequent Subculturing

J. Wells, R. J. Berry and A. H. Laing

INTRODUCTION

Two different methods of measuring *in vitro* chemosensitivity, namely six-day growth *in vitro* and true survival of cell reproductive capacity as measured by clonal growth, have been compared for six fresh human tumour explants which yielded high plating efficiencies.

1 MATERIALS AND METHODS

The procedure for setting up the primary cultures is shown in Fig. 1, tumour cells being obtained either from solid biopsies or from ascitic or pleural fluid. The culture fluid was medium 199 (BDH) with 15% human AB serum together with antibiotics, and additional L-gluta-

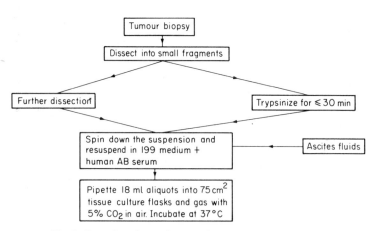

Fig. 1. Procedure for setting up primary tumour cell cultures.

TABLE 1

	In vivo	*In vitro* (MBC)
Mustine	42 mg/50L	0·84 μg/ml
Thiotepa	30 mg/50L	0·60 μg/ml
Methotrexate	5 mg/50L	0·10 μg/ml
5 FU	1 g/50L	20 μg/ml
Vinblastine	15 mg/50L	0·3 μg/ml

The maximum drug concentration used *in vitro* for a given drug was chosen to approximate to the maximum concentration likely to be achieved in the body fluids of a patient undergoing chemotherapy.

Therefore for each drug a unit called the *Maximum Body Concentration* (MBC) was arbitrarily defined.

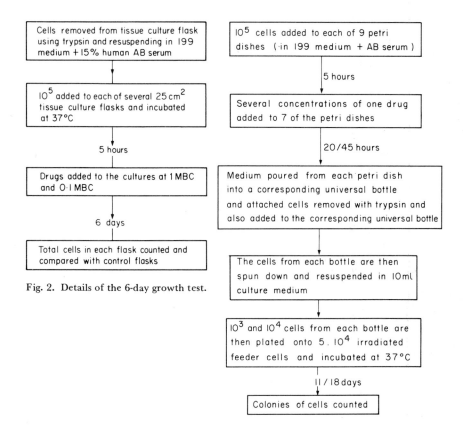

Fig. 2. Details of the 6-day growth test.

Fig. 3. Details of the survival curve procedure.

mine (88 mg/L). The trypsin was 0·1% (w/v) Bacto-trypsin 1:250 (Difco).

Table 1 specifies the units of drug concentration used and Figs 2 and 3 indicate the two test procedures.

2. RESULTS

Figure 4 shows the results of the six-day growth test for six cell lines (cells designated "B" were incubated for eight instead of six days). The drug concentration used was 1 MBC except for the cells designated "L", "K", "Q" and "S" which were tested at a concentration of 0·1 MBC of vinblastine. In general, there appears to be little change in sensitivity with time in culture, most cells having reached their maximum growth potential. The cells designated "B" however, did not reach their maximum growth potential *in vitro* until after the second subculture. One can see that after the maximum growth potential was reached, there was an increase in sensitivity to all drugs used. This is therefore independent of the mode of action of any one particular drug.

The survival curves for clonal growth after exposure to mustine are shown in Fig. 5. All plating efficiencies were in excess of 20% except for the cells designated "Q" which had a plating efficiency of 10%. Of the six cell lines tested, four have been subsequently retested after further subculturing, and all show increased sensitivity to this drug. This change in sensitivity is not reflected in the six-day growth test.

True clonal survival curves obtained after exposure to vinblastine (Fig. 6) are of quite different shape, as the limited length of exposure to this phase specific drug meant that a proportion of the cell population was totally unaffected by it. The apparent increase in survival with increasing drug concentration can be ascribed to non-specific effects (Sartorelli and Creasey, 1969) of the same drug in slowing the entry of cells into the sensitive mitotic phase. In determining sensitivity to this drug, it is more appropriate to consider the minimum effective concentration as indicative of the degree of chemosensitivity (i.e. the region between the left-hand end of the plateau and 100% survival). The data show a possible increase in sensitivity on serial subculture for three of the four lines which were re-tested.

3. DISCUSSION

The cells designated "Q" in Fig. 5 were very resistant to the alkylating agent mustine, a drug which is still often referred to as

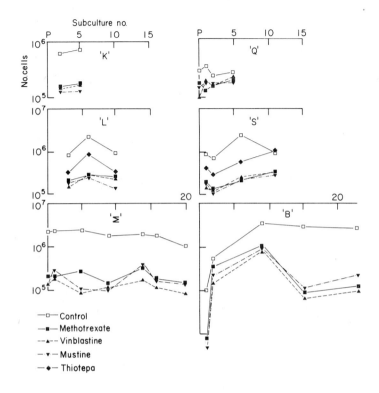

Fig. 4. The effect of several drugs at 1 MBC on the change in cell number from the seeding concentration of 10^5 cells/flask during 6 days growth at different passages following explantation (0·1 MBC Vinblastine for "L", "K", "S" and "Q"). Details of the tumour specimens tested are shown in the table below.

Code	Primary site	Presentation
B	Bronchus (carcinoma)	Solid biopsy (from lung)
Σ	"	"
K	Skin (melanoma)	Solid biopsy
L	Breast (carcinoma)	Pleural fluid
S	Stomach (carcinoma)	Solid biopsy
Q	Testis (seminoma)	Pleural fluid

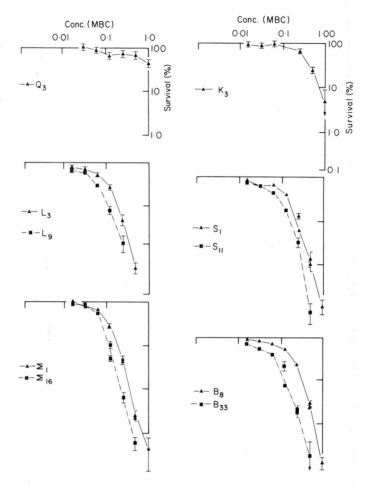

Fig. 5. Reproductive survival of explanted human tumour cells after exposure to different concentrations of mustine. Specimens are coded as in Fig. 4. The suffix is the number of passages before testing.

being radiomimetic. When one considers that this cell line was the most resistant to mustine, and the most radiosensitive cell line handled during the course of the work presented here, the term radiomimetic would seem inappropriate and misleading.

Figure 6 shows that vinblastine is apparently effective at concentrations lower than 1/100th of the maximum which is likely to be achieved in the body fluids of a patient being treated with this drug at currently accepted therapeutic dose levels. This probably means

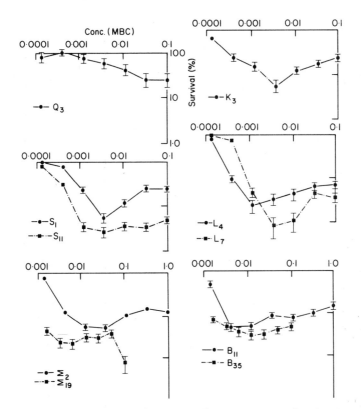

Fig. 6. Reproductive survival of explanted human tumour cells after exposure to different concentrations of vinblastine. Other details as for Figs 4 and 5.

that effective drug concentrations are maintained *in vivo,* despite elimination of the drug, for far longer than in the case of many other chemotherapeutic agents.

It can be seen that there is poor correlation between the growth test and true cell reproductive survival under the experimental conditions described here. The most obvious explanation for this difference is that the two test procedures measure different things. The growth test, although the simpler test of the two to perform, is undoubtedly complex if one wishes to analyse the results in detail. Further study of the cell kinetics involved in the growth test may be of value and both tests must be compared with clinical results.

There is evidence to suggest that at least for some explanted tumours, the cells become more chemosensitive on serial subculture even after reaching their maximum *in vitro* growth potential. This change in sensitivity may be associated with a mechanism which is independent of the specific mode of action of any one particular drug.

REFERENCE

Sartorelli, A. C. and Creasey, W. A. (1969). *Ann. Rev. Pharmacol.* 9, 51.

ACKNOWLEDGEMENTS

We would like to express our gratitude to George Breckon and Christine Horlor for their advice and help in establishing the karyotypes of the tumour cells reported in this paper.

J. Wells was aided by a grant from Eli Lilly & Co. Ltd.

Chapter 4

EFFECTS OF IONIZING RADIATION AND OTHER PHYSICAL TREATMENTS ON SHORT TERM CULTURES

(Moderator: R.J. Berry)

1. Introduction to the Effects of Ionising Radiation and Other Physical Treatments on Short-term Cultures

J. S. Mitchell

This section provides a useful opportunity to consider and try to understand the basis of a number of related developments which are relevant to practical applications in the treatment of patients with cancer. There appear to be four main aspects to be discussed:

(1) The first problem is the reappraisal of cell survival dose curves and their detailed interpretation in terms of molecular biology and the biochemical mechanisms of action. One must refer to the analytical treatment of target theory and dose-effect relations of Hug and Kellerer (1966) in their book "Stochastik der Strahlenwirkung" and in particular to their theorem (page 43 and Table 1, page 63) concerning the "relative steepness", S, of a dose effect curve, defined as $S = \bar{D}^2/\sigma^2$ where $\bar{D}$ is the mean inactivation dose and σ^2 the variance of the inactivation dose, showing that the mean number of elementary absorption events necessary to produce the observed effect in the object under consideration, is at least equal to S. It is of interest that this theorem can be generalised to include effects of chemical agents and of hyperthermia.

(2) One must raise the question of the relevance of *in vitro* measurements to *in vivo* studies and especially to the complex clinical problems of the treatment of malignant tumours. It is clear that in general host responses including immunological factors, are absent *in vitro* and that the possibility of changes in the biological properties of freshly grown human cells *in vitro* must be examined in detail concerning all the possible relevant factors. It is necessary to determine values of D_{37} and D_q for freshly grown human cells, normal and malignant, *in vitro* and to examine evidence for differences between *in vitro* and *in vivo* values (cf., e.g. Dawson *et al.* 1973).

The essential measurement made in determining cell survival curves is clone counting: each clone arises from one surviving cell which can proliferate. Evidence from measurements of chromosome and DNA distributions appears to give increasing support for the validity of the concept of "clonal proliferation of aneuploid cells" as a model of solid tumours. Though this is reassuring, the complexity of the *in vivo* tumour system must be emphasised.

Observations of radiobiological effect which depend on counting the total number of cells in a population—which may include differentiated and non-proliferating cells—must be distinguished from clone-counting experiments. It seems to me that, noting the reduction of growth rate after irradiation, it is desirable to measure the appropriate dose-response curves for total cell populations *in vitro* after different doses at given times after irradiation. Measurements of the uptake of ^{125}IUdR in confluent cultures of freshly grown human tumour cells are related to this second type of dose-response curve; under these conditions, Mrs Mary Lloyd working with Dendy in Cambridge found no split dose effect, but much further experimental study is necessary.

(3) Despite the difficulties, it is very important to try to develop *in vitro* methods for short-term assay of the radiosensitivity and if possible, of the radiocurability of malignant tumours in individual patients. Perhaps there is a better prospect of achieving this than previously. At least, a start is being made.

Among the problems to be studied are the effects of fractionation and of continuous irradiation and the apparent lack of correlation between the early regression and the eventual cure after radiotherapy of human malignant tumours. Factors to be studied obviously include cell kinetics, cell loss and reoxygenation. I personally think it is particularly important from a practical point of view to examine and understand the effects of continuous irradiation with low linear energy transfer (LET) radiations.

(4) It is still true that ionising radiations are the only agents, apart from surgery, which have cured substantial numbers of patients with cancer. Many attempts have been made to improve the results of radiotherapy by the use of different types of radiations, especially fast neutrons and of hyperbaric oxygen and various types of chemical radiosensitisers. At the present time, there is widespread interest in other physical treatments, especially hyperthermia when used alone and in combination with ionising radiations and/or chemical agents (*see* Congress of Radiation Research, Seattle, 1974 and von Ardenne, 1970). It is, of course, well known that these methods have been studied and used clinically for many years, including applications of diathermy alone (*see*, e.g. F. Westermark, 1898, and N. Westermark, 1927) and of combinations of radiotherapy and diathermy heating (C. Müller, 1912). For many years

the value of surgical diathermy in the treatment of some inoperable tumours has been recognised. Another clinical point to be mentioned is that normal tissues which have been heavily irradiated at least some months previously do not tolerate local heating and may undergo necrosis as a result. On the experimental side, my colleagues (Cater, Silver and Watkinson, 1964) reported on the value of combined therapy with 220 kV roentgen rays and subsequent 10 cm microwave heating in curing some rats with transplanted hepatoma. However, recently, detailed *in vitro* studies of the mechanisms of action of hyperthermia on malignant and normal proliferating cells have been carried out by Wüst *et al.* (1973) (*see* Wüst and Prang, 1973) and Ben-Hur and Elkind (1974), Gerweck, Gillette and Dewey (1974) and Leeper and Henle (1974) have examined interactions between hyperthermia and ionising radiations. Following X-irradiation, hyperthermia up to 42° enhances the initial rate of repair of single-strand breaks of DNA but slows the repair of the DNA complex (Ben-Hur and Elkind, 1974). Kim *et al.* (1974) presented evidence showing radiosensitisation of hypoxic HeLa S-3 cells in culture by hyperthermia. It would be interesting to do *in vitro* experiments with the combination of fast neutrons and hyperthermia, especially since local hyperthermia produced no enhancement of the effects of fast neutrons on the transplanted Ridgeway osteogenic sarcoma in mice, in contrast to the large enhancement observed after fractionated X-irradiation (Hahn *et al.* 1974). Further, little work appears to have been done on simultaneous local hyperthermia and X-irradiation. *In vitro* studies with freshly grown human cells should not be too difficult and the results might provide useful leads for renewed attempts at the clinical applications of hyperthermia.

REFERENCES

Ardenne, M. V. (1970). "Theoretische und experimentelle Grundlagen der Krebsmehrschritt-Therapie 2". stark erw. Aufl. Berlin: VEB Verlag Volk und Gesundheit.

Ben-Hur, E. and Elkind, M. M. (1974). *Radiat. Res. 59*, 484.

Cater, D. B., Silver, I. A. and Watkinson, D. A. (1964). *Acta radiol. Ther. Phys. Biol. 2*, 321.

Congress (5th Int.) of Radiation Research, Seattle, Washington, July 13-20 (1974). *Radiat. Res. 59*, No. 1: Abstracts of papers presented.

Dawson, K. B., Madoc-Jones, H., Mauro, F. and Peacock, J. H. (1973). *Europ J. Cancer, 9*, 59.

Gerweck, E., Gillette, E. L. and Dewey, W. C. (1974). *Radiat. Res. 59* 139, Abstract B-35-1.

Hahn, E. W., Canada, T. R., Alfieri, A. A. and McDonald, J. C. (1974). *Radiat. Res. 59*, 141, Abstract B-35-5.

Hug, O. and Kellerer, A. M. (1966). "Stochastik der Strahlenwirkung". Springer-Verlag Berlin, Heidelberg, New York.

Kim, J. H., Kim, S. H. and Hahn, E. W. (1974). *Radiat. Res. 59*, 140, Abstract B-35-3.

Leeper, D. B. and Henle, K. J. (1974). *Radiat. Res. 59*, 140, Abstract B-35-2.

Müller, C. (1912). *Münch. med. Wsch. 59*, 1546.

Westermark, F. (1898). *Zbl. Gynäk. 22*, 1335 (*loc. cit.* Cater *et al.* 1964).

Westermark, N. (1927). *Skand. Arch. Physiol. 52*, 257. (*loc. cit.* Cater *et al.* 1964).

Wüst, G. P., Norpoth, K., Witting, U. and Oberwittler, W. (1973). *Z. Krebsforsch. 79*, 193.

Wüst, G. and Prang, L. (1973). *Z. Krebsforsch. 79*, 204.

2. Current Aspects of Cell Survival Curve Theory

A. INTRODUCTION

Figure 1 shows a typical X-ray cell survival curve, in which the logarithm of the surviving proportion of cells is plotted against the X-ray dose. The main features of this curve can be summarised as follows.

(1) At low doses there is an inefficient portion, or "shoulder", followed by a straight exponential region (or at least nearly straight) at high doses.

(2) The "straight" portion of the curve extrapolates back to intersect the vertical axis at a multiple of unity which is sometimes equal to 2 but usually greater. This *extrapolation number* can be as high as several hundred. It represents, of course, the size of the shoulder. Also, the intercept of the straight part of the survival curve with the horizontal axis through 100% survival occurs at a dose called D_q, the "quasi-threshold dose" (Alper *et al.* 1962). This parameter too represents the size of the shoulder and is usually between 100 and 300 rads for mammalian cells *in vitro* and may be up to 500 rads *in vivo*.

Fifty years ago the simple idea was held that there may be a fixed number of identical target volumes in each cell and that when every one of these had received a "hit", or deposition of energy amounting to, say, one ion pair (60 eV) or one primary ionization, i.e. ion cluster (100 eV), then that cell would not survive. This is the "multi-target" theory. The extrapolation number would then equal the number of formal targets. The idea had its attraction for survival curves with an extrapolation number of 2, because the two targets just might be the two strands of DNA forming the double helix. But it was soon found that the extrapolation number varied greatly from one cell line to another, and with different conditions in a given cell line. Such variations could not really be thought to represent violent changes in the number of critical targets. The intercept was therefore called extrapolation number and not target number (Alper *et al.* 1960).

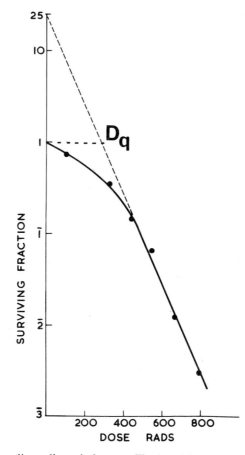

Fig. 1. A mammalian cell survival curve. The logarithm of the surviving fraction is plotted vertically against the X-ray dose horizontally. The extrapolation number is 25 and the value of "D_q" is 280 rads (horizontal dashed line). (Adapted from Dewey, 1971.)

(3) As the accumulation of cellular injury proceeds, just one more "hit", i.e. one more deposition of an ion cluster into a target volume of a given size, will kill the cell. This is the basis for the exponential increase of cell killing as the X-ray dose increases.

On the straight part of Fig. 1, the dose which will reduce the surviving proportion from a fraction "f" to $f/e = 0.37f$ is called the *mean lethal dose, D_o*. The *slope of the cell survival curve* in the exponential region is thus $1/D_o$. D_o represents, in classical target theory, the dose of X-rays required to deposit an average of one lethal event into each target volume. Therefore if D_o is determined experimentally, the expected average target volume can be calculated directly, using very simple assumptions. If D_o lies between 100 and 200 rads, as it commonly does for X-rays on mammalian cells, this dose deposits an *average* of 100 to 200 primary ionisations (clusters) per cubic micron, and the average volume per ion cluster has a diameter of about 0·2 microns.

(4) The *initial part* of the cell survival curve, at very low doses, may in principle be due to either the accumulation of injury in several target volumes or to a pool of radioresistance which is "used up" after doses of several hundred rads (such as m-RNA capable of repairing radiation injury), or to both effects. The existence of a shoulder implies that co-operation between two or more energy depositions is necessary to kill the cell. Whether the slope at very small doses is zero or not for mammalian cells has been controversial but results reported at the 6th L. H. Gray Conference (Alper, 1975) suggested that the initial slopes were usually finite, being 1/10th to 1/3rd as steep as the slope of the exponential region, for radiation of low ionising density (i.e. low "Linear energy transfer" or LET) such as X-rays or gamma rays from cobalt-60. In radiotherapy, doses of 200-300 rads per fraction are usually used and these are in the shoulder region of the survival curve. Different cell lines, and one cell line at different phases of the cell cycle, exhibit greater differences in this shoulder region than they do in the exponential region of the cell survival curve. Therefore the shape of this initial region is in practice a more important parameter than D_o and also than D_q or extrapolation number.

(5) For radiation which is more densely ionising along each particle track however (i.e. "high LET" *radiation* such as charged nuclei from a cyclotron, or protons and other nuclei released in tissue when irradiated by a beam of fast neutrons), the shoulder on the cell survival curve may disappear. This is because one charged particle track passing through the cell is now highly likely to deposit a large amount of energy in neighbouring small volumes. There is no need to accumulate separate depositions of energy; several ion clusters are formed close together by the one particle track (Fig. 2).

As the LET of the radiation used increases from X-rays, through deuterons, to helium nuclei, the shoulder of the cell survival curve is first reduced and then lost, with little change in the final slope $1/D_o$. Then, as LET is increased still further, the exponential portion becomes steeper (Fig. 3). At high LET there is simple exponential inactivation, i.e. "one hit in one target" killing (Barendsen *et al.* 1963).

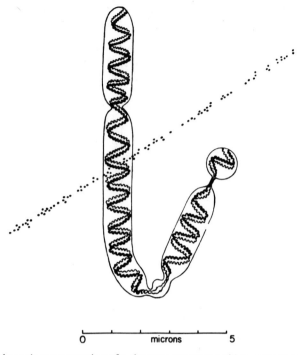

0   microns   5

Fig. 2. Schematic representation of a chromosome traversed by a proton track generated in tissue by neutrons. Each dot represents an ion pair. This is "high LET" radiation. (Johns, 1964.)

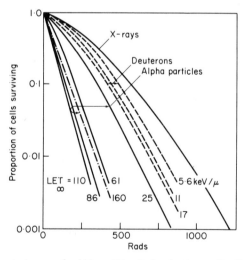

Fig. 3. Cell survival curves for kidney T1 cells for the types of radiation indicated.

The increase of LET causes the single-hit component of injury to grow larger relative to the multiple-target or "shoulder" type of injury.

(6) At *different phases of the cell cycle,* the X-ray cell survival curves differ greatly (Fig. 4, Sinclair, 1968). In the most resistant phase (late S) a large shoulder can be seen, so that accumulation of

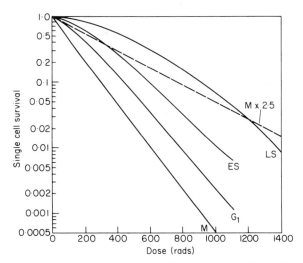

Fig. 4. Cell survival curves for synchronised Chinese hamster cells at different phases of the cell cycle. (M = mitosis, G_1 = G_1 phase, ES = early S phase, LS = late S phase.)

injury and co-operation between different energy deposition events must be occurring. In the most sensitive phases however, M and G_2 in Chinese hamster cells, the slope is steeper and the shoulder has disappeared. This means that the "one hit in one target" component of injury is predominant, possibly because the DNA is condensed at that time and presents a smaller sensitive target volume. Recently attempts have been made to relate these changes in X-ray survival curve shape in terms of DNA target volumes of varying degrees of condensation (Chadwick and Leenhouts, 1975).

(7) Some radiosensitising or radioprotecting drugs do not change the shape of the cell survival curve, but only modify the X-ray dose axis (e.g. oxygen versus nitrogen).

(8) Other types of radiosensitiser appear to reduce the "shoulder size", e.g. bromodeoxyuridine which intercalates into DNA and spoils its repair capability.

B. Cell Survival Curve Equations

If only one hit is required to inactivate one target volume in the cell to cause killing, the proportion of cells *surviving* is given by

$$S = e^{-D/D_o} \tag{1}$$

where D is the dose of radiation and D_o is the mean lethal dose, i.e. the dose required to deposit, on the average, one physical energy event or "hit" into each volume of the size of the sensitive target. The probability of *killing* for one target, is thus

$$1 - e^{D/D_o}$$

and if there are m identical targets, the probability of cell killing becomes

$$\left(1 - e^{-D/D_o}\right)^m$$

and the corresponding *survival* probability is

$$S = 1 - \left(1 - e^{-D/D_o}\right)^m \tag{2}$$

This is the old multi-target theory of cell killing which is still sometimes used but is seldom valid (Zimmer, 1961).

Figure 5 shows that equation (2) certainly predicts a straight exponential portion at high doses; but an initial region at low doses which is too flat. This is quite wrong when compared with experimental results. For example, if the dose at D_q is considered, then the cell survival at that dose always comes out to be about 65-70% according to this theory and yet nearly all experimental X-ray cell survival curves come out significantly below this level, even down to 30% in some cases.

Therefore an empirical correction has been made to this equation to allow for the initial slope, by multiplying by a single hit component (Sinclair, 1966; Dutreix *et al.* 1973):

$$S = e^{-D/D_1} \left[1 - (1 - e^{-D/D_m})^m\right] \tag{3}$$

where D_1 and D_m are the mean lethal doses for the one-hit and multi-target components respectively. The final slope $1/D_o$ is then given by

$$1/D_o = 1/D_1 + 1/D_m.$$

Unfortunately equation (3) does not give very good fitting to experimental results either. The discrepancy was detected in radiotherapy, where radiation is fractionated into a large number of small doses. If a large one-hit component is present (i.e. if the slope of the

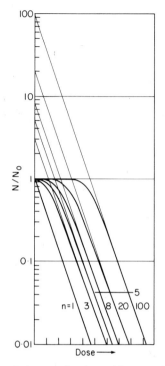

Fig. 5. Calculated cell survival curves for the multi-target, single-hit-in-each-target model (equation 2).

survival curve near the origin is steep) then this part of the survival curve will be nearly linear. Consequently no differences in the dose-sparing effect of the radiation would be expected as the dose per fraction was changed within this dose range. The total dose nd (when n fractions of d rads each were given) would then remain constant for different sizes of fraction. Rather low doses per fraction are involved (of 100-300 rads each) so that numerous dose fractions have to be given to produce a measurable degree of injury; for example 20-40 fractions.

The analysis by Dutreix *et al.* (1973), which relies upon the one-hit-times-multi-target equation (3) above, suggested that no change in total dose nd was required as the number of fractions n was increased above about 16, in order to produce a given degree of skin reaction.

Ellis's nominal standard dose (NSD) relationship, on the other hand, predicts a rather large increase of total dose with fraction number beyond 20 and even beyond 30 dose fractions (Ellis, 1969).

The implication of this is that the "cell survival curve" should continue to grow less steep as the dose per fraction is decreased. The one-hit component in the equation (3) would be a too severe modification to the multi-target equation (2), if Ellis is right and Dutreix *et al.* are wrong.

We therefore carried out experiments with the aim of distinguishing between these two approaches and elucidating the shape of the cell survival curve at low doses per fraction. These experiments will be described below but first let us turn to a different type of cell survival curve model: that for a single target volume but one that requires several hits.

C. The Multi-hit-in-one-target Model (Fowler, 1966)

A different sort of basic model starts from the idea of multiple hits in one target volume. Instead of having many independent target volumes each needing one deposition of energy, the multiple hit model assumes that in each cell there is a certain target volume into which a certain amount of energy has to be deposited: for example three ionisations. If three ionisations are required, the calculated survival curve is never perfectly straight, continuing to bend at higher doses, although one could hardly distinguish the bend experimentally (Fig. 6). Instead of the curve extrapolating back to three, as it would

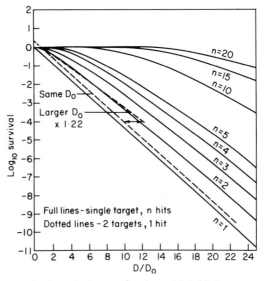

Fig. 6. Calculated cell survival curves for the multiple-hit-in-one-target model.

with the one-hit-in-each-of-multi-targets model, it extrapolates back to a figure between 30 and 100 (Fig. 6). Similarly if there are just two energy events required, the curve is very nearly straight over many decades and can extrapolate back to more than 10. Using this simple idea of some sensitive site in which only perhaps two or three depositions of energy are required we can get nearer to explaining shapes of cell survival curves. The essential point is that the different energy deposition events are assumed to be *inter-dependent* and not *independent*. The case of two such energy deposition events is of special interest, as will be seen below.

D. Experimental Investigation of Shape of Epithelial Cell Survival Curve

In recent experiments in our laboratory, using mouse skin desquamation (which can be interpreted as depletion of cells in the basal layer of the epithelium) we have been able to give as many as 64 X-ray dose fractions, as small as 107 rads each (Douglas *et al.* 1975). All fractions were given within eight days so that proliferation in the basal layer was negligible (Denekamp, 1973). The results are shown in Fig. 7 as the full line, together with the predictions of Dutreix *et al.* and of Ellis shown dotted. It is clear that, for large numbers of

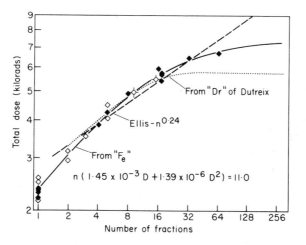

Fig. 7. Total X-ray dose required to produce the same degree of skin reaction using different numbers of fractions when proliferation can be neglected. Points—present results. Full line-derived from survival curve of the form $S = \exp- (\alpha D + \beta D^2)$. Dotted curve—results of Dutreix, Wambersie and Bounik (1973). Dashed curve—from Ellis's Nominal Standard Dose formula (Ellis, 1969).

small fractions, Dutreix's assumption, based on equation (3), was not confirmed. The total dose required to produce a given degree of skin reaction continued to rise instead with fraction number. (Dutreix's interpretation however becomes more valid when applied to a lower level of injury, i.e. to a smaller equivalent single dose.)

We found that when the reciprocal of total dose (i.e. $1/nD$ if n fractions of D rads were given) was plotted against the size of dose per fraction D, a remarkable fit of the experimental points to a straight line was obtained (Fig. 8). Such a fit can only occur if the

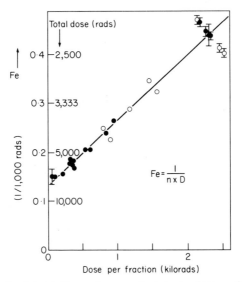

Fig. 8. Reciprocal of total X-ray dose required to produce a given degree of skin reaction (from Fig. 7) versus size of each dose fraction.

corresponding cell survival curve has a term proportional to $(\text{dose})^2$ but no term proportional to $(\text{dose})^3$. Further, since the line in Fig. 8 intercepts the zero dose axis at a finite dose (about 7500 rads), there is also a term proportional to dose. The intercept at zero dose, in fact, indicates the limiting maximum dose required in an infinite number of vanishingly small dose fractions, i.e. in continuous irradiation, when the effect of proliferation is not taken into account.

The corresponding cell survival curve is shown in Fig. 9:

$$S = e^{-(\alpha D + \beta D^2)} \tag{4}$$

and its implications are discussed below.

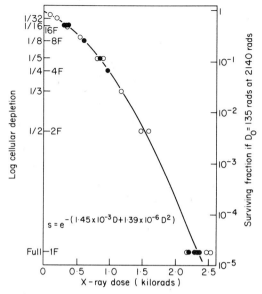

Fig. 9. The cell survival curve for epithelial cells derived from the present results shown in Figs 7 and 8.

The fact that the plot of reciprocal total dose versus dose per fraction (Fig. 8) is a straight line may be convenient for radiotherapy applications because it fits the experimental data over a wider range (1 to 64 fractions) than does Ellis's NSD equation (4-30 fractions; see Fig. 7).

E. BIOPHYSICAL INTERPRETATIONS

Equations of the form $\alpha D + \beta D^2$ (equation 4) have recently been found to fit a large number of mammalian cell survival curves extremely well. This type of equation has been used for chromosome aberrations for many years. It has been developed by Neary (1965), Rossi (1970) and Chadwick and Leenhouts (1973). Two "breaks", or damaged molecules, are assumed to be necessary to cause the biological effect observed. They are however not independent; they must be within a certain distance of each other, called the "site diameter" or "interaction distance" and they must both occur within a short interval of time. The similarities with the "multi-hit-in-one-target" model described above are obvious, but only two hits are necessary because the experimental results are consistent with a D^2 term but not a D^3 term.

Using Neary's (1965) model for chromosome aberrations and inserting the parameters determined from the experimental results shown in Figs 7, 8 and 9, with the absolute cell survival values matched against the skin clone experiments of Emery *et al.* (1970) and of Withers (1967), together with an assumed value for the "average LET" of the 240 kV X-rays, it can be calculated that the size of each of the two "target sub-lesions" that must interact to cause cell death in the mouse skin experiments was less than 46 Å and that the interaction distance was about 0·3 μm. The latter dimension is consistent with a pair of strand lesions in different molecules; possibly two chromosomes or one DNA strand and part of a membrane which must interact (e.g. misrepair or cross-link) to cause a lethal lesion. The rather large interaction distance does not agree with the assumption of Chadwick and Leenhouts that the two lesions are in sister strands of the same DNA double helix. It does however agree with the values for interaction distance found by Rossi and Kellerer and is also consistent with the simplest D_o = (reciprocal of target volume) calculation described in note (3) of the introduction.

Cell survival curves for synchronised cells (e.g. Fig. 4) can be considered in terms of the relative importance of the one-hit coefficient α and the two-hit coefficient β in the cell survival equation (4). The α coefficient changes only slightly through the cell cycle, increasing a little at the end of the cell cycle (as DNA becomes condensed in chromosomes). The β coefficient, on the other hand, rises significantly during the S phase when the interaction distances might be greater (and the cell made less sensitive) during DNA synthesis. Much more work is however required on these biophysical interpretations.

CONCLUSIONS

In conclusion, it now seems more appropriate to try and fit experimental data to a formula of the type

$$S = e^{-(\alpha D + \beta D^2)} \tag{4}$$

than to the previously popular multi-target equation (2), even if the latter is multiplied by a single-hit component (equation 3). Equation (4) appears to represent the initial and shoulder regions much more reliably than equations (2) or (3). In the present model (equation 4) the resulting cell survival curves continue to bend downwards with increasing dose, but the difference from a straight exponential line cannot be detected over 3 or 4 decades of survival even for large shoulders. For small shoulders, simulating low extrapolation numbers of about 2, the deviation from the straight part of the exponential curve would be even more difficult to detect.

The α and β coefficients can be interpreted in biophysical terms using Neary's (1965) model and are providing new information on the nature of the target for cell killing by radiation. Further discussions on this point will be published in the Proceedings of the 6th L. H. Gray Conference (T. Alper, ed. 1975).

ACKNOWLEDGEMENTS

It is a pleasure to thank the Editors and publishers of the following books and journals for permission to reproduce the figures:

British Journal of Radiology, for Fig. 1; Dr H. E. Johns and C. C. Thomas, Springfield, Illinois, for Fig. 2; *Radiation Research,* for Figs 3 and 4; *Physics in Medicine and Biology,* for Fig. 5; Oliver and Boyd, Edinburgh, for Fig. 6; and Dr T. Alper and the Institute of Physics, for Figs 7, 8 and 9.

REFERENCES

Alper, T., Gillies, N. and Elkind, M. M. (1960). *Nature, Lond. 186,* 1062-1063.
Alper, T., Fowler, J. F., Morgan, R. L., Vonberg, D. D., Ellis, F. and Oliver, R. (1962). *Brit. J. Radiol. 35,* 722.
Alper, T. (1975). Proc. 6th L. H. Gray Memorial Conf. (Pub: Inst. Phys., London).
Barendsen, G. W., Walter, H. M. D., Fowler, J. F. and Bewley, D. K. (1963). *Rad. Res. 18,* 106.
Chadwick, K. H. and Leenhouts, H. P. (1973). *Phys. Med. Biol. 18,* 78.
Chadwick, K. H. and Leenhouts, H. P. (1975). The effect of an asynchronous population of cells on the initial slopes of dose effect curves. In Proc. 6th L. H. Gray Conference (Tikvah Alper, ed.: Inst. of Physics).
Denekamp, J. (1973). *Brit. J. Radiol. 46,* 381.
Dewey, D. L. (1971). *Brit. J. Radiol. 44,* 816-817.
Douglas, B. G., Fowler, J. F., Denekamp, J., Harris, S. R., Ayres, S. E., Fairman, S., Hill, S. A., Sheldon, P. W. and Stewart, F. A. (1975). In Proc. 6th L. H. Gray Memorial Conference. (Tikvah Alper, ed.: Inst. of Physics).
Dutreix, J., Wambersie, A. and Bounik, C. (1973). *Eur. J. Cancer, 9,* 159-167.
Ellis, F. (1969). *Clin. Radiol. 20,* 1.
Emery, E. W., Denekamp, J. and Ball, M. M. (1970). *Rad. Res. 41,* 450.
Fowler, J. F. (1966). Distribution of hit-numbers in single targets. *In* "Biophysical Aspects of Radiation Quality", p. 63. Tech. Rept. Series No. 58, I.A.E.A., Vienna.
Johns, H. E. (1964). *In* "The Physics of Radiology". 2nd edn, Chapter 18, p. 651. C. C. Thomas, Springfield, Ill.
Neary, G. J. (1965). *Int. J. Radiat. Biol. 9,* 477.
Rossi, H. H. (1970). *Phys. Med. Biol. 15,* 255.

Sinclair, W. K. (1968). *Rad. Res. 33,* 620-643; Fig. 4, p. 632.
Withers, H. R. (1967). *Brit. J. Radiol. 40,* 187.
Zimmer, K. G. (1961). "Quantitative Radiation Biology", Oliver & Boyd, Edinburgh, Fig. 9, p. 27.

3. X-ray Survival Curves of Freshly Explanted Human Tumour Cells from a Variety of Origins

J. Wells, R. J. Berry and A. H. Laing

A. Introduction

There are no reports in the literature of survival curves for reproductive capacity of human tumour cells obtained as soon as possible after satisfactory growth has been established *in vitro* following the explantation. One of the reasons for this is the extremely poor plating efficiency obtained when spontaneous tumours are first cultured *in vitro*. This paper reports X-ray survival curves obtained for these cultures by using the "feeder layer" technique.

B. Materials and Methods

The procedure for setting up the primary cultures has already been described on page 158. The irradiation procedure shown in Fig. 1 was carried out at the first subculture to yield a sufficiently high plating efficiency for any given explant. 250 kVp X-rays with a half value layer of 1·3 mm copper were used at a dose rate of 370 rads/min. The "feeder layer" technique not only increased the plating efficiencies of the test cells but also ensured that the plating efficiency of the irradiated cells was independent of the number of dead cells produced. The upper limit for X-ray dose was chosen so that no possible toxic effects of the action of X-rays on the plastic would affect cell survival (Petterson *et al.* 1974) and so that the necessity for large cell numbers was eliminated, thus also eliminating the detrimental effect of large cell numbers on the plating efficiency of the irradiated cells (Masuda and Wakisaka, 1973).

C. Results and Discussion

The results are shown in Fig. 2. All plating efficiencies were in excess of 20% and the shapes of the cell survival curves are all very similar except for the cell line designated "Q". This cell line has yielded a

7*

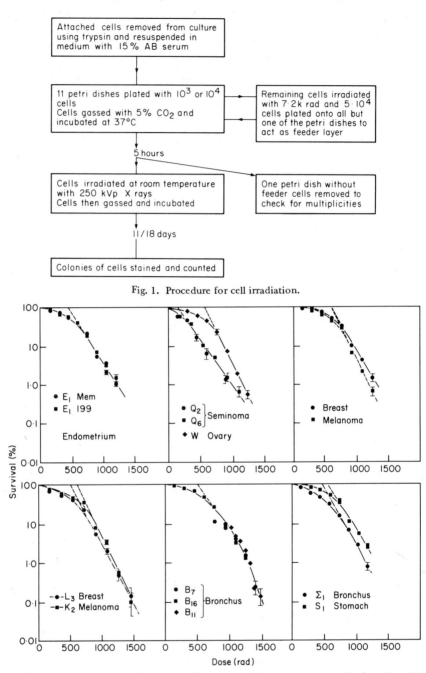

Fig. 1. Procedure for cell irradiation.

Fig. 2. Reproductive survival curves for explanted human tumour cells after X-irradiation. Further details about some of these specimens are given in the legend to Fig. 4 (p. 160). The seminoma and bronchus were tested after different numbers of passages. The "E" cells were established in MEM medium but results show that their radiation sensitivity was the same in MEM and 199.

survival curve with a small "shoulder" as indicated by a D_q value of 150 rads. The shape of this cell survival curve is similar to many other cell survival curves for cells of human and animal origin obtained *in vitro*. (Whitmore and Till, 1964.) The remainder of the cell survival curves have unusually large "shoulders" as indicated by D_q values in the range of 400-600 rads. The slopes of the exponential regions are similar with values for D_o within the range 100-200 rads and this compares favourably with previous *in vitro* results (Whitmore and Till, 1964).

The large values for D_q are similar to those obtained *in vivo* in studies of radiation effects upon normal tissues (Serge *et al.* 1964; Hornsey and Vatistas, 1963; Fowler *et al.* 1964). For two of the tumour lines, repeat survival curves were obtained after prolonged subculturing *in vitro*. Unlike the change in chemosensitivity on serial subculture *in vitro* (see p. 161), no real change in radiosensitivity was observed once freshly explanted human tumour cells had developed their full growth potential *in vitro*.

In conclusion, although the tumours studied represented clinically "radiosensitive" and "radioresistant" types, the survival curves obtained were with one exception remarkably similar. They had D_o values within the range 100-200 rads and D_q values within the range 400-600 rads. The exception was a cultured seminoma which showed a similar slope but a far smaller "shoulder" on the survival curve with a D_q of 150 rads.

ACKNOWLEDGEMENTS

We would like to express our gratitude to George Breckon and Christine Horlor for their advice and help in establishing the karyotypes of the tumour cells reported in this paper.

J. Wells was aided by a grant from Eli Lilly and Co. Ltd.

REFERENCES

Fowler, J. F., Lindop, P. J. and Berry, R. J. (1964). *Brit. J. Radiol. 37*, 401.
Hornsey, S. and Vatistas, S. (1963). *Brit. J. Radiol. 36*, 795.
Masuda, K. and Wakisaka, S. (1973). *Int. J. Radiat. Biol. 23*, 99.
Petterson, E. O., Oftebro, R. and Brustad, T. (1974). *Int. J. Radiat. Biol. 25*, 99.
Serge, E., Friedlander, G. and Noyes, H. P. (1964). Eds. *Annual Reviews Inc.*, Palo Alto, Calif. 347.
Whitmore, G. F. and Till, J. E. (1964). *Annual Review of Nuclear Medicine*, Vol. 14.

4. The In Vitro Effect of Hyperthermia on the Rate of Incorporation of Nucleic Acid Precursors into Tumour and Normal Tissues

G. P. Wüst

There are many clinical observations and experimental findings on the influence of local or body hyperthermia on tumour growth. At the present time hyperthermia is used alone or in conjunction with chemotherapy on patients with malignant tumours without any knowledge of the biochemical foundation of the effects of hyperthermia. It is clear that more information is required on both the biochemical and the molecular effects of elevated temperatures if this technique is to be applied successfully.

An *in vitro* screening test which we use for testing cytostatic agents was carried out at elevated temperatures and unexpectedly led to a remarkable inhibition of the utilisation of tritiated (^{3}H) thymidine and tritiated (^{3}H) uridine. The method follows that of Rajewsky (1966). Fresh tissue was removed under sterile conditions. The material was cut into slices about 400 μ thick using a mechanical tissue chopper. 10-15 tumour slices were put into Eagle's basal medium which was enriched with carbogen (O_2/CO_2 = 95/5 Vol. %) for 10 minutes. The incubation with ^{3}H thymidine (3 μCi/ml at 3-5 Ci/mM) or ^{3}H uridine (3 μCi/ml at 3-5 Ci/mM) lasted for 1 hr, 4 hr, and 6 hr at 37°, 39° and 41° C. The incubation was stopped by cooling down to 4° C and the samples were washed in inactive thymidine (10^{-4} molar). The impulses were counted in a Packard tri. carb. liquid scintillation spectrometer (model 3003) and were expressed in counts per minute per mg tumour dry weight.

Figure 1 shows the incorporation rate of ^{3}H thymidine and ^{3}H uridine in Jensen sarcoma and in tumour GW-39 under varying conditions of temperature of the medium. There is a decrease in the incorporation rate at temperatures of 39° C and 41° C. The same applies to human tumours. In Fig. 2 results are shown for a penis carcinoma, a parotid carcinoma, metastasis of a mammary carcinoma and a larynx carcinoma. Again there is a decrease in the rate of incorporation of nucleic acid precursors as a result of higher

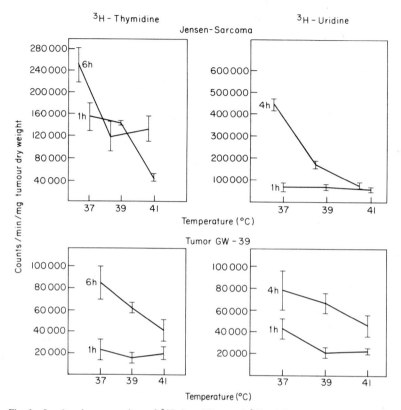

Fig. 1. *In vitro* incorporation of ³H thymidine and ³H uridine into the Jensen sarcoma and tumour GW-39 at normal and elevated temperatures.

temperatures. In a further series of experiments we investigated "fast proliferating" tissue of rats and mice in the same manner. The incorporation rate of liver and spleen of embryonic rats and mice is—as would be expected—high, and is the same as in tumours or higher. Once again the incorporation of nucleic acid precursors was inhibited at higher temperatures. The incorporation rate of nucleic acid precursors is relatively low in partially hepatectomised liver of rats, but there is still the same tendency of inhibition under higher temperature conditions.

However, we found no change in the utilisation of nucleic acid precursors in normal tissues of adult rats at elevated temperatures. Liver, spleen, kidney and skeletal muscle were all studied (Fig. 3).

A temperature of 39° C or 41° C has no effect on nucleic acid precursor incorporation into the liver of chicken embryos. This is

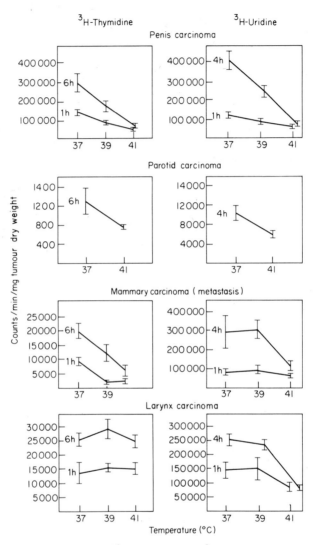

Fig. 2. *In vitro* incorporation of ^{3}H thymidine and ^{3}H uridine into human tumours at normal and elevated temperatures.

very interesting because the basal temperature of the chicken is about 41° C and the basal temperature of rats and mice is about 37° C. To have an effect on the utilisation of nucleic acid precursors, the temperature must presumably be above the basic temperature of the chicken, that means, above 41° C, but we have not yet tested this.

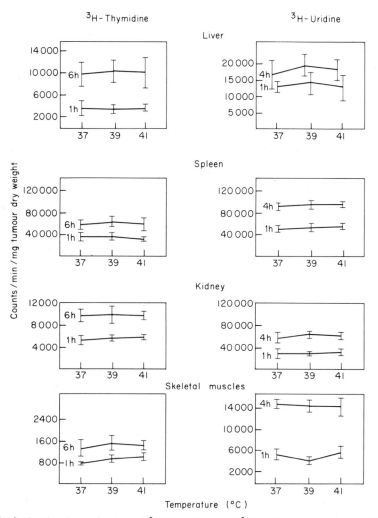

Fig. 3. *In vitro* incorporation of ³H thymidine and ³H uridine into normal adult rat tissues at normal and elevated temperatures.

In order to study the mechanism of thermosensitive insertion of tritiated nucleosides, we assayed the incorporation of ³H thymidine into acid soluble and precipitable cell fractions of the Walker-256-carcinosarcoma *in vitro* at 37°C, 39°C and 41°C. Figure 4 shows that the activity incorporated into the acid soluble fraction was reduced at elevated temperatures at both 1 hr and 6 hr (Buchholz, 1974).

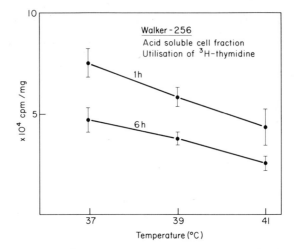

Fig. 4. Incorporation of ^{3}H thymidine into the acid soluble cell fraction of Walker 256 carcinosarcoma.

To obtain more information about the percentage of the total activity in TTP, TDP, and TMP at $37°$ C, $39°$ C and $41°$ C we studied the fractionation of labelled thymidine nucleosides in the acid soluble fraction using thin layer chromatography on PEI cellulose. At 1 hr the peak corresponding to TTP which appears on the left in the $37°$ C profile has already been markedly reduced (Fig. 5) and after 6 hr at $41°$ C (Fig. 6) it has disappeared. The changes which occur in

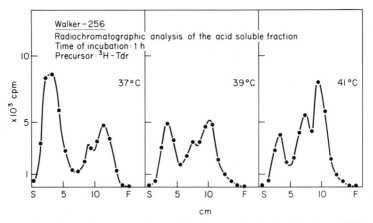

Fig. 5. Radiochromatographic analysis of the acid soluble fraction in a Walker 256 tumour after 1 hr incubation with ^{3}H thymidine at different temperatures.

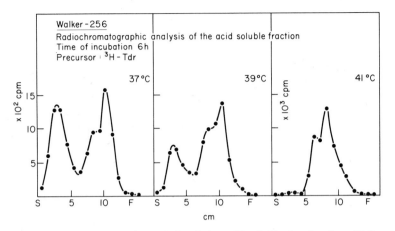

Fig. 6. Radiochromatographic analysis of the acid soluble fraction in a Walker 256 carcinosarcoma after 6 hr incubation with ^{3}H thymidine at different temperatures.

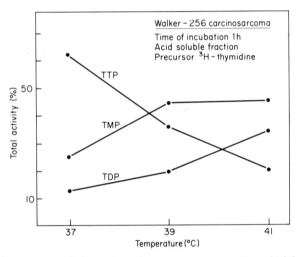

Fig. 7. The percentage of the total activity present as mono-, di-, and triphosphate in the acid soluble fraction from a Walker 256 carcinosarcoma after 1 hr incubation with ^{3}H thymidine at different temperatures.

the levels of TTP, TDP and TMP during the first hour are summarised in Fig. 7 (Buchholz, 1974).

We complemented these *in vitro* observations with *in vivo* investigations on tumour-bearing rats, which were heated to 41° C. There was a decrease in the utilisation of ^{3}H thymidine in both the acid soluble fraction and in the acid precipitable fraction. The ratios of thymidine nucleotides were also altered in the *in vivo* experiment. We found no thymidine-triphosphate in five overheated tumours whereas all non-treated tumour tissue contained measurable amounts of all the labelled nucleotides.

The results quoted here for inhibition of ^{3}H thymidine incorporation at elevated temperatures are supported by those of Gericke *et al.* (1971) and Mondovi *et al.* (1969a) who found a specific heat sensitivity of DNA synthesis. The present work also extends the idea to inhibition of ^{3}H uridine incorporation. Thermal sensitivity can be regarded as a phenomenon of fast proliferating cells and the inhibition of incorporation is generally proportional to the height and duration of the temperature. The differences in inhibition between different tumours might be explained in terms of differential thermosensitivity. This view is supported by work of Bender and Schramm (1966) in tissue culture, who showed an individual thermosensitivity in neoplastic cells of different origin.

The effect of hyperthermia described above is probably not caused by a primary attack on the DNA-polymerase since this mechanism should be accompanied by an increase in the TTP pool as recently shown by Schneider (1970) rather than a decrease. An influence of elevated temperature on nucleoside phosphorylation is more probable leading to our observed decrease in ATP and ADP and a change in the ATP/ADP quotient *in vitro*.

We think the decrease in thymidine activity in the acid soluble fraction under hyperthermia is a secondary effect of the reduced TTP pool. Mondovi *et al.* (1969b) doubt this explanation, referring to their own experiments, in which the temperature sensitivity of cancer cells could not be influenced by the addition of ATP and ADP to the incubation medium. On the other hand the transport of ATP and ADP through the membrane of mitochondria (Klingenberg and Pfaff, 1968) and the regulation of intracellular redox equilibrium have proved temperature sensitive (Dallner, 1963; Rapoport, 1967). It is thus clear that we are still a long way from understanding the precise mechanism by which hyperthermia acts and further efforts are needed in this field.

REFERENCES

Bender, E. and Schramm, T. (1966). *Acta Biol. Med. Germ.* *17*, 515.
Buchholz, B. (1974). In Vitro Unteruchungen zur Thermosensitiblitat der Verwertung radioacktiv markierter Nukleoside durch Tumor- und Normalzellen. Inaugural-Dissertation, Münster/Westfalen, Deutschland.

Dallner, G. (1963). *Acta Pathologica at Microbiologica Scandinavia, Supplementum 166*, 34.

Gericke, D., Chandra, P., Orii, H. and Wacker, A. (1971). *Naturwissenschaften*, *58*, 155.

Klingenberg, M. and Pfaff, E. (1968). *In* "The Metabolic Roles of Citrate" (T. W. Goodwin, ed.). Academic Press, New York and London.

Mondovi, B., Strom, R., Rotilio, G., Finazzi Agro, A., Cavaliere, R. and Rossi Fanelli, A. (1969*a*). *Europ. J. Cancer*, *5*, 129.

Mondovi, B., Finazzi Agro, A., Rotilio, G., Strom, R., Moricca, G. and Rossi Fanelli, A. (1969*b*). *Europ. J. Cancer*, *5*, 137.

Rajewsky, M.F. (1966). *Biophysik*, *3*, 71.

Rapoport, S. (1967). "Grundlagen der Krebs-Mehrschritt Therapie" (M. v. Ardenne, ed.), p. 328. VEB Voluk und Gesundheir, Berlin.

Schneider, F., Warnecke, P. and Harlin, R. (1970). *Drug Res. 12*, 1942.

GENERAL DISCUSSION

Dendy reported some experimental data obtained by Mrs Mary Lloyd in Cambridge. The methods followed those presented on p. 24. Cultures were established within about 2-5 days, and when healthy they were fed and then irradiated with a range of doses of 60-Cobalt γ rays. After a 24-hr interval to allow for recovery processes the cultures were exposed to ^{125}IUdR for 24 hr and assayed according to the method on p. 144. Figure 1 shows the dose response

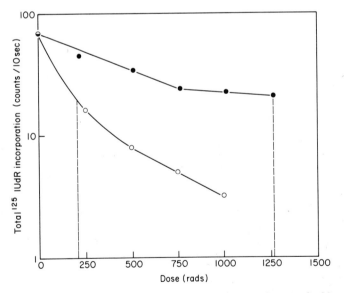

Fig. 1. Reduction in ^{125}IUdR uptake with dose of radiation for two freshly cultured human tumour specimens. ○ Specimen 48 = Ascites fluid from carcinoma of bronchus. ● Specimen 49 = Solid malignant melanoma.

curves for just two specimens which have been selected because they had two features in common. First the numbers of cells in the control tubes at the end of the experiment were very similar, $1 \cdot 5 \times 10^5$ per tube for specimen 48, and 2×10^5 cells per tube for specimen 49, and secondly the uptake of label in the control tubes was very similar. So if we can assume that the cell cycle times and duration of S phase were similar (see p. 70) there were approximately the same proportion of cells cycling for the two specimens. The two curves are quite different and there is a very big difference in the dose of radiation required to reduce ^{125}IUdR uptake to 30% of the control value ($D_{30\%}$).

Table 1 is a summary of all results to date. There is a big range of values of $D_{30\%}$ and a malignant melanoma was the most resistant specimen investigated. When repeat tests were made on samples taken from the same patient, the $D_{30\%}$ values were fairly similar and the spread was much less than the spread for different specimens.

TABLE 1

Dose of radiation required to reduce ^{125}IUdR uptake to 30% of the control value ($D_{30\%}$) for various human tumours in short term culture. Two independent experiments were performed on specimens 45 and 58 and three on specimen 47

Sensitivity of Human Tumour Cells in Culture to 60—Co γ Radiation

Specimen No.	Specimen	Control activity (counts/10 sec)	Dose in rads for 30% control activity ($D_{30\%}$)
34	Pleural aspirate ca breast	120	410
35	Pleural effusion ca bronchus	258	510
39	Ascites fluid ca cervix	15	840
40	Brain secondary	12·6	480
42	Ascites fluid ca ovary	9·2	660
45(a)	Ascites fluid ca ovary	157·7	420
(b)		334	310
47(a)	Pleural effusion ca breast	22·6	390
(b)		56·1	290
(c)		78·1	240
48	Ascites fluid ca bronchus	67·3	200
49	Solid malignant melanoma	62	1260
50	Pleural fluid ca breast	13·4	665
58(a)	Pleural fluid ca cervix	107·7	780
(b)		52·4	1070

Berry said these curves for ^{125}IUdR uptake, which measured DNA synthesis in this population, were very like the curves for radiation inhibition of DNA synthesis studied by a variety of isotopic methods (e.g. Lajtha *et al.* 1958). There is no correlation for radiation as a damaging agent between the retention by the cells of ability to synthesise DNA, and cell reproductive survival as measured by a clonal end point. They have opposite dose rate dependences and very different dependences upon ionisation density.

Dendy agreed entirely with regard to the immediate effect of radiation on rate of DNA synthesis, but emphasised that the parameter measured here was the total DNA synthesised between 24 and 48 hr after irradiation. There is some evidence for bacteria (Cramp and Elgat, 1972) that one full generation time after irradiation, DNA synthesis may begin to correlate with reproductive integrity.

Twentyman made a number of comments about the methodology Wells described.

(1) Cultures were irradiated only 5 hr after trypsinisation and plating but Berry himself had described work in which partial synchronisation was brought on by trypsin. Would it not be better to irradiate the cells growing as a monolayer and trypsinise them after irradiation? Berry replied that the 5-6 hr point was a good time in the cells they had studied because it was at the middle of the wide fluctuations seen with time after trypsinisation. Brockas added that trypsinisation of irradiated cells would complicate the repair mechanisms operating because of the effects of trypsin on the cell.

(2) Were the plated out cells taken from plateau phase cultures? The behaviour of cells in the first 24 hr after plating is very dependent on the state of the cultures from which they are taken. So to determine anything from an *in vitro* test the proliferative state of the cells must be related to what might be expected in the tumour. Wells said the cells were plated from cultures that were towards the end of the log phase and agreed that work was needed on cells in plateau phase.

(3) There is a lot of conflicting data which suggests that the size of the shoulder is very dependent on whether the cells are in log phase or plateau phase. Some people find an increased shoulder, some people find a change in D_o on moving from log to plateau phase. Berry replied that on going into plateau phase, what tends to happen is that the extrapolation number if anything comes down and the shoulder becomes smaller. This would underestimate the effect seen here which is a rather large shoulder.

In reply to Freshney, Wells said all the cells in their clonal cultures were epithelial and although tumour cells could not be specifically identified, for all the explants reported the modal chromosome number was above 55. Berry added that they could be certain about a melanoma because the cells in culture were black.

Smets asked if it had been possible to compare the radiosensitivity with the clinical response for any cases. Laing replied that seminoma in the clinical situation is one of the few tumours where radiotherapists can cure secondary disease because it is so sensitive. It is outstandingly sensitive and appears to be so *in vitro* too. However, Berry re-emphasised that it was not "sensitive" in terms of the final slope of the survival curve, having a very similar D_o to the other specimens tested. It was "sensitive" only in that the shoulder was small ($D_q = 150$ rad), but since radiotherapy is delivered by multiple dose fractions the effect of the shoulder portion of the survival curve is very relevant to the treatment. Figure 1, p. 172, was from a relatively freshly explanted melanoma (Dewey, 1971). It had a large D_q, and is the only continuously cultured line one can recall from the literature where there was a large shoulder on the survival curve, like the fresh explants seen here.

Dickson made a number of important points. First several people have shown that the results obtained at elevated temperature depend on the incubation conditions, and upon the way the viability of the cells is tested, after heating

(Johnson, H. J., 1940; Mondovi, B., *et al.* 1969; Dickson, J. A. and Shah, D. M., 1972). It is necessary to heat the cells and *then* assess the uptake of thymidine, uridine or leucine. Otherwise you cannot show whether or not the cells will recover. When cells are heated at either 42°C or 43°C in the presence of labelled thymidine, uridine or leucine, there may be a gross decrease in the uptake of label. However, after the heat is taken away the cells can recover, not simply in terms of isotope uptake, but to the extent that they are lethal if put back into the animal (Dickson, in press).

The second point is that animals with tumours cannot be cured by heating them to 41°C and this applies to human beings also. The operational temperature for heating tumours by whole body hyperthermia is believed to be 41·5°C minimum and possibly 42° maximum (Dickson, 1974). With local hyperthermia, by regional perfusion for example, tumour temperatures in excess of 42°C can be used (Cavaliere *et al.* 1967).

Finally recent work indicates that the initial lesion in heat damaged cells is in RNA, and the effect on DNA is probably secondary (Dickson and Shah, 1972; Palzer and Heidelberger, 1973; Strom *et al.* 1973). Following hyperthermia, there is a disparity between the synthesis of DNA and the synthesis of RNA, and this has been shown for example in recent work by Heidelberger using different drugs to block RNA and DNA pathways. The fact that RNA synthesis or repair seems to be critical for cell recovery and multiplication following heating can be shown in several ways, including tissue culture and bio-assay systems which demonstrate that after RNA has ceased to be synthesised, cells won't grow in the animal system (see above refs.).

Wüst said they used the lower temperature range from 39-41°C because of the difficulty and danger of heating human patients to 42°C. Dickson said they were heating patients at 42°C under general anaesthesia with monitoring of temperature, cardiac rhythm and rate, blood pressure, and intravenous fluid replacement. Pettigrew *et al.* (1974) had also heated a large series of patients at 42°C. Although the patients are very tired after this treatment, there have been no serious side effects, and no patients have died in Dickson's series. In Pettigrew's series one patient died from ventricular fibrillation when the temperature rose to 43°C due to thermometer failure.

In reply to Fowler, Dickson said the time of heating was important, there being an exponentially decaying relationship between temperature and its duration of application. For heat susceptible cancers, it has been found that for each centigrade degree rise in temperature above 42°C, the heating time required to cure the tumour can be approximately halved (Johnson, 1940). However, for most cases below 41·5°C no effect on animal tumours can be demonstrated unless heating continues for very prolonged periods and the animal just will not stand this. Neither human beings nor animals can tolerate total body temperature above 42°C for long (Pettigrew *et al.* 1974; Dickson, 1974). At 42°C a current problem with human beings is that we do not yet know how long we should be heating for, although there are now several indications that the time required in whole body hyperthermia will be in the region of 20 hr (Dickson, in press). It may be feasible to do this all at one time, but at the moment the heating is fractionated into three sessions in the region of 6-8 hrs.

Berry said tumours with bad blood supplies, and many of them do have impaired blood supplies, are unable to carry heat away as well as many of the normal tissues in the vicinity and this has a potential selective advantage in hyperthermia which must not be forgotten.

In conclusion Berry said there appear to be rather better prospects for assisting the clinician in defining treatment for individual patients with chemotherapy than with radiotherapy. It is not possible to do so yet but a tremendous amount of work is tending in that direction (see Chapters 3 and 7). As for ionising radiation however, we can only explore mechanisms or make predictions for treatment of classes of tumours. We have not touched at all on problems of tumour cell population kinetics *in situ* although Fig. 4, p. 175, shows clearly that the position of a cell in the cell cycle makes a tremendous difference to its radiosensitivity. The limiting radiation sensitivity of normal tissues has not been considered and we know little about the way *in vitro* measures can possibly predict what is happening *in vivo*. Hyperthermia on its own, or perhaps in combination with radiotherapy or chemotherapy is probably going to be introduced at the clinical level before we have much chance to do laboratory studies. We can only hope there will be a chance to look at the mechanisms involved and to suggest ways in which the technique can be improved if it proves to have clinical utility.

REFERENCES

Cavaliere, R., Ciocatto, E. C., Giovanella, B. C., Heidelberger, C., Johnson, R. O., Margottini, M., Mondovi, B., Moricca, G. and Rossi-Fanelli, A. (1967). *Cancer, 20,* 1351.

Cramp, W. A. and Elgat, M. (1972). *Rad. Res. 51,* 121.

Dewey, D. L. (1971). *Brit. J. Radiol. 44,* 816.

Dickson, J. A. (in press). *In* "Selective Heat Sensitivity of Cancer Cells" (A. Rossi-Fanelli, ed.). Springer-Verlag, Berlin.

Dickson, J. A. and Shah, D. M. (1972). *Europ. J. Cancer, 8,* 561.

Dickson, J. A. (1974). *Cancer Chemotherap. Rpts, 58,* 294.

Johnson, H. J. (1940). *Amer. J. Cancer, 38,* 533.

Lajtha, L. G., Oliver, R., Berry, R. and Noyes, W. D. (1958). *Nature, Lond. 182,* 178.

Mondovi, B., Agro, A. F., Cavaliere, R. and Rossi-Fanelli, A. (1969). *Europ. J. Cancer, 5,* 129.

Palzer, R. J. and Heidelberger, C. (1973). *Cancer Res. 33,* 421.

Pettigrew, R. T., Galt, J. M., Ludgate, C. M. and Smith, A. N. (1974). *Brit. Med. J. 4,* 679.

Pettigrew, R. T., Galt, J. M., Ludgate, C. M., Horn, D. B. and Smith, A. N. (1974). *Br. J. Surg. 61,* 727.

Strom, R., Santoro, A. S., Grifo, C., Bozzi, A., Mondovi, B. and Rossi-Fanelli, A. (1973). *Europ. J. Cancer, 9,* 103.

Chapter 5

BEHAVIOUR OF HORMONE-DEPENDENT TUMOURS IN CULTURE AND THE RESPONSE OF TUMOURS TO HORMONES

(Moderator: P. K. Bondy)

1. Behaviour of Hormone-dependent Tumours in Culture and the Response of Tumours to Hormones

F. J. A. Prop

The title of this section covers an enormous field, the study of which could be extremely useful for clinical application in the context of predictive tests. I am unable to cover the whole subject, however superficially, within the limits of this introduction and have therefore chosen one organ, the mammary gland and its tumours. In doing this most of the problems that may be met in this field should be covered since the mammary gland is a most complicated hormonal target organ and mammary tumours are about the most reluctant to permit themselves to be properly cultured.

1. THE PROBLEM

(a) Can we, by means of cultures of mammary tumours, provide the clinician with information regarding the individual hormonal sensitivity of each of those tumours so that he can "tune" his therapy to this information?

(b) If we have the cultures available, can we extend the work to test the sensitivity to chemotherapeutic drugs?

(c) Finally, we may ask whether this latter sensitivity is influenced by addition of hormones. As hormones may act upon the mitotic activity of the tumour cells and several cytostatic drugs attack a stage of the mitotic cycle, this seems a reasonable approach.

If we should succeed in realising a series of practical tests along these lines we may provide good guidance to the clinician for his therapy.

2. WHAT IS THE PRESENT STATE OF AFFAIRS?

Several decades ago there was an adage that it is as difficult to keep alive human mammary tumour *in vitro* as it is to kill it *in vivo,* and there is still a hard core of truth in that. Killing *in vivo* is still an unobtained goal, though somewhat easier than it used to be, and keeping alive mammary tumour cultures has improved somewhat.

From the cultural point of view the main problem if we wish to develop methods for clinical use is that they should approach 100% success. Success means not only that we get cells in culture from the explant, but that the cultures are representative of the tumour *in vivo* from which they were made. It is disappointing that most authors do not provide data on this latter aspect and that journals accept papers without asking for such important details.

In recent years there has been much activity in the field of hormone testing on mammary tumours. A sample of the publications on the subject that came to my attention in 1973 and early 1974 (Bishun *et al.* 1973; Riley *et al.* 1973; Hoge *et al.* 1973; Aspegren and Hakanson, 1974) resulted in four papers all dealing with actions of steroids on mammary tumour cultures. Results were contradictory and at best it can be said that some correlation existed between culture results and the presence of steroid binding as revealed by biochemical techniques. Cell culture techniques or histiotypic organ culture methods were used and in all the papers the experimental set-up was generally very simple and straightforward. It was striking that in the publication lists, reference to papers dealing with results obtained with animal mammary glands and their tumours was almost completely absent. In this latter field much experience has been accumulated that can and *should be* usefully applied in experiments with human tumours. Probably other investigators are very aware of the advantages that lie in carefully studying papers on the culture of animal mammary material and applying the experience acquired in this field to human culture methods. Up till now, not much has reached the publication stage from this latter group of investigators—maybe because they are more reluctant to publish preliminary results. Anyway, from what has been published it is clear that much of the work being done urgently needs a better theoretical foundation. In particular, for a successful approach to the human tumour problem, we have to take into account the experience gained from experiments with animal material.

From a technical viewpoint the published results suggest that the yield of cells from the tumours—generally not specified, so one has to rely on impressions only—is not very high. The pictures often show an abundance of fibroblasts interspersed with some epithelial islands. Sometimes a picture shows purely epithelial cells, but nothing is stated about whether the cultures are representative of the tumours from which they come.

In cell cultures we have the possibility of observing individual cells. With organ cultures *in vitro* there is often a period of time when nothing is known about the changes occurring within the cultures, since no measurements are made until the explants are homogenised for biochemical determination. From long experience I know that the survival of human mammary tumour cells in these organ cultures is unpredictable so that in the same flask we may find pieces that are completely necrotic, pieces that show excellent survival, and pieces with incomplete survival. If we also take into consideration the heterogeneity of the tumour material, then it becomes clear that lack of sufficient material and time may make it impossible to prepare enough cultures for the results to be statistically reliable. This also applies if mechanical choppers are used as they are much more damaging to the material than careful manual dissection.

Very short term "cultures" as often used for biochemical experiments, carry the great risk that we are measuring material that is a mixture of cells in all stages of damage, death, repair and survival. Though for years a protagonist of the use of organ culture methods, for tumour studies directed towards clinical application, I am now strongly in favour of monolayer cell culture methods within certain limits to be discussed in the next section.

3. RELEVANCE OF RESULTS OBTAINED WITH ANIMAL TISSUE FOR THE HUMAN CARCINOMA PROBLEM

I want now to elaborate on what insight and understanding cultures of animal material have yielded that might be usefully applied in the study of human tumours of the mammary gland.

The following maxim in my opinion is a sound foundation for experimentation, in the animal field as well as in the human field.

Hormone action on tumour cultures can be studied fruitfully, only if we are able to stimulate cultures of the normal original target tissue to react to hormones in a way that can be understood in terms of normal hormone effects on that tissue.

This maxim is based on the idea, not new, but never fundamentally contradicted, that tumour cells should be considered as defective cells and what we generally study in tumours are the more or less derelict remnants of normal processes. If the tumour cells show new features, these should be interpreted in terms of normal processes become deviant because of defective controls (exceptions may be cases where viral genetic material has stealthily crept into the genome). Therefore, if we cannot freely manipulate the normal cells *in vitro* by hormones, how can we expect to manipulate the tumour cells?

This poses a real problem in the case of the human mammary tumour. Though we can stimulate mouse mammary glands *in vitro* to react specifically to hormones, like morphogenesis or milk secretion, nobody has yet succeeded in doing so with normal human mammary gland—at least not from the resting state.

Much has been learnt from experiments with animal material *in vitro* about the very diverse parameters that determine the "program" cells will perform. Looking at the cell as a kind of "computer", the parameters are of "hardware" as well as "software" type.

a. Species, Race, Strain

The differences in hormone requirements for stimulation of the mammary gland in different species are considerable. Even between two sublines of an inbred mouse strain there can be differences. Figure 1 (Prop, unpublished) shows that milk secretion is stimulated

Milk Secretory Activity				
C$_3$H / Crgl	4	18	12	21
/ AvL	0	18	6	23
7 week virgins	ACst	BCst	ACst + GH	BCst + GH

Fig. 1. Milk secretory activity expressed in arbitrary units in mammae of two substrains of C$_3$H 7-week old virgin mice that were cultivated for five days in media containing: ACst = insulin and corticosterone; BCst = insulin, Prolactin and Corticosterone; ACst + GH = ACst + growth hormone; BCst + GH = BCst + growth hormone. The growth hormone can partially substitute for prolactin only in the C$_3$H/Crgl mice.

about twice as much by growth hormone in combination with insulin and hydrocortisone in an American C$_3$H subline, as it is in a subline at an Amsterdam institute.

Between different inbred mouse strains there are considerable differences in mammary morphology, in sensitivity to, and in requirement of hormones. How much more difference we may expect in this respect between individuals in a human population that is heterogeneous to the extreme!

b. Age of Donor: Degree of Differentiation

Hormones and other, often unknown factors, determine the degree of differentiation and so the reactivity to hormones *in vitro*. Mammae from 3-4 week-old mice fail to react to hormone *in vitro* unless—as Ichinose and Nandi (1964) found—the donor mice have been "primed" *in vivo* by injection with hormones some days prior to explantation.

Figure 2 (Prop, 1966) shows that depending on age—5, 6 and 7 weeks—the reactivity of mouse mammary glands to hormones *in vitro* shows a gradual shift. So the hormone combination: insulin + prolactin + hydrocortisone provokes an abnormal type of growth in

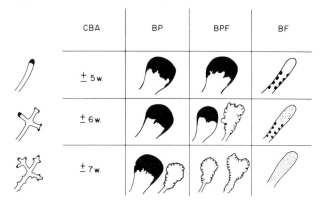

Fig. 2. Reactivity to hormones *in vitro*, for animals of different ages. Far left: the degree of development of the virgin mammary gland at different ages. BP = medium containing insulin, prolactin and progesterone. BPF = same medium with additional hydrocortisone. BF = the same without progesterone. Mammary glands were cultivated in these media for 5 days. The reactions: e.g. 5 weeks BP; intraductal massive epithelial proliferation; 5 weeks BF: formation of small intraductal epithelial buds; 7 weeks BPF: lobulo-alveolar development; 7 weeks BF: milk secretion.

the ducts of mammary glands from 5 week-old mice, whereas from the sixth week of the donor's life onwards this hormone combination causes milk secretion.

c. Past History of Stimulations (Memory)

This is related to section (b). Here we have the fact that pregnancy or pseudo-pregnancy alters the glands, resulting in a different system which also reacts differently. This is also species dependent, whereas the mouse mammary gland undergoes a regression nearly to the pre-pregnancy state after each lactation, this is not true to the same extent in humans.

d. Recent Hormonal History and Present Hormonal Status

These factors determine the program that the cells are performing at the moment of explantation. It is easier to let the cells continue with that program *in vitro*, than to make them switch over to another program by stimulation with a set of hormones different from the combination they were subjected to *in vivo*. Any attempt to induce a change will take time (Lockwood *et al.* 1966).

e. Physio-chemical Conditions in Medium and Completeness of the Medium

Very little is actually known about whether our usual media are really optimal for our purposes. For example as early as 1954 Mary Pikovski (1954) proposed a pH of 9·3 for optimal cultivation of mouse mammary tumours!

Generally with regard to media, there are two trends. One is to use fully synthetic media in which all substances are known. These media may offer a false security, as the big unknown factor is the absence of substances that may nevertheless, be essential. The alternative is to use serum supplemented media. Experience suggests that they are often superior for the survival and well being of cells.

f. Hormone Composition of the Medium and Its Hormonal Completeness

Generally the mammary gland will be programmed by sets of synergistic hormones (Lyons, 1958). Replacing one hormone by another in the combination may change the program in such a manner that the result is completely different, e.g. from milk secretion to proliferative activity (Prop, 1961 and Fig. 3). Each hormone in a set, if added separately, is often completely inactive, but if it fits into a program that is already under way, it may prolong the program for a limited time while the complete set will guarantee continuity of that program.

The above "programming" parameters mostly stem from observations made on mouse mammary gland material. As stated before, it has not yet been possible to induce hormone reactions in normal human mammary gland *in vitro* from the resting state. However, the following example shows that similar parameters may be valid for

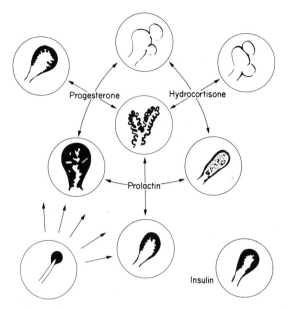

Fig. 3. Effects of different hormone combinations on organ cultures of normal mouse mammary glands *in vitro* from 6-7-week-old mice. Lower left: state of development at the moment of explantation. Lower right: After 5 days *in vitro* in a medium containing insulin: slight epithelial proliferation. The seven circles in the middle represent cultures that all had insulin + one or more of the hormones indicated by the arrows. The figures symbolise: cystic development (top right) milk secretion (middle right) massive epithelial intraductal proliferation (middle left) and lobulo-alveolar development (centre).

human mammary gland as well. Cultures of a lactating human mammary gland (it is very rare to obtain one) were made with several hormone combinations (Prop, 1968). The combination insulin + prolactin + hydrocortisone caused an abundant rather explosive milk secretion, whereas the combination insulin + prolactin + progesterone suppressed the secretion, resulting in a low cuboidal alveolar epithelium. This functional difference between hydrocortisone and progesterone agrees with the *in vivo* reaction but is only effective *in vitro* if the medium is "completed" with insulin and prolactin.

g. *The Degree of Intactness of the Tissue in Culture*
The more intact the tissue can be kept *in vitro,* the more readily it will show comparable features with *in vivo* situations. An important aspect often neglected, is that every explantation is accompanied by

HTSTC–8

a great deal of *wounding*. Cells confronted with wounding will, to counter the emergency, switch over from whatever program they are performing just before explantation to a *wound-healing reaction*. The following is a nice illustration of this. A combination of hormones, insulin and hydrocortisone, causes, in total mammary gland cultures from 6-7 week-old virgin CBA mice, a state of cystic dysplasia in which the ducts and cysts are lined with an extremely thin epithelium devoid of mitotic activity, as shown by the absence of uptake of tritiated thymidine in autoradiographs. At the surface of the same cultures, however, there is considerable uptake of thymidine and mitotic activity in epithelium that is growing out over the surface of the culture, i.e. the wounded area. After some 3-5 days in culture, the latter cells may constitute over 50% of the epithelial population (Prop, unpublished). These cells would produce an enormous background activity if we attempted to study the thymidine uptake of the culture by the usual biochemical homogenisation methods.

The wound healing reaction has an even greater influence on the results when the usual 1 mm^3 cubes in histiotypical so-called "organ cultures" are studied as the ratio wounded surface/volume is larger.

In most monolayer cell cultures wound healing is a predominant feature. The cells are generally confronted with virtually an infinite wound, i.e. the bottom of the culture vessel. In most common culture procedures this wound is kept infinite by transferring as soon as the wound tends to be healed, i.e. when a dense layer covers the whole vessel bottom, so as to keep the cells proliferating.

Although a few workers studied this problem many years ago (Fischer, 1922; Fischer and Parker, 1929; Fischer, 1946) it is only recently that much work has been done on the inhibition of growth at high cell densities, shifting attention from growth to more functional aspects in high density cultures and to the interaction between different cell types, e.g. epithelial and stromal fibroblastic cells. As an illustration, Visser, Wiepjes and Prop (in press) found that in normal mouse mammary epithelium, so called "domes" only occur if the epithelial cell density over a large surface in the culture exceeds $2 \cdot 0 \times 10^5$ cells/cm^2; tumour cells show the same effect but with a different threshold density. There is no doubt that "domes" do secrete and they are considered to be the two-dimensional equivalents of secreting alveoli (McGrath *et al.* 1972) although the evidence for this supposition is not yet conclusive. Although a kind of transformed clone sometimes arises that does not form "domes" even at very high densities, the existence of a threshold cell density generally holds equally for normal and for tumour epithelium. Since the mouse mammary tumours are mostly highly differentiated adenomatous tumours, this may not be too surprising. It is probable that the cells only consider their wound healing task finished when the threshold cell density has been reached and then switch over to more functional secretory activity. An interaction between epithelium and fibroblasts presumably operates, since "domes" do not occur if a layer of fibroblasts overgrows the epithelial layer, even though the epithelial layer remains intact under the fibroblasts.

Visser *et al.* (1972) showed that there is a hormone dependent interaction between epithelium and fibroblasts. Primary mouse mammary cell cultures prepared according to the sequential enzymatic method of Wiepjes and Prop (1970) (*see also,* Prop and Wiepjes, 1973) consist of epithelial and fibroblastic cells. In sufficiently dense cultures the epithelial cells form a monolayer that covers the whole of the base of the culture vessel. The great majority of the fibroblasts lie on top of this monolayer, though some fibroblasts may be trapped between the epithelial layer and the bottom of the vessel. Upon addition of several hormone combinations, the fibroblasts accompanied by part of the epithelium, rearrange themselves into multilayered "ridges". Between these "ridges" there are more or less circular spaces containing a thin, purely epithelial, monolayer; sometimes these spaces are devoid of cells. The formation of these "ridges" is reversible, so if the hormones are withdrawn the original less-organised two-layer structure is re-established. This effect does not occur in purely epithelial cultures nor in purely fibroblastic ones. Combination of a purely epithelial culture with normal human fibroblasts obtained from a hare lip operation in a young child, resulted in cultures that, with the proper hormone stimulation, showed the "ridge" effect (unpublished). A human mammary carcinoma culture with a large proportion of fibroblasts and only sparse clumps of tumour cells, showed the "ridge" effect during hormone treatment (unpublished).

In experiments with human tumours *in vitro* all the factors described so far for animal material should be considered, particularly:

(1) the synergism of hormones
(2) the wound healing effect that may interfere with hormone action
(3) the cell density effect
(4) the interaction between stroma and epithelium.

4. ,HOW FAR DO HUMAN MAMMARY TUMOURS IN CULTURE
REPRESENT THE ORIGINAL TUMOURS?

In organ cultures there is a real hazard that some categories of cells will die, but it is difficult to check or to evaluate quantitatively. There is a wide range between complete survival of the whole cell population, through partial survival without affecting the proportions of the different cell types, via partial survival with altered proportions and survival of stromal cells only to complete necrosis.

The problem is also complex, in cell monolayer cultures.

(1) The method of preparing cultures from the original explant is the first cause of selection, e.g. the "spilling" method will bring into culture the more loosely attached cells and the most motile cells in the tumour if they will attach to the culture substrate. Different enzymatic methods may eliminate the cells with more delicate cell membranes, simply because they cannot resist the severe enzymatic attack. In the same way—*mutatis mutandis*—with mechanical methods to free the cells from their stromal support, the cells with the lower mechanical resistance will be the victims. Each method has its own drawback and we must be constantly aware of the danger that from the outset we may cultivate a selected population.

(2) It is usually recognised that in primary cultures, fibroblasts tend to overgrow the epithelial population. Far less attention is given to the fact that there is a tendency for the less aneuploid tumour cells to grow faster than the more aneuploid cells, especially those of high ploidy. During the culture period a shift in the overall population may occur.

(3) Further, we may assume that the culture situation is favourable for further cell transformation, particularly in the tumour cells that have low "quality" control mechanisms, making work with short term cultures even more imperative.

In view of the danger that the cell population can be altered during preparation and culture, there is urgent need for methods to check that the cultures are representative of the original. Wiepjes and Prop (paper in preparation) have made imprints on microscope slides from freshly cut surfaces of human mammary tumours and determined the nuclear DNA microcytophotometrically in the resulting cell preparation after Feulgen staining. Measurements were made at random for the rounded epithelial nuclei, omitting the elongated fibroblastic nuclei and the white blood elements. After sequential enzyme treatment of the tumour, the resulting cell suspension was cultured for some days and the cells that had spread onto the bottom of the culture vessel were used for the same Feulgen measurement of DNA. The resulting histograms of the cultured cells were compared with those of the original imprints.

One cannot be absolutely certain about the epithelial character of the rounded nuclei and the fibroblastic character of the elongated nuclei from the Feulgen stained preparations, because they do not show any other characteristics, but subsequent staining of the slides with light green revealed that a high percentage of roundish nuclei belonged to cells with epithelial characteristics. There are, however, a minority of epithelial cells with oblong-shaped nuclei that are thus excluded from measurement.

The results (Figs 4 and 5) show that there is generally a larger fraction of cells in the diploid or near diploid range in the cultures

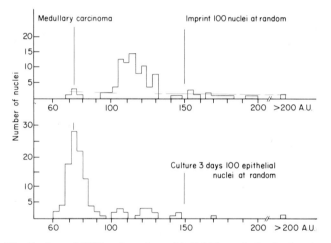

Fig. 4. Distribution of DNA values for epithelial like cells in the imprint and 3-day monolayer culture of a medullary carcinoma.

than in the imprints. This may be due to the more rapid proliferation of this cell family, but it is also possible that these cells have a firmer hold on the stroma in the original tumour so that they are less easily transferred to the glass when making the imprints.

Further analysis of the histograms shows that the cultivated cell population may show every picture from a rather close resemblance with the imprint, to a completely different picture. Generally the latter picture is that of a growing diploid population, so this confirms that the method presented may be valuable in checking the culture's

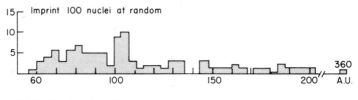

Infiltrating comedocarcinoma

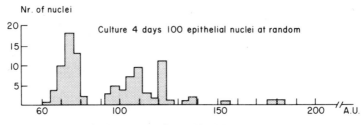

Fig. 5. Distribution of DNA values for epithelial-like cells in the imprint and 4-day monolayer culture of an infiltrating comedocarcinoma.

representativity. Figure 6 indicates the importance of checking cultures for cell types. Two histograms are shown for cultures from the same tumour; the upper one shows the DNA distribution in a five-day culture of tumour cells after the normal sequential enzyme treatment; the lower histogram shows the DNA distribution in a six-day culture of material released from this comedo carcinoma by slight pressure and made into a cell suspension by a short treatment with pronase. This latter culture is nearly devoid of the near-diploid cell family that dominates the culture after the sequential method and may be much more firmly attached to the tumour stroma. As an intermediate step, we now also make a DNA histogram of the cells in the suspension obtained by sequential enzyme treatment of the tumour before culturing (Fig. 7). Thus we may check step by step if and where the loss of certain cell categories occurs.

Finally, the DNA histogram method will be used to evaluate hormone actions and effects of chemotherapeutic drugs.

5. OUTLOOK FOR THE NEAR FUTURE

There are a wealth of good culture methods available, but we need more criteria for checking that the culture is representative of the original tumour. This involves not only ensuring that all cell types in the right proportions are present, but also checking that whatever remains of the functional state in the tumour cells is represented in

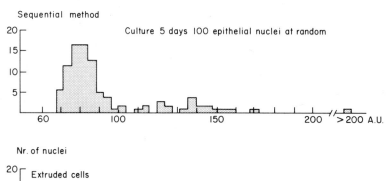

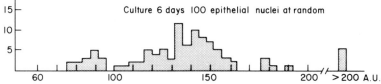

Fig. 6. Distribution of DNA values for epithelial-like cells from a comedocarcinoma. Upper—5-day culture following sequential enzymic treatment. Lower—6-day culture of extruded cells.

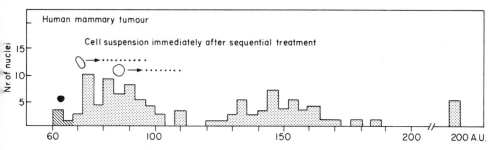

Fig. 7. Histogram of DNA distribution in a cell suspension after sequential treatment and before culturing. The types of nuclei prevailing in the different regions of DNA classes are indicated. • small blood nuclei; ◊ elongated fibroblastic nuclei; ○ rounded epithelial nuclei.

the cultures. In this latter respect, the cell density problem and the interaction between tumour cells and stromal cells are of importance.

Apart from some morphological aspects of cell degeneration and death, the criteria for hormone or chemotherapeutic drug sensitivity will generally be biochemical. In this respect cytochemical and autoradiographic methods, and sometimes immunofluorescence microscopy, are in the first rank of importance as they demonstrate *ad oculos* what is happening to individual cells in a very inhomogeneous cell population. These methods can be applied equally well on monolayer cell cultures as on sections of "organ cultures". Homogenisation methods may, as has been said before, have only limited value in this respect, as too much is done blindly without taking the inhomogeneity of the tumour sufficiently into account.

The methods are available. What is essential is that research is organised and collaboration between disciplines is established.

First the clinician, primarily concerned with the patient's well being, should provide the material, the criteria and the data needed to evaluate the profit and/or damage to the patient by the treatment. Secondly, there is the cell biologist or experimental cytopathologist, by which is meant the experimenter who tackles problems regarding the abnormal cell with the methods and approach of the cell biologist. He is the difficult member of the team because he tells the clinician as well as the biochemist with whom he is working, not to think in terms of schemes which are too simple. He sees the cell not as a simple unit always behaving in more or less the same way, but as a highly flexible and adaptable unit that behaves differently under different circumstances. He is the one who, in conjunction with the clinical pathologist, knows the morphology and the heterogeneity of the cells that constitute the tumour. Finally there is the biochemist (cytochemist, histochemist) who, with his knowledge of what *can* be going on in the cells, must provide data about what is actually wrong in that special tumour cell, what we may do to eliminate or to suppress its activity, and what our drugs, hormones or other treatments are doing to the dynamics within the cell.

Tissue culture in all its methodological aspects is a very attractive method for predictive tests for clinical use. Its major drawback, as I hope to have shown, is that it is highly artificial and not everybody is sufficiently aware of that. If we can get reliable data by simpler, less sophisticated techniques, we should do so, but there remain many problems—more, in fact, than available specialist manpower or the capacity of existing laboratories permit to be studied—that can be brought nearer to a solution *only by tissue culture*. For the moment the problems of hormone sensitivity and sensitivity to chemotherapeutic drugs are in this category, but this may well change if only we can show their usefulness for clinical problems.

REFERENCES

Aspegren, K. and Hakanson, L. (1974). *Acta Chir. Scand. 140*, 95.
Bishun, N., Mills, J., Williams, D. C. and Raven, R. W. (1973). *Cytologia, 38*, 651.

Fischer, A. (1922). *J. Exp. Med. 36*, 393.
Fischer, A. and Parker, R. C. (1929). *Archiv. f. exp. Zellforschung, 8*, 325.
Fischer, A. (1946). "Biology of Tissue Cells", Cambridge Univ. Press, Stechert & Co., New York and Nordisk Forlag, Copenhagen.
Hoge, A. F., Hartsuck, J. M., Kollmorgen, G. M. and Schilling, J. A. (1973). *Amer. J. Surgery, 126*, 722.
Ichinose, R. R. and Nandi, S. (1964). *Science, 145*, 496.
Lockwood, D. H., Turkington, R. W. and Topper, Y. J. (1966). *Biochem. Biophys. Acta, 130*, 493.
Lyons, W. R. (1958). *Proc. Roy. Soc. Ser. B. Biol. Sci. No. 936*, 149.
McGrath, C. M., Nandi, S. and Young, L. (1972). *J. Virol. 9*, 367.
Pikovski, M. A. (1954). *Exp. Cell Res. 7*, 52.
Prop, F. J. A. (1961). *Pathol. et Biol. (Paris) 9*, 640.
Prop, F. J. A. (1966). *Exp. Cell Res. 42*, 386.
Prop, F. J. A. (1968). *Exc. Medica Internat. Congress Series* (M. Margoulies, ed.), No. 161, 508.
Prop, F. J. A. and Wiepjes, G. J. (1973). Sequential enzyme treatment of mouse mammary gland. *In* "Tissue Culture; Methods and Applications" (P. F. Kruse and M. K. Patterson, eds.), p. 21. Academic Press, New York and London.
Riley, P. A., Latter, T. and Sutton, P. M. (1973). *Lancet*, October 13, 818.
Visser, A. S., de Haas, W. R. E., Kox, C. and Prop, F. J. A. (1972). *Exp. Cell Res. 73*, 516.
Wiepjes, G. J. and Prop, F. J. A. (1970). *Exp. Cell Res. 61*, 451.

DISCUSSION

Freshney emphasised that there is a limitation on the availability of epithelial cells in cultures from mammary carcinoma and from some other forms of solid tumour. A number of groups, including Lasfargues (1973) and themselves have digested fragments of tumour with collagenase. This is potentially a very useful tool for handling many of the common solid tumours with a very strong stromal fibroblastic content. By prolonging the exposure to collagenase, fragments of mammary carcinoma may be exposed for 5 days, there is progressive breakdown of the matrix of the tumour and the last fragments to break down are little nodules which are probably malignant epithelium. It is also possible that by retaining collagenase in the medium during subculture all the cells which adhere and form a monolayer are epithelial cells. The method applies equally well to normal mammary tissue and malignant mammary carcinoma. Prop said that during the long time required for collagenase treatment, the properties of the cells might change and their usefulness for clinical tests would be affected. They have developed a method published by Wiepjes and Prop (1970) using sequentially collagenase for some hours followed by pronase. Less damage is caused to the cell membrane than with proteolytic enzymes alone and successful cultures are obtained from over 80% of the mammary tumours received.

Morasca suggested that the stage of tumour is important. For a small primary tumour most of the tissue is quite normal mammary gland and there may be so little tumour that the pathologist has difficulty with the histology. If the tumour has reached a later stage of disease, it is much easier to get good cells and in these circumstances a simple spilling technique gives better results than either collagenase or trypsin. Prop agreed that if a spilling method can be made to work it is valuable because it does not interfere with cell surfaces or constituents. But for some tumours selection of those cells which are very loosely attached or actively moving around may occur. Less motile cells may remain in the original tissue and be removed with it.

Stoker said that in papers about cultures of breast cancer cells, authors hardly ever refer to anything except epithelial cells or fibroblasts (one good, one bad). Their experience so far is that in cultures prepared by the spillage technique, the cells propagated most successfully seem to be neither one thing nor another. Islands of these intermediate cells can also be recognised amongst fibroblasts after collagenase treatment. They are somewhat elongated but are easy to differentiate from fibroblasts because the edges of the islands are very smooth. They tend sometimes to be arranged in circular structures as though they are trying to form some sort of organ, but it would be extremely useful to know more about these intermediate cells and their origin. Freshney suggested that one candidate for this cell type is capillary endothelium which could be expected to form organoid structures and would be released from both normal and malignant tissues.

Ambrose has suggested that fibroblasts might be identified by their high uptake of ^{3}H-proline which they need for collagen synthesis. Prop and co-workers have developed this idea and tried to identify fibroblasts by an immunofluorescence technique using anti-collagen serum. So far it has not been possible to make the method sufficiently sensitive.

Bondy asked if it is important in these studies to separate the epithelial cells from stroma. The stromal cells and the epithelial cells interact, yet certain of the stromal cells, for example the fat cells will respond very actively to certain hormones, such as adrenaline which probably have no effect on the epithelial cells. We are in a dilemma because if the stroma is removed then the epithelium does not grow like normal epithelium or like "normal" cancer, and if we do not remove it we may get confusion from the background.

Freshney said it might well be very important to measure the effect of fibroblastic stroma on the response of the mammary carcinoma in culture no matter what response one is measuring. However, he thought it was better to try and look at a pure culture first, in other words to aim for pure cultures of fibroblasts, pure cultures of mammary carcinoma and then start mixing them. Perhaps by a synthetic approach like this we can learn something about interaction, just as in the early days of embryonic induction studies.

Prop thought there must be a compromise which would be largely a matter of policy. But he suggested that for clinical tests we are already introducing quite a lot of artificial circumstances so it is preferable to have the stroma present and remain as close as possible to the normal conditions the cells are in. If such a test proves to be clinically useful, it can be improved as our scientific knowledge increases.

REFERENCES

Lasfargues, E. Y. (1973). *In* "Tissue Culture Methods and Applications" (Kruse and Patterson, eds.), p. 45. Academic Press, New York and London.
Wiepjes, G. J. and Prop, F. J. A. (1970). *Exp. Cell Res. 61*, 451.

2. The Possible Use of Histoculture for
In Vitro Culture of Human Biopsies

Doreen Lewis and R. C. Hallowes

Apart from diagnostic applications, two types of study may be performed on human biopsies: those relating to cell or molecular biological aspects and those relating to the treatment of patients.

Cell and molecular biologists have so developed their art that cells can be just carriers of the particular pathway being studied. The cells behave in a predictable and controllable manner and morphological variation has been selected against. In breast cancer, however, morphological variations are numerous and many different cell types are found in the tissue. This complex has to be unravelled if it is to be analysed by techniques currently available to biologists.

The clinician who tries to use biopsy tissue for non-diagnostic purposes must ensure two things. First, the tissue must not be so altered by technical procedures that the results are no longer relevant to tissue that remains within the patient. Secondly, the results must be derived from a defined cell population and not from random cell populations within the biopsy. Separation techniques may select the wrong cells and may also destroy either important cell-cell relationships or cell components.

We have tried two types of culture methods in the study of biopsy tissue, organ and tissue culture, and recently, have added a third method called histo-culture. In organ culture, cubes or slices of tissue are interfaced between a chemically defined culture medium and a controlled atmosphere (see p. 35). Slices 200 μm thick were chosen as these were easy to handle, gave some indication of the cellular content that we were culturing and have been shown by previous workers to allow good metabolic and gaseous exchange across the tissue. We referred the counts to mg wet weight of tissue because although not the ideal method it is quick and convenient. Initially we compared our counts per min against total DNA or total protein. We found that the responses were similar to those obtained using wet weight but we wasted large amounts of tissue in the process.

Table 1 indicates the results of this study. We analysed 22 tumours and they fell into 4 distinct groups without the need for complicated statistics. When we came to compare our results with clinical findings

TABLE 1

Effect of Insulin and Oestradiol on DNA Synthesis in 200 μm thick explants of Human Breast Cancer

Number of cases	9	3	3	7
(a) Insulin	+	+	+	±
Degree of Insulin stimulation	1·87 (1·24-2·75)	1·32 (1·22-1·46)	1·66 (1·37-1·96)	None
(b) Oestradiol	—	±	+	±
Degree of Oestradiol inhibition or stimulation	0·59 (0·28-0·80)	None	1·63 (1·39-1·87)	None

The explants were cultured for 0-20 hr in 199 + 1-20 μg/ml insulin with and without 10^{-3} μg/ml oestradiol; then 2 μCi/ml ^{3}H-thymidine was added and the explants harvested at 24 hr. Uptake of ^{3}H/mg wet weight of tissue was determined and the results expressed as (a) was uptake greater in medium that contained insulin compared with no added insulin? and (b) did oestradiol affect uptake in medium that contained insulin?

we were faced with a problem. The tissue had been generously donated by consultant pathologists from five separate hospitals but we found that there was little agreement between the methods used for staging or grading the clinical or pathological findings. All we could say after a lot of hard work was that no patients in the first group showed widespread metastases or poorly-differentiated cancers and no patients in the last group showed well localised growths or well-differentiated cancer. More confusion followed as shown in Fig. 1. Considering the top graph first, this shows the uptake of tritiated thymidine in counts per mg wet weight during 20-24 hr of culture in a range of insulin concentrations; the optimum rate of synthesis occurred at 20 μg per ml. The second graph shows the incorporation of thymidine during 20-24 hr culture in either 10 or 20 μg of insulin and a range of corticosterone concentrations. As can be seen there is no significant difference between either of the insulin doses on the effect of corticosterone on DNA synthesis. In the last graph we incubated cells of the same breast cancer either in medium that contained 10 μg of insulin plus 5 μg of corticosterone or 20 μg of insulin plus 5 μg of corticosterone and a range of prolactin concentrations from 1-20 μg per ml. With 10 μg of insulin the

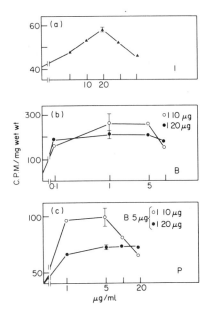

Fig. 1. Effect of concentration of insulin, corticosterone and prolactin on DNA synthesis in 200 μm thick explants of human breast cancer.

(a) effect of insulin at medium concentration 1-80 μg/ml on DNA synthesis during 20-24 hr culture

(b) explants were cultured either in medium that contained 10 or 20 μg insulin (I) per ml plus a range of corticosterone concentrations from 0·1 to 10 μg/ml. Rate of DNA synthesis was determined during 20-24 hr culture.

(c) explants were cultured either in medium that contained 10 or 20 μg insulin (I) and 5 μg corticosterone (B) per ml plus a range of prolactin concentrations from 1 to 20 μg/ml. Rate of DNA synthesis was determined during 20-24 hr culture.

tumour appeared prolactin responsive to a greater extent than when cultured in 20 μg per ml! At this stage we decided to return to work with mammary cancers induced in rats, and we now used tissue culture.

Tissue culture of breast cancer was tried in the hope that the proliferative stimulus provided by cells colonising the plastic would reveal the underlying growth factors required. This approach (see p. 36) is working well in our studies of dimethyl-benz(a)anthracene-induced breast cancers in rats. Figure 2 shows the specificity of the response of the rat mammary epithelial cells to separate and combined hormones. 67-69 hr was the time chosen for the analysis so that results were derived from epithelial cells and not fibroblasts as determined by autoradiographical and ultra-structural studies. Figure 3 shows that the epithelial cells are capable of differentiating

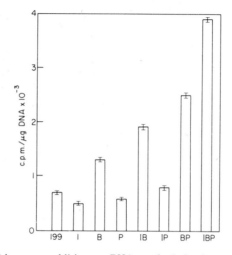

Fig. 2. Effect of hormone addition on DNA synthesis in tissue cultures derived from DMBA-induced rat mammary carcinomas.

Primary cultures from rat mammary carcinomas were cultured for 67 hr in medium that contained 5 μg/ml of the following hormones, insulin (I), corticosterone (B), prolactin (P). 0·2 μCi/ml ³H-thymidine was added and the cultures harvested at 69 hr. The uptake of ³H-thymidine per μg DNA was determined. The histograms represent the mean ± SEM.

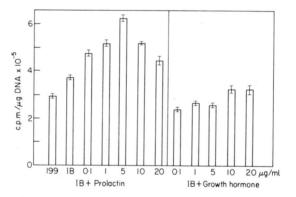

Fig. 3. Effect of a range of concentrations of prolactin and of growth hormone on DNA synthesis in tissue cultures derived from DMBA-induced rat mammary carcinomas.

Primary cultures from rat mammary carcinomas were cultured for 67 hr in medium that contained insulin and corticosterone (IB) at 5 μg/ml plus a range of prolactin or growth hormone concentrations from 0·1 to 20 μg/ml. 0·2 μCi/ml ³H-thymidine was added and the cultures harvested at 69 hr. The uptake of ³H per μg DNA was determined. The histograms represent the mean ± SEM.

between prolactin and growth hormone by giving increased response to increases in amounts of prolactin but not to growth hormone. This agrees with our organ culture studies on the same tumours which showed that prolactin stimulates DNA synthesis whereas growth hormone does not (Lewis and Hallowes, 1974).

We have tried unsuccessfully to apply this approach to cultures of human breast cancer. Although we can get small amounts of epithelium to grow from most if not all biopsy samples, our biochemical methods are not sufficiently sensitive to select for the relatively small numbers of these cells that grow amongst the other cell types found in the cell suspensions and which also proliferate in culture conditions.

Can organ culture and tissue culture be combined so that the cancer cells are encouraged to proliferate without destroying either the cell-cell relationships or cell components? Sherwin and Richters in Los Angeles have used a technique they call histoculture to try to achieve this (p. 36). Using their histoculture technique Sherwin and Richters have studied the effect of gas concentration on cells (Sherwin and Richters, 1975), the *in vitro* behaviour of lung carcinoma (Sherwin *et al.* 1967), the effect of lymphocytes on breast carcinoma (Richters and Sherwin, 1971) and the effects of chemo-

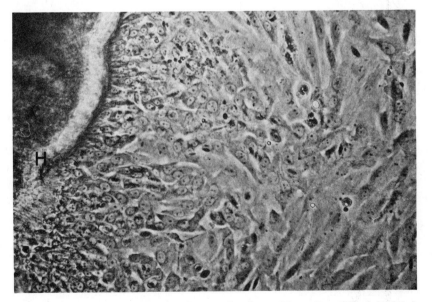

Fig. 4. Fibroadenoma. Epithelial cells spreading from a histoculture (H) on the 5th day after plating onto a collagen-coated Petri dish. Medium 199 plus 5% foetal calf serum. ×100.

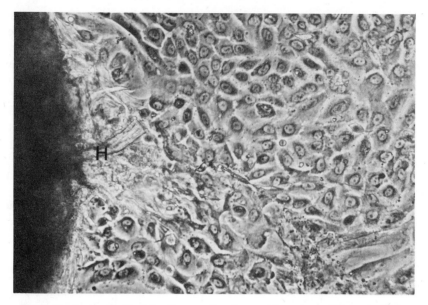

Fig. 5. Carcinoma. Epithelial cells spreading from a histoculture (H) on the 13th day after plating onto a collagen-coated Petri dish. Medium 199 plus 5% foetal calf serum. ×100.

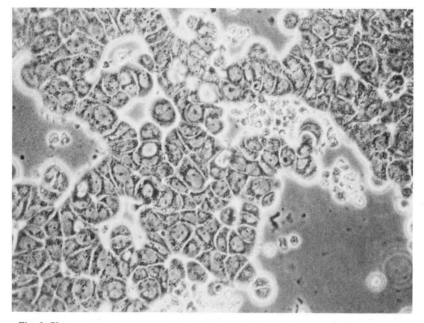

Fig. 6. Phase contrast appearance of a histoculture from a human breast carcinoma. This photograph was kindly loaned by Professors R. P. Sherwin and A. Richters.

therapeutics and cytotoxics on cells. They are currently studying human breast cancer and Figs 4, 5 and 6 show the cultural appearances of cells derived from the histocultures. Time-lapse cinematography of these histocultures has demonstrated that the breast cancer cells are capable of cell division, absorption, secretion and organised growth, and that they retain a three-dimensional structure that appears identical with that seen in the original biopsy specimens.

Unfortunately this technique is not readily applicable to handling large numbers of slices on a routine basis. Morasca has described the setting up of 100 Rose chambers. I enquired how long this took: it took two technicians $4\frac{1}{2}$ hr. We have therefore modified the technique (p. 36) and are studying the growth of cells within and growing out from the slices by time-lapse cinematography, stereoscan and autoradiography. We hope thereby to characterise the various cell types upon and growing out from the slices and compare these with similar studies on cell suspensions from biopsies, malignant effusions, milk, etc. This is a necessary stage to ensure that both cell biologists and clinical scientists are studying the correct group of cells from biopsy specimens.

We intend to use the methods being developed in the selection of patients with carcinoma for endocrine therapy, and Fig. 7 shows in a greatly oversimplified form how this might be carried out. We think that slices of tissue will be used rather than cell cultures because of the problems of cell separation, but cell culture work will be necessary to establish first, what new event is induced in epithelial cells by growth regulators and secondly, what metabolic processes

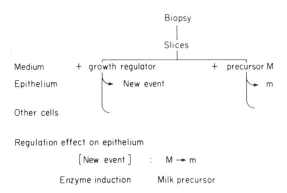

Fig. 7. Schematic design for determination of regulator dependence of epithelial cells in a heterogenous tissue. M → m denotes ability of epithelial cells to convert M to m.

can be used to determine the number of viable epithelial cells from amongst a heterogeneous population of other cells. There is already evidence that this type of approach is practical. It has been shown that oestrogens can induce the formation of an enzyme peroxidase in the uterus (Churg and Anderson, 1974) and androgens can induce the enzyme alcohol dehydrogenase in the kidney (Ohno *et al.* 1970). It has also been shown by Young (Young *et al.* 1973) that casein and/or lactoferrin can be localised to human mammary cancer cells in histological sections and by Dermer and Sherwin (1975) that mammary cancer cells can incorporate glucosamine in specific glycoproteins.

ACKNOWLEDGEMENTS

We gratefully acknowledge the help of Professors Sherwin and Richters in setting up the histoculture method and for access to their material. A gift of ovine prolactin PS-11 from the National Institutes of Health, Bethesda is also gratefully acknowledged.

REFERENCES

Churg, A. and Anderson, W. A. (1974). *J. Cell Biol., 62,* 449.
Dermer, G. B. and Sherwin, R. P. (1975). *Cancer Res. 35,* 63.
Lewis, D. and Hallowes, R. C. (1974). *J. Endocr. 62,* 225.
Ohno, S., Stenius, C., Christian, L., Harris, C. and Ivey, C. (1970). *Biochem. Genet. 4,* 565.
Richters, A. and Sherwin, R. P. (1971). *Cancer, 27,* 274.
Sherwin, R. P. and Richters, A. (1965). *Exp. Cell Res. 37,* 697.
Sherwin, R. P., Richters, V. and Richters, A. (1967). *Cancer, 20,* 1.
Young, S., Pang, L. S. C. and Goldsmith, I. J. (1973). *J. Clin. Path. 7,* 94.

3. Organ Culture—A Model for Defining the Hormone Dependency of Human Benign Prostatic Hyperplasia

A. C. Riches, P. A. M. Shipman, Valerie Littlewood,
L. Donaldson and G. H. Thomas

Studies of factors affecting cell kinetics and hormone dependency of human tumours cannot be carried out *in vivo* in most instances as many of the techniques involved use isotopes and cytotoxic drugs. Attempts to devise culture models for these studies thus have obvious advantages. Maintenance of tissue architecture may well be important in view of the interactions between stromal and epithelial components (Franks *et al.* 1970) and thus organ culture models could well be useful. Tissues can also be maintained in defined environments which is an obvious advantage in studies on hormone dependency of tumours.

Previous work has clearly demonstrated that in the rat prostate the effects of testosterone are mediated through metabolites which are thought to control cell differentiation and proliferation (Baulieu *et al.* 1968; Wilson, 1970). Results with human benign prostatic hyperplasia (BPH) have not been as clear cut and withdrawal of androgen support is not accompanied by marked morphological changes in culture (McMahon and Thomas, 1973; Harbitz, 1973; McRae *et al.* 1973).

In order to define the hormone dependency of a tissue in culture, it is thus necessary to develop techniques for studying differentiation and proliferation. Attempts to define the behaviour of BPH in organ culture using parameters of differentiation and proliferation are described.

A. ORGAN CULTURE MODEL

The method used for these studies was similar to that introduced by Trowell (1954, 1959) and incorporating modifications by Riches, Littlewood and Thomas (1972). Explants were placed on a millipore filter supported on a stainless steel grid in a petri dish containing 3 ml of Eagles Minimum Essential Medium supplemented with 10%

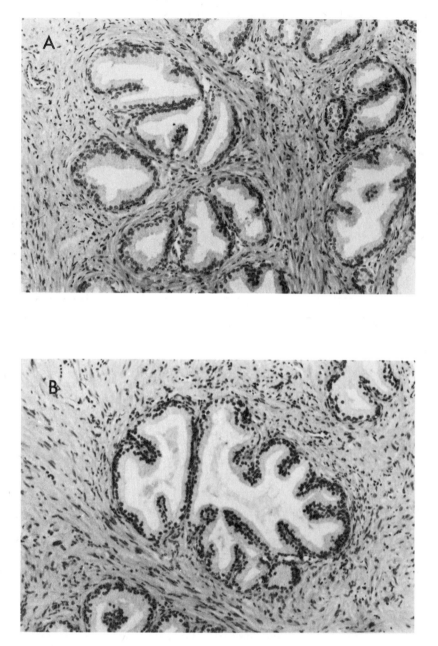

Fig. 1. *A* Section from a biopsy specimen of human benign prostatic hyperplasia (x130). *B* Section from a 4-day culture of human benign prostatic hyperplasia taken from the same biopsy specimen (x130).

calf serum, the dishes were placed in a McIntosh and Fildes jar and gassed with humidified 95% O_2 and 5% Co_2. The media was changed at two daily intervals.

Human neoplastic prostate was obtained from open (retropubic and transvesical) prostatectomy, placed in a sterile container and stored at 4° C until culture. Tissue slices, weighing about 15-20 mgm of about 1 mm thickness, were prepared from 1 cm square blocks cut from the biopsy specimen. The cultures were maintained for 2-4 days with good preservation of tissue architecture (Figs 1A and 1B).

Rat prostates, from eight to nine-week old wistar rats were removed and carefully teased into 2 mm diameter portions thus avoiding cutting the prostate which is known to cause regenerative hyperplasia (Lasnitzki, 1965).

B. Indices of Differentiation

1. ANALYSIS OF TISSUE COMPONENTS

A modified form of the method described by Chalkley (1943) was used to determine the relative volumes of the three basic tissue components: stroma, space and alveolar epithelium.

For each section 40 microscope fields were scored using a modified Chalkley point array graticule (Smith, Thomas and Riches, 1974). This number was found to give a reasonable estimate of the mean with an acceptable standard error.

The composition of the biopsy specimens and BPH explants cultured for 2 and 4 days and rat prostates cultured for 4 days were measured. In both cases there was good preservation of the components (Tables 1 and 2). The percentage epithelium decreased slightly in cultured rat prostate but remained constant in BPH explants.

TABLE 1

Analysis of Tissue Composition
Rat Prostate

| | % composition | | |
	Epithelium	Stroma	Space
Biopsy	26·3 ± 1·2	37·4 ± 4·7	36·3 ± 3·7
day 4	17·0 ± 0·4	40·0 ± 2·1	43·2 ± 2·0

TABLE 2

Analysis of Tissue Composition
Human Benign Prostatic Hyperplasia

	% composition		
	Epithelium	*Stroma*	*Space*
Biopsy	11·8 ± 0·9	69·5 ± 1·4	18·4 ± 0·7
day 2	10·2 ± 0·5	77·8 ± 1·0	12·0 ± 0·7
day 4	11·1 ± 0·5	76·1 ± 0·9	12·7 ± 0·7

2. ANALYSIS OF EPITHELIAL COMPONENTS

Using a Zeiss projection microscope, the image of a section was projected on to a blank sheet of paper and the outlines of about 30 alveoli were drawn. The epithelium was classified into three types: squamous/cuboidal, columnar and stratified. Using a map measurer, the total length of each epithelial type was measured and expressed as a percentage. This thus gave an index of morphological types present in the epithelium.

In the rat, the percentage columnar epithelium decreased from 72% to 33% in culture with a corresponding increase in squamous/cuboidal epithelium, which is indicative of a castration response (Table 3). In the BPH, the changes were more complex. Although the

TABLE 3

Analysis of Epithelial Composition
Rat prostate

	% composition		
	Squamous/cuboidal	*Columnar*	*Stratified*
Biopsy	17·5 ± 8·4	72·1 ± 3·7	10·1 ± 4·7
day 4	42·7 ± 4·1	32·7 ± 2·9	24·6 ± 2·7

TABLE 4

Analysis of Epithelial Composition
Human Benign Prostatic Hyperplasia

	% composition		
	Squamous/cuboidal	*Columnar*	*Stratified*
Biopsy	17·2 ± 3·3	52·8 ± 4·0	24·6 ± 2·9
day 2	16·5 ± 2·5	35·7 ± 2·5	45·4 ± 1·9
day 4	14·5 ± 2·4	36·6 ± 2·5	48·5 ± 1·6

percentage of columnar epithelium decreased in culture, there was no increase in squamous/cuboidal epithelium but an increase in stratified epithelium (Table 4).

C. INDICES OF PROLIFERATION

1. METAPHASE ARREST STUDIES

Metaphase arrest drugs provide a useful method for measuring cell production rates both *in vivo* (Smith, Thomas and Riches, 1974; Bertalanffy, 1964) and *in vitro* (Riches, Littlewood and Thomas, 1972).

After an appropriate time in culture, 4 μgm of vincristine sulphate was added to the culture medium and the metaphase arrested cells examined histologically (Fig. 2). Explants of BPH were cultured for

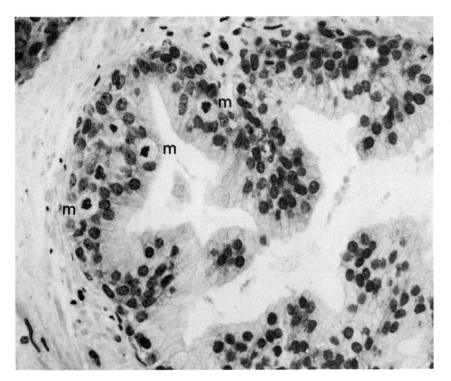

Fig. 2. Section from a 4-day culture of human benign prostatic hyperplasia after treatment with the metaphase arrest drug vincristine (×420). The arrested metaphase figures can be seen (m).

2 days and removed at 2, 4 and 6 hr after vincristine administration. The 4-hr metaphase index was also measured at 2 and 4 days in culture.

Between two to three thousand alveolar epithelial cells were counted and the number of metaphases recorded. Appropriate corrections for section thickness were used (Abercrombie, 1946; Philp and Buchanan, 1971).

The number of metaphases increased linearly with time (Fig. 3) although a long lag phase was apparent. The cell production rate can

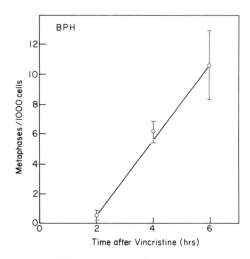

Fig. 3. Metaphase accumulation per 1000 cells with time in explants of human benign prostatic hyperplasia cultured for 2 days.

be estimated from the gradient of the line and is 2·5 cells per 1000 cells per hour, giving a turnover time of about 16·5 days. The number of metaphases accumulated after 4 hr can only be used as an index of proliferative activity and the hourly rate cannot be estimated from the one value. This index of proliferation can be used, however, to compare cell production at 2 and 4 days in culture (Table 5). The index at 4 days is much greater than at 2 days for the BPH explants. Cellular proliferation of the alveolar epithelium thus increases with time in culture.

2. 5-[^{125}I]-IODO-2′-DEOXYURIDINE STUDIES

5-[^{125}I]-iodo-2′-deoxyuridine (^{125}IUdR) is a specific DNA precursor (Hughes *et al.* 1964) and has been extensively used in kinetic studies

TABLE 5

Metaphase Accumulation in BPH Explants

number	metaphases/1000 cells/hour	
	2-day	4-day
P1	3·60	—
P2	1·95	—
P3	1·70	—
P4	2·00	—
P5	3·45	—
P7	0·44	—
P17	1·95	2·82
P18	0·75	2·38
P19	1·07	2·78
P20	—	2·05
P21	0·38	3·50
P22	0·25	3·52
P23	0·25	2·18
P24	0·38	2·88
	1·40 ± 0·32	2·76 ± 0·19

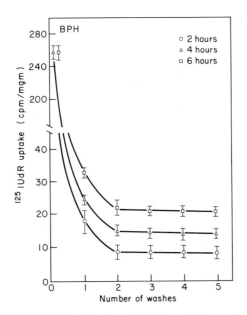

Fig. 4. Uptake of ^{125}IUdR (cpm/mgm) into explants of human benign prostatic hyperplasia cultured for 2 days after successive washes in 70% alcohol.

(Dethlefsen, 1974, Micklem, 1972). ^{125}IUdR has the advantage over tritium and carbon 14 labels that the activity can be assayed on whole organ samples without extensive biochemical and sample preparation. Washing of the tissues with 70% alcohol removes 98-99% of the unbound activity (Micklem, 1972; Pritchard and Micklem, 1972; Fidler, 1970). Re-utilisation of label is much less of a problem with ^{125}IUdR compared with ^{3}H-thymidine (Dethlefsen, 1971; 1974; Clifton and Cooper, 1973).

Two μCi of ^{125}IUdR were added per culture and after an appropriate time explants were removed, blotted, weighed and then fixed in alcoholic Bouins for 24 hr and washed in 70% alcohol, after 3 washes the activity remained constant (Fig. 4). Uptake into BPH explants cultured for 2 days (Fig. 5) and rat explants cultured for 4

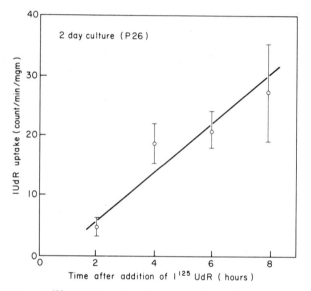

Fig. 5. Uptake of ^{125}IUdR (cpm/mgm) into explants of human benign prostatic hyperplasia cultured for 2 days with time after addition of ^{125}IUdR.

days was linear for at least 8 hr after ^{125}IUdR administration. The standard errors for the BPH uptakes were rather large. Much of this variation could be due to the inhomogeneity of the percentage of epithelium between explants. In a further series the added advantage of ^{125}IUdR was utilised and histological sections were prepared from the fixed specimen after isotope counting. A comparison between the percentage epithelium measured using the Chalkley method and

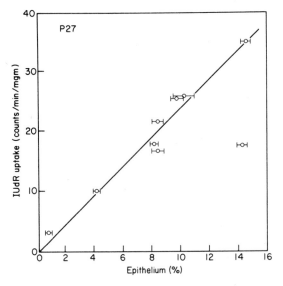

Fig. 6. Uptake of ^{125}IUdR (cpm/mgm) into explants of human benign prostatic hyperplasia cultured for 4 days and the percentage epithelium in each explant.

the uptake of ^{125}IUdR on day 2 and day 4 (Fig. 6) showed a very good correlation (day 2 r = 0·90, P < 0·001; day 4 r = 0·83, 0·01 > P > 0·001).

Effects of Insulin and Testosterone on Proliferation

The uptake of ^{125}IUdR has been measured at 2, 4 and 6 days in culture for the BPH explants and rat prostate explants. The pattern of activity was somewhat different for the two series.

In the rat, the uptake decreases with time in culture and by day 4 and 6 the uptake is small, whereas in the BPH explants the uptake increased with time in culture reaching a maximum around day 4 and decreasing by day 6 (Fig. 7).

The effect of insulin (3·0 μgm/ml) and testosterone (10^{-7} mole/l) were also examined. There was a marked increase in the uptake at day 4 for the rat prostate which decreased again by day 6. Insulin plus testosterone appeared to maintain the proliferative activity of rat prostate for an extended period in culture (Fig. 7). The uptake pattern for BPH explants was similar to that of controls without insulin and testosterone although the uptake was increased on day 4 and day 6 (Fig. 7).

Preliminary studies using vincristine to monitor the proliferative index of BPH alveolar epithelium demonstrated an increased cell

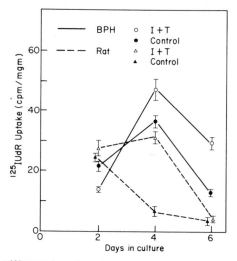

Fig. 7. Uptake of ^{125}IUdR (cpm/mgm) into explants of rat prostate and human benign prostatic hyperplasia cultured for 2, 4 and 6 days in the presence and absence of insulin (3·0 μgm/ml) + testosterone (10^{-7} mole/l).

TABLE 6

Metaphase Accumulation in BPH Explants After Culture with Insulin + Testosterone

| | *metaphases/1000 cells (4 hours)* | |
	2-day	*4-day*
Control	1·0	8·7
insulin + testosterone	4·5	19·0

production rate with insulin and testosterone (Table 6). The 4 hr index of controls increasing between 2 and 4 days in culture as has been demonstrated previously (Table 5). The index for insulin and testosterone also increased between day 2 and day 4 and was greater than the control values on these two days.

The Responses of Prostatic Tissue in Organ Culture

Organ culture would seem to provide a useful model for studying human BPH. Parallel studies using rat prostate have been carried out so that some comparison between *in vivo* and *in vitro* data can be undertaken, which is difficult with human BPH studies. Analysis of the percentage composition at 2 and 4 days in culture has demonstrated quantitatively that the explants maintain their structure. These results agree with the results described by Harbitz (1973), McMahon and Thomas (1973) and McRae et al. (1973). The simple epithelial analysis demonstrates clearly the effects of culturing rat prostate without androgen support. The percentage columnar epithelium decreases and is replaced by squamous/cuboidal epithelium, changes which are consistent with the descriptions of other workers (Lasnitzki, 1965; Lostroh, 1968). The changes seen in the BPH explants were different. Although the percentage of columnar epithelium was reduced, it was replaced by a dramatic increase in stratified epithelium. This would tend to suggest that BPH is less sensitive to withdrawal of hormone support, and the metaplasia that occurs is more indicative of a repair mechanism.

An approach to the cellular kinetics of BPH was possible using the metaphase arrest drug vincristine. It is important when using stathmokinetic drugs to define the appropriate dose and time relationships for metaphase accumulation (Riches, Littlewood and Thomas, 1972; Smith, Thomas and Riches, 1974) and apply appropriate corrections for metaphase loss (Aherne and Camplejohn, 1972). Although accurate values for the turnover time could not be calculated, both the ^{125}IUdR studies and the metaphase arrest studies showed a similar pattern of activity in culture.

The changes in proliferative activity in the rat prostate in culture were similar to those described by Simnett and Morley (1967) in the mouse. They found that the metaphase index decreased with time in culture and was lower than in vivo values for young mice (3 weeks old). In contrast there was a marked increase in the metaphase index between day 1 and day 4 in culture for older mice (24, 44 weeks old), which was larger than in vivo values. The metaphase index is much lower in old mice than young mice. BPH appears to follow the proliferative response of old mice. It is thus important to consider this factor in attempts in defining hormone dependency. Simnett and Morley (1967) suggested that the response for proliferation is high in a young mouse. When these factors are removed in culture the proliferative response is less. In the old mouse inhibitors may play an important role, which are not present on removal to culture. This results in a surge of cells moving from the G_o population into cycle.

Combinations of insulin and testosterone had a stimulatory effect on the proliferative activity for both rat and BPH explants. The pattern was more marked in the rat explants where with hormones added, the proliferative response was maintained for longer periods in culture. Lostroh (1968) demonstrated a synergistic stimulatory effect of insulin and testosterone on prostates of gonadectomised mice in culture. For the BPH explants, only a small stimulatory effect was apparent. It may well be that in the presence of the proliferative surge around day 4 in culture, any attempts to define the role of hormones is meaningless. Although at longer time intervals a more marked response was shown. Preliminary studies with vincristine showed a similar response to the ^{125}IUdR uptake studies.

Human BPH would thus seem to demonstrate some of the characteristics of a hormone dependent tissue. It has become clear in these studies that both the age of the tissue and the time in culture may be important factors in defining the responses to hormones of BPH. Further studies using the indices of proliferation and differentiation described, may well shed more light on the hormone dependency of this tissue.

REFERENCES

Abercrombie, N. (1946). *Anat. Rec. 94*, 239.
Aherne, W. and Camplejohn, R. S. (1972). *Exp. Cell Res. 74*, 496.
Baulieu, E. E., Lasnitzki, I. and Robel, P. (1968). *Nature, Lond. 219*, 1155.
Bertalanffy, F. D. (1964). *Lab. Invest. 13*, 871.
Chalkley, H. W. (1943). *J. nat. Can. Inst. 4*, 47.
Clifton, K. H. and Cooper, J. (1973). *Proc. Soc. exp. Biol. Med. 142*, 1145.
Dethlefsen, L. A. (1971). *Cell. T. Kinet. 4*, 123.
Dethlefsen, L. A. (1974). *Cell T. Kinet. 7*, 213.
Fidler, I. J. (1970). *J. nat. Can. Inst. 45*, 773.
Franks, L. M., Riddle, P. N., Carbonell, A. W. and Gey, G. O. (1970). *J. Path. 100*, 113.
Harbitz, B. T. (1973). *Scand. J. urol. Nephrol. 7*, 6.
Hughes, W. L., Commerford, S. L., Gitlin, D., Kreuger, R. C., Schultze, B., Shah, V. and Reilly, P. (1964). *Fed. Proc. 23*, 640.
Lasnitzki, I. (1965). *Europ. J. Can. 1*, 289.
Lostroh, A. J. (1968). *Proc. Nat. Acad. Sci. 60*, 1312.
McMahon, M. J. and Thomas, G. H. (1973). *Brit. J. Cancer, 27*, 323.
McRae, C. U., Ghanadian, R., Fotherby, K. and Chisholm, G. D. (1973). *Brit. J. Urol. 45*, 156.
Micklem, H. S. (1972). *Cell T. Kinet. 5*, 159.
Philp, J. R. and Buchanan, T. J. (1971). *J. Anat. 108*, 89.
Pritchard, H. and Micklem, H. S. (1972). *Clin. exp. Immunol. 10*, 151.
Riches, A. C., Littlewood, V. and Thomas, D. B. (1972). *J. Anat. 114*, 299.
Simnett, J. D. and Morley, A. R. (1967). *Exp. Cell Res. 46*, 29.
Smith, S. R., Thomas, D. B. and Riches, A. C. (1974). *Cell T. Kinet.* (in press).
Trowell, O. A. (1954). *Exp. Cell Res. 6*, 246.
Trowell, O. A. (1959). *Exp. Cell Res. 16*, 118.
Wilson, J. D. (1970). *In* "Some Aspects of the Aetiology and Biochemistry of Prostrate Cancer" (K. Griffiths and C. G. Pierrepont, eds.). Alpha Omega, Cardiff.

4. Selection of Patients with Carcinoma of the Breast for Endocrine Therapy

D. I. Beeby, G. C. Easty, J.-C. Gazet and A. Munro Neville

Approximately 5% of the female population of the United Kingdom will develop breast cancer (Barker and Richmond, 1971). Although the majority of cases present at an early stage of apparently localised disease and receive vigorous local therapy, the overall cure rate is only 20-24% (Ratzkowski *et al.* 1973): thus a substantial number of women reach an advanced stage of breast cancer. About 30% of these show some clinical improvement for up to two years as a result of some form of endocrine therapy.

The selection of patients who are likely to respond to hormone therapy is still largely empirical. As a result a number of women are submitted to the mortality and morbidity of surgery or the side effects of therapeutic hormone preparations without benefit. Despite extensive research into the endocrine status of individual patients, tissue hormone receptor sites, and direct effects of hormones on cultured tissue, no predictive test of clinical value has yet emerged.

In recent years direct hormonal influences on cultured tissue from biopsy specimens of human breast cancers have been studied in several centres (Chayen *et al.* 1970; Stoll, 1970; Barker and Richmond, 1971; Burstein *et al.* 1971; Salih *et al.* 1972a, 1972b, 1973; Willcox and Thomas, 1972; Riley *et al.* 1973; Aspegren and Hakansson, 1974). For the most part organ cultures have been preferred to cell suspensions or monolayers. Most workers have noted either no effects, or predominantly inhibitory effects, of hormones on cell metabolism and proliferation. However, Burstein *et al.* (1971) found small degrees of enhancement of DNA synthesis in cell suspensions in 40% of hormone responsive tumours, and Chayen *et al.* (1970) noted that 44% of breast cancers in organ culture fail to survive without added oestrogen. Salih *et al.* (1972a, 1972b, 1973) have demonstrated a substantial increase *in vitro* in pentose shunt dehydrogenase activity due to hormones in 50% of breast carcinomas submitted to investigation, and comparisons of the clinical response of some of those patients' tumours to endocrine therapy with the results of their *in vitro* tests showed a high degree of correlation.

We have used short term organ cultures of 30 primary and 4 secondary human breast carcinomas, maintained in most cases for 24 hr but latterly for 72 hr, to test the effects of various hormones added to the culture medium.

The method employed was based on that described by Trowell (1959) (see p. 37) and the hormones used together with the relevant concentrations are shown in Table 1.

TABLE 1

A List of the Hormones Used Together with the In Vitro *Concentrations at which They Were Tested*

	µg/ml		
OESTRADIOL-17β	3,	0·3,	0·03
TESTOSTERONE			
TAMOXIFEN	3,		
Triphenylethylene compound with antioestrogenic properties			
PROLACTIN	1,	0·1,	0·01

We have assessed the hormonal effects by histology, by estimation of pentose shunt dehydrogenase activity both histochemically and biochemically, and by estimations of tritiated base incorporation into DNA or RNA.

As a rule the tissues showed good preservation of their morphology after 24 hr in culture, but looked less healthy after 72 hr.

The histochemical principle used in this study was that of reduction of a colourless tetrazolium salt by the enzyme system in unfixed sections to produce localised deposits of highly coloured formazan dye. As recommended by Chayen *et al.* (1970), we used phenazine methosulphate as a hydrogen carrier in this system to prevent loss of this ion into other biosynthetic pathways which would bypass the tetrazolium salt. Polyvinyl alcohol was used to bind the soluble enzymes within the tissues and prevent their loss into the incubating fluid during the histochemical reaction.

We compared two tetrazolium salts, the monotetrazole MTT and the ditetrazole, NT. Of the two, MTT has the better redox potential, better tissue penetrating ability, and forms a finer formazan deposit than NT. The fineness of the deposit is dependent upon chelation of the formazan within the tissues in the presence of cobalt. This process does not occur with NT formazan, and consequently the deposits tend to coalesce into large crystals which obscure tissue localisation (Pearse, 1972). Most breast carcinomas are highly heterogeneous in nature, and contain variable amounts of stroma in addition to cancer cells. Histochemistry provides a method of visual assessment of regional enzyme activity which is especially useful in tissue of this type. When we compared histochemical and adjacent H and E stained sections we found more marked enzyme activity in the tumour cell areas than in the stromal cells. However, more stromal cell dehydrogenase activity was revealed by MTT because of its greater sensitivity, than by NT, and for this reason regional variations were less pronounced.

The variations which we observed between different sections of a breast tumour were usually no greater than the variations between areas of individual sections. Because of these variations we found precise comparative estimations between sections difficult. Nevertheless, we are satisfied that we have seen no case in which the tumour dehydrogenase activity in slices, cultured with any hormone, exceeds that in the fresh specimen or cultured control.

Our quantitative dehydrogenase determinations were made by measuring the rate of conversion of NADP to NADPH by this enzyme system in tissue homogenates. We used a fluorimetric method which proved reproducible and reliable. Dehydrogenase activity and tritium incorporation were expressed per microgram of DNA in the tissue.

We used the tissue DNA content as an index of its cell mass, and have thus excluded from our estimations the weight of the metabolically inert tissues.

Even so, breast tumours tend to contain a heterogeneous population of cells, including variable numbers of fibroblasts, fat cells, and lymphocytes as well as cancer cells. In view of this we carried out experiments to determine the range of dehydrogenase activity or tritium incorporation which could be encountered in replicate samples. The variability is shown in Table 2 which records mean absolute values and the standard deviations.

The range of dehydrogenase activity in those tissues cultured with hormones is demonstrated in Fig. 1. This shows 76 samples from 20 carcinomas. The activity in each case is expressed as a multiple of the dehydrogenase activity in a cultured control from the same tumour. Most tissues show approximately the same dehydrogenase activity as their cultured controls and the majority of the remainder fall within the range which might be expected amongst replicate samples.

The one sample which appears separately on the enhanced activity side of the scale shows a six-fold increase, and the three samples, all

TABLE 2

Variations in Dehydrogenase Activity, ^{3}H-Uridine Uptake and ^{3}H-Thymidine Uptake between Replicate Samples of Human Mammary Carcinomas

Mammary carcinomas	Dehydrogenase activity (Moles × 10^{-5} per min μgm DNA)		Uridine uptake (cpm/μgm DNA)	Thymidine uptake (cpm/μgm DNA)
Prior to culture	1.	30 ± 10	—	—
	2.	40 ± 8	—	—
After culture	3.	50 ± 33	1366 ± 729	345 ± 143
	4.	40 ± 9		

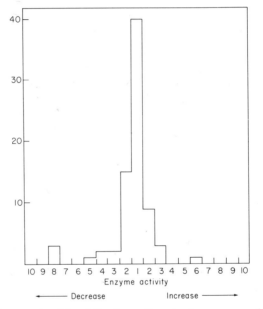

Fig. 1. Dehydrogenase activity following culture in the presence of hormone for 76 samples from 20 carcinomas expressed as a multiple of (increase) or a fraction of (decrease) the activity in a control culture from the same specimen.

from different tumours, on the inhibited activity side of the scale show an eight-fold decrease. These differences are not substantial enough to be regarded with confidence as being significant and are certainly not comparable with the 10 to 40-fold variations estimated by Salih *et al.* on the basis of their histochemistry. Furthermore, all of these tumours fall within the normal range when assessed in terms of uridine and of thymidine incorporation.

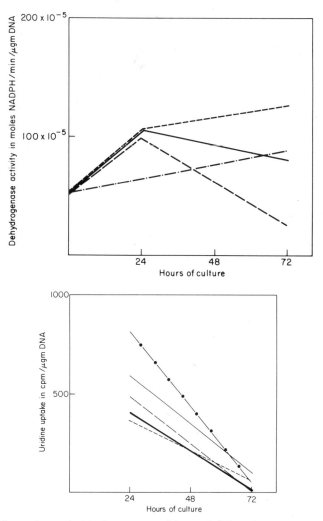

Fig. 2. Comparison of dehydrogenase activity and ^{3}H uridine uptake in a breast carcinoma cultured for 24 and 72 hr. ^{3}H uridine was added to all specimens for the last 6 hr of culture.

Top	——— Control and Prolactin	Lower	——— Control
	·············· Tamoxifen		——— Prolactin
	— — — Oestradiol		·············· Tamoxifen
	—·—··—·— Testosterone		— — — Oestradiol
			—·—··—·— Testosterone

In the assessment by each parameter a small number of samples fall outside the range of the majority, but there is no correlation for any tumour in this small group between its dehydrogenase activity, RNA synthesis and DNA synthesis.

Statistical analysis of variance has failed to reveal any significant hormonal effects throughout the series. Similarly, no dose-response effects have been observed.

In one experiment, we demonstrated that tissue allowed to die in distilled water retained 16% of its dehydrogenase activity after 24 hr. In a further experiment we compared the dehydrogenase activity and uridine uptake at 24 and 72 hr of culture (Fig. 2). Although the dehydrogenase activity remained relatively constant throughout this period, the uridine uptake, which is an established index of metabolic activity, fell significantly. We interpret this as an indication that the enzyme can be retained in stable form within dead and senescent cells, a finding which reinforces Yagil and Feldman's (1969) work on enzyme stability *in vitro*. This raises doubts about the sensitivity of pentose shunt dehydrogenase activity as an indicator of short term metabolic changes.

From this series we have also concluded that the hormonal effects which occur in 24 to 72-hr cultures are too small to be reliably detected by the techniques applied here.

Possibly cell suspension cultures assessed in terms of thymidine incorporation into DNA as used by Burstein *et al.* (1971) and Aspegren and Hakansson (1974), may eventually yield more satisfactory results. It is likely that as techniques in xenografting human tumours into experimental animals improve, this may provide a method of long-term tissue culture which will prove of considerable value in the development of predictive tests.

REFERENCES

Aspegren, K. and Hakansson, L. (1974). *Acta Chir. Scand. 140*, 95.
Barker, J. R. and Richmond, C. (1971). *Br. J. Surgery, 58*, 732.
Burstein, N. A., Kjellberg, R. N., Raker, J. W. and Schmidek, H. H. (1971). *Cancer, 27*, 1112.
Chayen, J., Altmann, F. P., Bitensky, L. and Daly, J. R. (1970). *Lancet, i*, 868.
Forrest, A. P. M. (1969). *In* "Recent Advances in Surgery", Churchill-Livingstone, p. 84.
Pearse, A. G. E. (1972). *In* "Histochemistry", Vol. II, Churchill-Livingstone Chap. 20.
Ratzkowski, E., Adler, B. and Hochman, A. (1973). *Oncology, 28*, 385.
Riley, P. A., Latter, T. and Sutton, P. M. (1973). *Lancet, ii*, 818.
Salih, H., Flax, H. and Hobbs, J. R. (1972a). *Lancet, i*, 1198.
Salih, H., Flax, H., Hobbs, J. R. and Brander, W. (1972b). *Lancet, ii*, 1103.
Salih, H., Flax, H., Hobbs, J. R. and Newman, K. A. (1973). *Lancet, i*, 1204.
Stoll, B. A. (1970). *Cancer, 25*, 1228.
Willcox, P. A. and Thomas, G. H. (1972). *Br. J. Cancer, 26*, 453.
Yagil, G. and Feldman, M. (1969). *Exp. Cell Res. 54*, 29.

5. The Limitations of Progesterone Sensitivity Testing of Endometrial Carcinoma Using Organ Culture

E. I. Kohorn

In 1968 Kohorn and Tchao (1968) reported a study of the effect of progesterone on endometrial carcinoma using organ culture. The results were similar to those of Nordqvist (1964) and demonstrated a frequent enhancing effect when low doses of progesterone were used, while large doses caused necrosis of the tumour cells. Nordqvist subsequently expanded his studies using uptake of tritiated uridine and thymidine (Nordqvist, 1970). Tumours were obtained by endometrial biopsy or at hysterectomy at the time of definitive therapy. The tissue was cut into pieces 1 mm^3 and these were placed on millipore paper, on 2% agar enriched with 10% calf serum. Progesterone at a concentration of 10 μg or 50 μg per ml was added

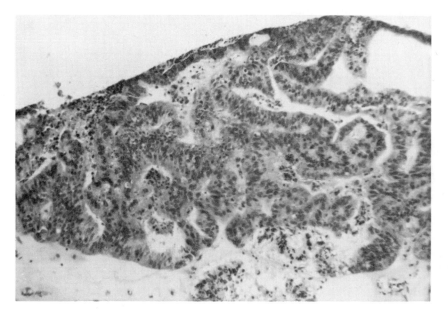

Fig. 1. An endometrial carcinoma in culture with a low concentration of progesterone (10 μg/ml).

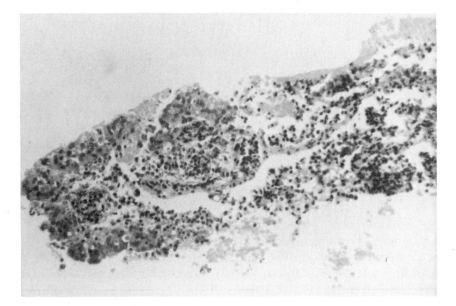

Fig. 2. At a higher concentration of progesterone (50 μg/ml) a culture from the specimen shown in Fig. 1 is destroyed.

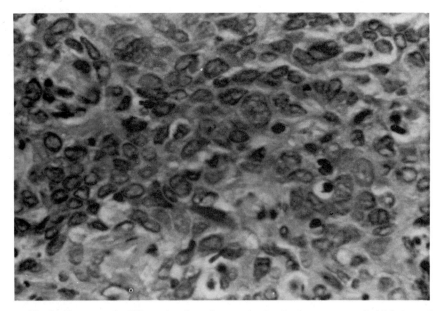

Fig. 3. For a poorly differentiated carcinoma growing in the presence of a high dose of progesterone, the appearance is similar to that of the original tissue and the control culture.

to the medium. The cultures were sustained in 95% oxygen and 5% CO_2 for 48-72 hr and then fixed in Bouin's fluid and stained with H and E with Periodic acid Schiff and assessed by light microscopy.

Figure 1 shows an endometrial carcinoma in culture with a low concentration of progesterone (10 μg per ml). The appearance is not significantly different from that of the control culture or the original biopsy. With a higher dose of progesterone (50 μg per ml) the culture is destroyed (Fig. 2). Figure 3 shows a poorly differentiated carcinoma growing in the presence of a high dose of progesterone and the appearance is similar to that of the original tissue and the control culture, demonstrating that high dose progesterone does not affect this poorly differentiated endometrial carcinoma in culture.

Biopsies from 46 patients have now been placed in organ culture. In 3 cases the patient had had radium application previously and none of these cultures survived. In 12 patients the original tissue was necrotic and none of the cultured tissue survived. Most of these patients had had previous diagnostic curettages or out-patient biopsies before the biopsy for culture was obtained. In five patients the cultured tissue did not survive. Thus only 26 cultures could be assessed. Among these, 5 showed necrosis with progesterone at both high and low concentrations, 6 showed necrosis with high dose progesterone and 15 showed no significant effect in culture.

It would thus appear that the biopsy for culture must be obtained at the time of initial endometrial biopsy, and biopsies obtained subsequent to this provide poor material for organ culture. Also, one must be sure that carcinoma tissue is being cultured, as the site of cancer is frequently focal.

Only one patient of these 46 developed metastases. She had anaplastic tumour and developed cerebral metastases. One other patient did not have an initial hysterectomy and her tumour responded to gestogen both *in vitro* and *in vivo*.

Although the method provides a good investigational tool, its clinical application is limited, because even if good primary biopsies are obtained, so very few of the patients develop metastases that a mass screening programme does not seem to be justified in this disease.

REFERENCES

Kohorn, E. I. and Tchao, R. (1968). *J. Obstet. Gynaec. Br. Commonw.* 75, 1262.

Nordqvist, R. S. B. (1964). *Acta Obstet. Gynaec. Scand.* 43, 296.

Nordqvist, S. (1970). *J. Endocr.* 48, 29.

GENERAL DISCUSSION

Morasca compared Hallowes' culture method with the older method of covering slices with a cellophane strip. This served two functions. One was mechanical, the other was that under a cellophane strip there is better differentiation of tissue with organoid structures and mitoses are very rare. Thus cells can be kept for a long time without significant growth and this may be very important for tumours, since we know a lot about growing cancer cells but very little about cancer cells in the resting stage.

Hallowes said in some cell systems, particularly in the rat mammary gland, when cells are cultured on sheets of polyester melinex, the melinex tends to float in the medium. Cells often get underneath the sheet and the cells that grow best are those trapped between the melinex and the bottom of the dish. Similar effects may occur in the comparison of small slices of tumour which have been stretched, or compressed very slightly under the dialysis tubing and pieces that are allowed to attach without compression to the base of the petri dish. The dialysis tubing is used to stop the pieces of tissue floating about; coating the bottom piece of glass in the Rose chamber with collagen might be an alternative way to help the attachment of pieces of tissue.

Hallowes continued that the surface of the medium should be just over the top of the slice so that surface tension effects hold it in place. In most incubators a very small amount of vibration from a fan, or vibrations in the room, keep the piece of tissue just hovering. Cells may then fall out and grow, but the substructure of the piece of tissue may be lost.

The question of cellular growth in these pieces of tissue is important, particularly if one wishes to do work similar to Armelin *et al.* (1974) who have added hormones sequentially to the totally resting population of cells. This has worked with the rat dimethyl benzanthracene system, so it should be possible in the human system when the technology has been worked out.

Prop said they found that in CMA mouse mammary gland cultures, prolactin activity was enhanced by additional growth hormone only at low doses of prolactin. At higher doses of prolactin they saw no effect (Fig. 1). Hallowes added that in normal mammary glands in organ culture neither prolactin nor growth hormone on their own has any effect on DNA synthesis, RNA synthesis or protein synthesis. They are equally effective as far as the synthesis of milk proteins, milk sugars and milk fats are concerned and this is not due to contamination of the growth hormone by prolactin and vice versa. The dose levels are not physiological but it is possible in secondary culture systems to remove the serum and work at physiological levels of hormones. The only problem is that in the Sprague Dawley rat strain physiological levels for circulating prolactin are high, 70-80 ng/ml mean and may rise to 200-300 ng/ml and this is very different from the human situation. In the tumour there was no inhibition and no synergism between growth hormone and prolactin.

In reply to questions about the morphology of the epithelial cells in cultured prostate after hormonal treatment *in vitro*, Riches said reversal of the castration effect with insulin and testosterone can be shown in the rat system, but when androgen support is removed from the BPH cultures the changes are far less marked than with the rat. The difficulty with organ culture is that one observes a proliferative response and changes in differentiation but the interpretation remains a problem. Particularly with the proliferative response it is important to consider non-specific hyperplasia as a possible repair mechanism after trauma.

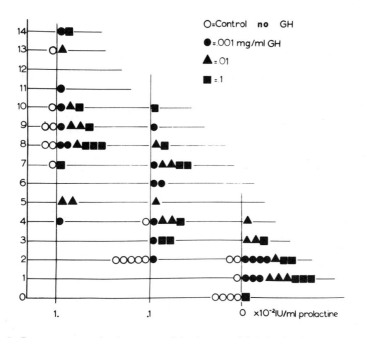

Fig. 1. Response to prolactin expressed in degrees of lobulo-alveolar development in culture for different concentrations of growth hormone (GH). There is an increase in sensitivity to low concentrations of prolactin, independent of the dose of GH used. This shows that the GH effect is not caused by prolactin contamination in the GH preparation (from Prop, 1963).

The presence of an epithelial outgrowth can be demonstrated with some explants. Finally, in any studies of proliferation one must look at the explants histologically. It may be misleading to examine biochemical changes alone and these must be coupled with morphological studies.

Masters said Salih and co-workers (Salih *et al.* 1972*a*, 1972*b*; Flax, 1973; Flax *et al.* 1973) had reported that 50% of 300 human breast tumours were hormone-dependent. However, Beeby, Miss Wilson and he have all had limited success with this particular technique and so far have been unable to demonstrate consistent quantitative differences, certainly not in a high percentage of the tumours. Miss Wilson suggested that a possible explanation for the lack of success with Salih and Flax's method may lie in a technical variable noted in Sheffield with regard to section thickness. The H and E sections on the duplicate slides can often be seen to be of different thicknesses, despite being cut at a nominal 8μ. Obviously the estimation of the amount of dye deposited will depend on the thickness of section. Because this variable would come to light if multiple sections were cut from each block, a quantitative study was done on multiple, theoretically identical sections, using a Quantimet 720. It was

9*

found that very large differences in optical density occurred between sections from the same block; thus a specimen that was visually assessed as testosterone and prolactin dependent was found to be independent, with no significant difference between blocks incubated in different hormones, when measured quantitatively. Bondy added that most clinical data have suggested that not more than a third of patients respond to hormonal manipulation, so a figure of 50% seems a bit high.

Bondy continued that the oestrogen binding data seem to be quite accurate in predicting those tumours which will not respond and the response rate of the operated or manipulated group is enriched perhaps two or threefold, if this information is available as compared to making decisions at random. The question of whether this is a practical thing to do is another matter.

Kohorn said another useful system is the combination of organ culture with electron microscopy. An organ culture was developed to test the effect of progestational agents in endometrial carcinoma (Kohorn and Tchao, 1968). Electron microscopy was then added to study the organelle changes caused by the effect of progestational agents on normal endometrium *in vitro* (Kohorn *et al.* 1970). Figure 2 shows an electronmicrograph of a nucleolar cannalicular system induced by progesterone in normal late proliferative endometrium in

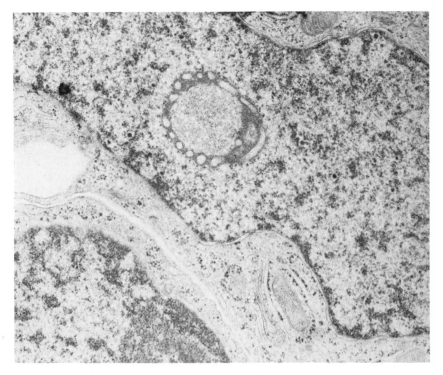

Fig. 2. Electron micrograph of a nucleolar cannalicular system induced by progesterone in normal late proliferative endometrium in organ culture.

organ culture. The steroid characteristics in the progesterone molecule responsible for this cannalicular system, have been defined (Kohorn *et al.* 1972). Only
progestational agents with an acyl, CH_3-CO-, group in the 17β position will
produce nucleolar differentiation. The substituted 19-nor-testosterone progestational steroids, which form the basis of most contraceptive pills, will not do so,
although these still produce glycogen and giant mitochondria. Further studies
with well differentiated endometrial carcinoma exposed to progesterone both *in
vivo* and *in vitro* have so far failed to show an effect.

Hallowes said that workers in the San Francisco Medical Centre had studied
breast cancer using organ culture and hormones and had analysed the results by
electron microscopic examination. They have no evidence so far of any change
in morphology that could be correlated with a hormone effect in the manner
described by Kohorn for endometrial carcinoma.

In summarising the session, Bondy considered the problem not as an
oncologist, but as an endocrinologist. He said Prop had put forward a number of
difficult questions which would continue to be difficult questions for some time
to come.

It would indeed be interesting to follow the ability of the cells to produce
certain specific secretions and this ability might be a way to study the effects of
manipulations, hormones or whatever, on the activity of the cells. Unfortunately, most mammary tumours, for example, do not seem to make casein and
probably do not make lactose. However, most cells, tumours included, do make
rather specific cell surface materials and it may be worthwhile to look rather
more widely in our search for markers. We might look for example at the various
mucopolysaccharides and other such substances which form the cell coat and
may be indicators of the state of health or disease of the cell.

Another point about the use of endocrines is that it is terribly seductive to
put cells into some sort of isolated test system, subject them to the influence of
a variety of endocrine or other types of substance, and deduce from this whether
or not these substances will work in patients with the particular tumour being
studied. Care is required in interpreting the results of *in vitro* work because of
the complex nature of the action of many of the substances studied, including
the endocrines, on other parts of the body besides the tumour. For example,
consider the ability of androgens to interfere with the formation of the nipple
connection in the embryonic mouse. Normally there is a bud of mammary tissue
which attaches to the nipple at the embryo surface, and when at a certain stage
in development, testosterone enters the system, this nipple pinches off and loses
its connection with the mammary anlage. As a result the male mouse does not
have a connection between the nipple and the mammary gland. This is quite a
specific reaction and occurs at a quite specific time in the development of the
animal. Testosterone itself is highly active in this system, more active than
dihydrotestosterone, and this is most surprising because the general feeling
among endocrinologists has been that before it can act, testosterone must be
reduced to dihydrotestosterone. The moral of this is that we may not know
what form of hormone to use in our tests. We may think we know what the
active form of a hormone is, but it may be that in a particular system, for
example, a cancer, what we consider to be an active form may be inactive. It is
dogma, for example, that you must have an 11β-hydroxyl group on a
corticosteroid to make it act. Substances such as cortisone are believed to be
totally inactive until they are activated in the liver for example, and yet we are
not aware that anybody has actually tested this in tissue cultures of cancer cells.

Although there is no evidence, maybe *in vitro* cortisone is much more active than hydrocortisone. This kind of thing must concern us if we try to translate what we know about the intact animal or about normal tissues to a discussion of abnormal tissues.

Thirdly, the effects of hormones may not be exerted on the tumour directly but by their ability to call forth some other response. For example, the effects of oestrogens on the secretion of prolactin may be important in treating mammary carcinoma and it is possible that the major effect of oestrogen *in vivo* is through this mechanism; but the ability of oestrogens to call forth or suppress prolactin varies in different species so that generalisations made from rats and mice may not be applicable to human beings.

The fourth thing causing confusion is the precise composition of the tissue culture. We really do not know what is put into these systems for two reasons. First there is very good evidence that some breast tumours, for example, are capable of forming oestrogens from cholestrol which means they are capable of forming oestrogens from acetate, which means that you cannot set up a totally oestrogen-free system. The amount of oestrogen formed during *in vitro* studies is very small (Miller and Forrest, 1974) but if it is formed at just the right place in the cell the local concentration might be adequate to produce an effect. Thus one must worry about whether a system set up in the absence of exogenous oestrogen is really oestrogen-free as far as the internal cellular milieu is concerned. Although this type of information is available for oestrogens, the situation with respect to other hormones is not known. So the question of whether the tumours are producing growth substances which affect them and which are, in a sense, autostimulatory, would be difficult to determine though it might alter seriously the results of our experiments. Secondly, granted that it is difficult to grow mammary tumours in tissue culture under any conditions, it is very much more difficult to grow them in the absence of added serum or comparable biological material. The type of biological material that is added may be very important. Serum contains some hormones, some steroids, perhaps some amino acid hormones such as thyroxin and certainly some polypeptide materials. In addition, there is evidence now that bovine serum has a very active growth factor for breast tumours *in vitro* although apparently calf serum does not. This point has no specific value here but indicates how difficult it is to know what we are doing when, in order to get any kind of activity in these systems, we have to add materials of unknown composition which may in themselves be far more powerful than any of the known materials we are testing in our experiments.

It is not a gloomy prospect but there is a long road ahead before we are really ready to get the answers we would like today.

REFERENCES

Armelin, H. A., Nichikawa, K. and Sato, G. H. (1974). *In* "Control of Proliferation in Animal Cells" (Clarkson and Baserga, eds.). Cold Spring Harbour Symposium.

Flax, H. (1973). *Brit. J. Surgery, 60,* 317.

Flax, H., Salih, H., Newton, K. A. and Hobbs, J. R. (1973). *Lancet, i,* 1204.

Kohorn, E. I. and Tchao, R. (1968). *J. Obstet. Gynaec. Br. Commonw. 75,* 1262.

Kohorn, E. I., Rice, S. I. and Gordon, M. (1970). *Nature, Lond. 228*, 671.
Kohorn, E. I., Rice, S. I., Hemperly, S. and Gordon, M. (1972). *J. Clin. Endocr. Met. 34*, 257.
Miller, W. R. and Forrest, A. P. M. (1974). *Lancet, ii*, 866.
Prop, F. J. A. (1963). *Acta Physiol. Pharmacol. Neerlandica, 12*, 172.
Salih, H., Flax, H. and Hobbs, J. R. (1972a). *Lancet, i*, 1198.
Salih, H., Flax, H., Brander, W. and Hobbs, J. R. (1972b). *Lancet, ii*, 1103.

Chapter 6

STUDIES ON THE IMMUNOLOGICAL STATUS OF PATIENTS USING SHORT TERM CULTURES

(Moderator: M. Moore)

1. Immune Reaction Against Human Tumour Cells *In Vitro*

M. J. Embleton

A variety of *in vitro* methods have been used to search for evidence of immunity to human tumours, using both serological techniques and cell-mediated immunity tests. Animal studies involving adoptive transfer of immunity have shown that tumour immunity is principally mediated by lymphoid cells (Klein *et al.* 1960; Old *et al.* 1962), so most interest has centred on assays for cell-mediated immunity. A number of different techniques have been developed, the major ones being leucocyte migration inhibition (Cochran *et al.* 1973), lymphocyte stimulation by mixed culture with tumour cells or "soluble" extracts (Stjernsward *et al.* 1973), and lymphocyte cytotoxicity (Hellström *et al.* 1971; Fossati *et al.* 1972, De Vries *et al.* 1972, Baldwin *et al.* 1973*a*, O'Toole *et al.* 1973).

Cytotoxicity tests depend upon the use of cultured tumour target cells. In recent years a number of long-term cell lines have been established, but most published studies have used short-term cultures (Hellström *et al.* 1971, Fossati *et al.* 1972, De Vries *et al.* 1972, Baldwin *et al.* 1973*a*). This paper describes some immunological studies carried out using short-term cultures of human tumours using a microcytotoxicity test based on the method developed originally by Hellström *et al.* (1971).

A. METHODS

1. TARGET CELLS

Monolayer cell cultures were established from surgically removed specimens of solid tumours and from suspended cells present in malignant effusions. Solid tumours were finely minced and suspended in culture medium, and fragments were allowed to settle so that the cell-rich supernatants could be decanted off. The remaining fragments were washed in Hank's balanced salt solution and treated with 0·25% trypsin or a mixture of 0·1% collagenase and 0·1% hyaluronidase at 37°C, to release further cells. Cells from malignant effusions were harvested by centrifugation and suspended in culture medium.

Cells were plated in plastic or glass bottles and allowed to form confluent monolayers, and were subsequently subcultured with 0·25% trypsin and passaged for between 2 and 5 generations. The media used were Hamm's F10 supplemented with 20% foetal calf serum for carcinomas of colon and rectum, and Waymouth's MB 752/1 with 20% foetal calf serum for other tumours which included melanoma, mesothelioma, and carcinomas of breast, pancreas and bronchus. Penicillin (200 IU/ml) and streptomycin (100 μg/ml) were used in all media.

2. MICROCYTOTOXICITY TEST

The basic technique is summarised in Fig. 1. Cultured cells were plated at 200 in 0·2 ml of medium per well, in Falcon 3040 plates or Cooke Microtiter plates. After 4 to 24 hr incubation at 37°C to allow cells to attach to the bottoms of the wells, the medium was replaced by 5×10^4 or 10^5 peripheral lymphocytes in 0·2 ml of

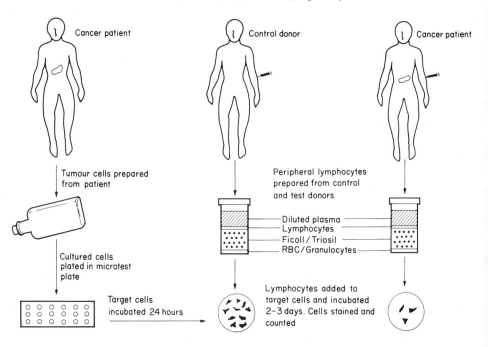

Fig. 1. Microcytotoxicity test for demonstration of lymphocyte cytotoxicity against human tumour cells.

serum free medium. The lymphocytes were prepared by centrifugation on gradients of Ficoll (6·35%) and Triosil (13·4%) as described previously (Baldwin *et al.* 1973*a*). After 45 min 0·1 ml of 50% foetal calf serum in medium was added and the cells were cultured for a further 2 days. Lymphocytes and dead cells were gently rinsed off and the remaining cells fixed and stained with Giemsa or crystal violet. Percentage cytotoxicity was calculated by the following formula:

$$\frac{\text{Mean No. of cells in wells treated with control lymphocytes} - \text{Mean No. of cells in wells treated with patients lymphocytes}}{\text{Mean No. of cells in wells treated with control lymphocytes}} \times 100\%$$

All results were evaluated statistically by the Student "t" test.

In some experiments the effector cells (both test and control) were pretreated with varying amounts of soluble tumour membrane extracts for 45 min, then centrifuged and resuspended in fresh medium before being added to the target cells. The soluble extracts were prepared by limited papain digestion of crude cell membranes followed by DEAE cellulose chromatography as previously described (Baldwin *et al.* 1973*b*) using methods developed for experimental rat hepatomas (Baldwin *et al.* 1973*c*).

B. RESULTS AND DISCUSSION

Details of experiments performed with two mammary carcinoma cultures are shown in Table 1. In both cases one sample of patients' lymphocytes reduced the number of target cells compared with

TABLE 1

Cell-mediated Cytotoxicity against Mammary Carcinomas M4 and M5

Target cells	Lymphocyte donor	No. cells after exposure to lymphocytes from:		Percentage cytotoxicity	$P <$
		Control	Patient		
M4	M4	42·1 ± 4·4	51·1 ± 4·5	−21·4	
M4	M4	97·5 ± 5·4	93·5 ± 7·7	4·1	0·35
M4	M5	97·5 ± 5·4	82·0 ± 5·3	15·9	0·05
M5	M4	50·0 ± 4·7	38·1 ± 3·6	23·7	0·05
M5	M5	50·0 ± 4·7	46·2 ± 5·4	7·5	0·35
M5	M5	24·6 ± 3·0	24·7 ± 3·1	−0·5	

control lymphocytes, but the other sample allowed equal or greater target cell survival than control lymphocytes. In both cases the "positive" results occurred when the patient donors were tested against a mammary carcinoma other than their own tumour. This raises the possibility that the patients' lymphocytes might be reacting against alloantigens in the allogeneic target cells, and illustrates one problem of interpretation which sometimes occurs with cytotoxicity tests. However, this fortunately does not appear to be a common problem as discussed below.

Another problem experienced with some target cells is an apparent lack of reactivity by patients, or perhaps an equal non-specific reactivity by control donors which masks the reactivity of cancer patients. Reports of reactivity by controls are somewhat variable and perhaps depend mainly on the type of cytotoxicity test employed, some methods of evaluation giving less specificity than others (Takasugi, 1973). An example of some studies showing apparent lack of reactivity by patients is shown in Table 2 which gives the mean numbers of mesothelioma target cells surviving after treatment with lymphocytes from patients who had been exposed to atmospheric asbestos particles. In five tests involving six separate groups of controls or patients with different pathological conditions, three results stand out as being significantly different from the others. These donors were a normal donor, and patients with asbestosis and pleural thickening. These figures are part of a larger study on mesothelioma cells in which about 10% of donors overall had lymphocytes which reduced target cell survival compared with others in the series or compared with medium controls, with no increased reactivity by mesothelioma patients. All lymphocytes were allogeneic with respect to the target cells, so the low overall rate of reactivity suggests that responses directed against alloantigens are not common. Also, donors giving low target cell survival equally affected all target cells they were tested against, so perhaps even with these donors alloantigens were not involved.

More successful results were obtained with studies on carcinoma of colon and rectum. Table 3 summarises results of 46 tests carried out with lymphocytes from colon carcinoma patients applied to allogeneic colon carcinoma target cells. Patients with growing tumours were positive in 18/30 tests, and those who had undergone surgical resection of their tumour 2 to 6 days previously reacted in 11/16 cases. Thus, there was no significant difference between the two groups, and together they showed a reactivity by 60% of patients. In two cases target cells survived better after treatment with

TABLE 2

Cell-mediated Cytotoxicity against Mesothelioma Cells by Patients with
Various Pathological Symptoms Following Asbestos Exposure

Group No.	Target cells	No. of target cells surviving with lymphocytes from patients with diagnosis:					
		Normal	Control	Asbestosis	Pleural thickening	Pleural plaques	Mesothelioma
1	MES-10B	26 ± 3	14 ± 5	35 ± 6	7 ± 1	34 ± 4	39 ± 6
	MES-SK	327 ± 11	322 ± 18	294 ± 8	183 ± 8	275 ± 11	258 ± 14
2	MES-12	33 ± 2	21 ± 3	5 ± 1	39 ± 3*	26 ± 2	37 ± 1
	MES-SK	77 ± 5	75 ± 4	43 ± 3	72 ± 5*	75 ± 2	80 ± 4
3	MES-10B	NT	62 ± 8	70 ± 4	43 ± 6	62 ± 5	54 ± 6
	MES-SK	NT	52 ± 1	68 ± 1	41 ± 2	70 ± 1	68 ± 2
4	MES-22	10 ± 1	10 ± 2	10 ± 1	10 ± 1	9 ± 1	10 ± 1
	MES-25	17 ± 1	16 ± 1	12 ± 1	10 ± 1	5 ± 1	9 ± 1
5	MES-21	13 ± 1	38 ± 2	29 ± 2	42 ± 2	45 ± 1	43 ± 1
	MES-22	11 ± 1	41 ± 3	41 ± 2	40 ± 1	49 ± 2	42 ± 2
	MES-26	9 ± 1	23 ± 1	23 ± 2	22 ± 1	26 ± 1	24 ± 2
	MES-SK	1 ± 1	32 ± 1	30 ± 1	66 ± 1	64 ± 2	65 ± 2

* Pleural fibrosis
Underlined values in this and subsequent tables are statistically significant

TABLE 3

*Cell-mediated Immunity Against Human
Colon and Rectum Carcinomas*

Target cell line	No. of positive reactions by lymphocytes prepared from patients:	
	Pre-operatively	Post-operatively
REC-1	1/3	1/2
REC-2	1/3	
REC-4	2/2	0/1
REC-6	0/2	1/1
DAC-3	3/3	
CO1	2/2	
CO3	2/5	1/2
CO4	0/1	
CO14	2/3	3/4
CO15	1/1	1/2
CO16		2/2
CO17	1/1	1/1
CO20	3/4	1/1
Total positive	18/30	11/16

patients' lymphocytes than controls, and in the remaining 15/46 tests there was no significant difference between patients or controls. It was not possible to determine whether the lack of difference in the latter group could be ascribed to unresponsiveness of patients, or high reactivity by controls.

Table 4 summarises cross-tests between colon carcinoma patients and cells from carcinomas of other organs, and between patients with

TABLE 4

Cross-tests Between Colon Carcinomas and Carcinomas of Other Organs

Target cells	Lymphocytes from donors with carcinoma of:	No. of positive reactions
Breast Carcinoma M18	Colon	0/1
Pancreatic Carcinoma Ca-1	Colon	0/2
Bronchial Carcinoma Lu-2	Colon	0/2
Colon Carcinoma Co14	Breast	0/3
Colon Carcinoma Co15	Breast/Lung	0/3
Colon Carcinoma Co17	Breast, Kidney	0/2
Colon Carcinoma Co20	Lung	0/1
Normal Colon HC-1	Colon	0/5
Normal Colon HC-1	Breast, Kidney	0/2

carcinomas of different organs and colon carcinoma target cells. No instances of cross-reaction were observed; however not all the patients tested were reactive against their own tumour type. Thus the data are not extensive or convincing enough to confirm the claimed tissue-type specificity of human tumour-associated antigens (Hellström *et al.* 1971) but they do show that cancer patients are not reacting against histocompatibility antigens on the target cells. This is further supported by data in Table 5 showing that prior blood

TABLE 5

Effect of Prior Blood Transfusion on Cell-mediated Cytotoxicity against Colon Carcinoma Cells

Effect of patients' lymphocytes	*No transfusion*	*Post- transfusion*
Cytotoxicity	19/34	8/12
No difference	13/34	4/12
Enhancement	2/34	0/12

transfusion does not markedly affect the cytotoxicity of colon carcinoma patients' lymphocytes for allogeneic colon carcinoma cells. Since transfused patients might reasonably be expected to become sensitised to histocompatibility antigens, these do not appear to be important in the microcytotoxicity test as described, so the test is probably measuring reactivity directed towards tumour-associated antigens (Hellström *et al.* 1971).

Having established a system for detecting tumour-directed immunity in a significant proportion of patients, experiments were designed to test the effect of solubilised tumour antigen preparations. Both patients and control lymphocytes were pretreated with varying amounts of soluble membrane extracts of colon carcinoma, normal colon mucosa or melanoma before being applied to colon carcinoma target cells. Pretreatment with these extracts had no effect on control lymphocytes, but as seen in Fig. 2 patients' lymphocytes were progressively inhibited following incubation with increasing amounts of colon carcinoma extracts (Colon carcinoma-1 and Colon carcinoma-2) prepared from pooled surgical specimens. Extracts of normal colon mucosa (Normal colon-1) or melanoma (Melanoma-16) had no effect on cytotoxicity by patients' lymphocytes. A third extract (Colon carcinoma-3) prepared from 6 hr post-mortem colon carcinoma metastases also inhibited specific cytotoxicity (Fig. 3) but had no effect on control lymphocytes. To

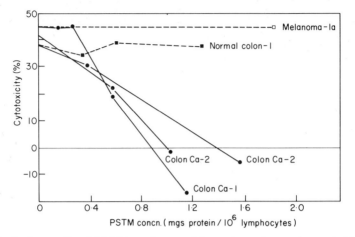

Fig. 2. Antigen-mediated inhibition of cytotoxicity against colon carcinoma Co14 cells.

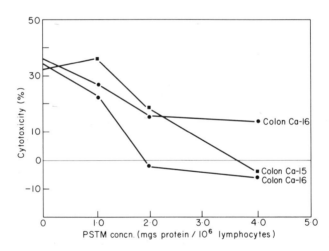

Fig. 3. Inhibition of cytotoxicity against colon carcinoma cells by antigen prepared from post-mortem derived metastatic colon carcinoma.

confirm the specificity of lymphocyte inhibition by colon carcinoma extracts, further experiments showed that the melanoma extract could inhibit melanoma patients' reactivity against auto-chthonous melanoma cells, but colon carcinoma preparations had no effect in the melanoma system (Fig. 4). Thus, the inhibitory effect seems to be associated with tumour antigen, at least by comparison between colon carcinoma and melanoma. In the case of colon carcinoma extracts, the inhibitory activity did not correlate with

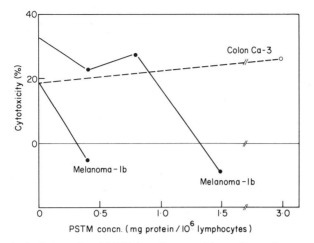

Fig. 4. Antigen-mediated inhibition of cytotoxicity against melanoma cells.

carcinoembryonic antigen (CEA) content since the ability to impair cytotoxicity was lowest in the post-mortem preparation (Colon Ca-3) which contained the most CEA (Table 6).

To characterise the antigen responsible for inhibition of lymphocyte cytotoxicity against colon carcinoma cells further, crude

TABLE 6

Lymphocyte Inhibitory Activity and Carcinoembryonic Antigen in Colon Carcinoma Extracts

Extract	Neutralisation index *	CEA (μg)
COLON Ca-1	0·5-1·0	>1·0
COLON Ca-2	1·0-1·5	8-12
COLON Ca-3	2·0-4·0	50-100

* mg protein required to neutralise 10^6 sensitised lymphocytes.

extracts were fractionated on Sephadex G200 to yield 4 fractions. Two of these fractions retained inhibitory activity (Table 7). One was a fraction of between 30,000 and 100,000 daltons containing the least amount of CEA but the most protein, and the other was a fraction greater than 150,000 daltons which had a small protein concentration but probably contained most of the CEA judging by its molecular weight. These data indicate that effective lymphocyte

TABLE 7

Inhibition of Lymphocyte Cytotoxicity against Colon Carcinoma Co 20 by Sephadex G 200 Antigen Fractions.

Fraction No.	Protein[1] concn.	CEA[2] concn.	Molecular wt. range $(\times 10^{-3})$	Percent cytotoxicity	Percent inhibition
None				37·6	
1	0·15	0·65	<30	25·6	32·0
2	3·00	0·40	30-100	0	100
3	1·50	0·92	100-150	25·2	32·9
4	0·50	ND	>150	6·7	82·1

[1] mg per 10^6 lymphocytes   [2] μg per 10^6 lymphocytes

inhibition was correlated neither with CEA nor simply the amount of "non-specific" protein. Further proof of the non-involvement of CEA is shown in Table 8 where purified CEA used at the same concentrations as present in the active unfractionated antigen had no effect on cytotoxicity. It is concluded, therefore, that these assays

TABLE 8

Effect of Purified CEA on Lymphocyte Cytotoxicity against Colon Carcinoma Cells.

Material tested	Concentration $(\mu g/10^6$ lymphocytes)	Percent cytotoxicity	Percent inhibition
NONE		22·8	
CEA	50	27·7	0
NONE		59·0	
CEA	100	66·0	0
NCA	100	61·2	0

detected a colon carcinoma-associated antigen which was distinct from CEA. Hollinshead *et al.* (1972) similarly concluded that colon carcinoma antigen eliciting delayed-type hypersensitivity in colon cancer patients was distinct from CEA, although probably still being an embryonic antigen (Hollishead *et al.* 1970) as previously suggested by Hellström *et al.* (1970).

In summary, it can be stated that the demonstration of cell-mediated immunity against human tumours using short-term cultures has problems of interpretation and problems of poor reactivity or specificity. In spite of this, however, it is possible to detect reactions against antigens associated with certain tumours, and by the use of inhibition tests to show specificity and partially characterise the antigens involved. The relevance to host immunity of the *in vitro* reactions has yet to be proven, but there is little doubt that their measurement is a valid phenomenon and represents a useful application of short-term cultures of human tumour cells.

ACKNOWLEDGEMENTS

Antigen extracts were prepared by Dr. M. R. Price, and CEA assays were performed by arrangement with Professor A. M. Neville. Purified CEA was provided by Dr. P. Burtin. This work was supported by the Cancer Research Campaign.

REFERENCES

Baldwin, R. W., Embleton, M. J., Jones, J. S. P. and Langman, M. J. S. (1973a). *Int. J. Cancer, 12*, 73.

Baldwin, R. W., Embleton, M. J. and Price, M. R. (1973b). *Int. J. Cancer, 12*, 84.

Baldwin, R. W., Harris, J. R. and Price, M. R. (1973c). *Int. J. Cancer, 11*, 385.

Cochran, A. J., Mackie, R. N., Thomas, C. E., Grant, R. M., Cameron-Mowat, D. E. and Spilg, W. G. S. (1973). *Br. J. Cancer, 28*, 77.

De Vries, J. E., Rümke, P. and Bernhein, J. L. (1972). *Int. J. Cancer, 9*, 567.

Fossati, G., Canevari, S., Della Porta, G., Balzarini, G. P. and Veronesi, U. (1972). *Int. J. Cancer, 10*, 371.

Hellström, I., Hellström, K. E. and Shepard, T. H. (1970). *Int. J. Cancer, 6*, 346.

Hellström, I., Hellström, K. E., Sjögren, H. O. and Warner, G. A. (1971). *Int. J. Cancer, 7*, 1.

Hollinshead, A., Glew, D., Bunnag, B., Gold, P. and Herberman, R. (1970). *Lancet, i*, 1191.

Hollinshead, A. C., McWright, C. G., Alford, T. C., Glew, D. H., Gold, P. and Herberman, R. B. (1972). *Science, N.Y. 177*, 887.

Klein, G., Sjögren, H. O., Klein, E. and Hellström, K. E. (1960). *Cancer Res. 20*, 1561.

Old, L. J., Boyse, E. A., Clarke, D. A. and Carswell, E. A. (1962). *Ann. N.Y. Acad. Sci. 101*, 80.

O'Toole, C., Perlmann, P., Unsgaard, B., Moberger, G. and Edsmyr, F. (1972). *Int. J. Cancer, 10*, 77.

Stjernswärd, J., Vanky, R. and Klein, E. (1973). *Br. J. Cancer, 28*, 72.

Takasugi, M., Mickey, M. R. and Terasaki, P. I. (1973). *Cancer Res. 33*, 2898.

DISCUSSION

Moore said that in studies of the cytotoxicity of peripheral blood lymphocytes from over 2,000 patients, Takasugi *et al.* (1973) had found that cytotoxicity was greater among normal individuals than it was among tumour bearing patients, not only for short term human cultures derived from various tumour types but for long term cell lines as well.

Embleton said these workers used smaller tissue culture plates called "Terasaki plates" which do give poorer specificity than the bigger plates used in the work he described. Also they compared lymphocyte treated wells with control wells containing medium alone. If any lymphocytes at all are added to the target cells in "Terasaki plates" there is decreased target cell survival compared with medium alone controls. However, if a series of lymphocyte donors is compared with each other rather than with medium controls, the reactivity is much less than the region of 100% which Takasugi et al. claim. Opinion varies on long term and short term cultures. Some groups using both believe that long term cultures result in less specificity than short term cultures, other groups say there is really no difference between them.

In reply to Mehrishi, Embleton said that all studies so far had been done on unfractionated cells. Attempts were now being made to fractionate human lymphocytes for these studies using several methods, including nylon columns and glass bead columns either uncoated or immunoglobulin coated. He continued that experiments with rat cells have shown that the killer cells are in the T cell population, rather than the B cell.

Replying to Moore who asked if the in vitro reactions gave tumour specificity as distinct from organ specificity, Embleton said they had not looked at enough normal tissues or embryonic tissues of various organs to say anything about organ specificity. As for tumour specificity the only instance where any specificity can be claimed is in the inhibition assays. There appears to be specificity at least between colon carcinoma and melanoma which may or may not be organ related. In experimental rat studies there does seem to be an organ specific embryonic antigen in mammary carcinoma.

Vose said they had taken peripheral blood leucocytes from patients with lung tumours in much the same way as Embleton had described, and tested them for cytotoxicity against a range of target cells derived from the lung (Table 0). A positive response indicated a statistically significant reduction of target cell survival compared with leucocytes from healthy donors. When these leucocytes were tested for cytotoxicity against normal lung cultures, 42% of the tests were positive although there was a wide spread for different cultures from 20% to 70%. The lung tumour patients' leucocytes showed a low reactivity to cells derived from malignancies other than the lung, but a very high reactivity for

TABLE 1

*Evidence for Organ-Related Cell Mediated Cytotoxicity in
Human Pulmonary Neoplasia**

Target cells	Leucocyte donor	Positive tested
Lung Tumour	Lung Tumour	65/79 (73%)
Lung Tumour	Malignant Condition	7/17 (41%)
Lung Tumour	Non-malignant Conditions	4/14 (29%)
Normal Lung	Lung Tumour	11/26 (42%)
Non Lung Malignancy	Lung Tumour	8/43 (18%)
13-14 week foetal lung	Lung Tumour	19/22 (86%)

* Adapted from Vose, Moore and Jack (1975).

foetal lung cells. In this situation part of the reactivity may be directed against normal lung components rather than against the tumour specific component and the leucocyte toxicity may be organ specific, rather than tumour specific.

REFERENCES

Takasugi, M., Mickey, M. R. and Terasaki, P. I. (1973). *Cancer Res. 33*, 2898.
Vose, B. M., Moore, M. and Jack, G. D. (1975). *Int. J. Cançer. 15*, 308.

2. Isolation of Labelled Glycoproteins from Organ Cultured Carcinoma of the Cervix

A. J. Brockas and G. Wiernik

A. INTRODUCTION

Tumour associated antigens have been demonstrated using cells or solubilised products from biopsies of carcinoma of the cervix by workers using a variety of immunological techniques, viz. lymphocyte mediated cytotoxicity (Vasudevan *et al.* 1970), leukocyte migration inhibition (Goldstein *et al.* 1971) and complement fixation (Hollinshead *et al.* 1972). Other groups (Disaia *et al.* 1971; Byfield *et al.* 1971) have utilised cultured cell lines derived from cervical carcinomas as a target for assessing the immunological potential of circulating lymphocytes and antibodies from patients with active tumour.

The present paper outlines the results of some of our preliminary work into the nature of these antigens and their clinical role, using soluble products from the whole tissue or from short term, 30-hr organ cultures.

B. MATERIALS AND METHODS

A brief outline only of the methods is given here and a more detailed description will be published elsewhere (AJB and GW in preparation).

1. Tissue and Blood Samples

Biopsies of cervical carcinomas were obtained at examination under anaesthesia before any radiotherapy and placed immediately into a holding medium of MEM without leucine (Gibco/Biocult Ltd.) containing Hepes (20 mM), Glutamine (2 mM), Penicillin (500 units/ml), Streptomycin (1 mg/ml) and Gentamycin (80 μg/ml) and Fungizone (5 μg/ml). Biopsies for routine histology were taken at the same time. Biopsies of normal cervix were taken from patients having hysterectomy for non-malignant conditions. Venous blood

(10-12 ml) was obtained from patients before any sedation, anaesthesia or radiotherapy and mixed immediately with a sterile heparin solution (preservative free, a gift from Union International Research Co. Ltd.) to a final concentration of 10 units/ml.

2. Culture of Samples

The procedure is summarised in Fig. 1. After 30 min in the holding medium, blood, mucin and necrotic tissue were removed, the remaining tissue was cut into 2 mm cubes and placed into culture in a medium consisting of MEM without leucine containing Glutamine (2 mM) Penicillin (100 units/ml) and Streptomycin (0·2 mg/ml). The medium and any exfoliated cells were removed after 5 hr and

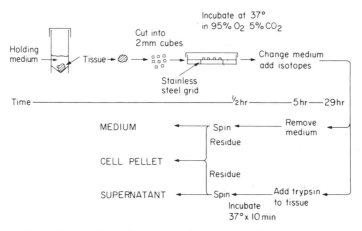

Fig. 1. Organ culture of cervical carcinoma and normal cervix biopsies.

replaced by fresh medium containing $(4, 5-{}^3H)$-leucine (1 μCi/ml), and $(U-{}^{14}C)$-glucosamine (0·4 μCi/ml). Twenty-four hours later the medium was removed, tested for sterility by incubation of an aliquot with dextrose broth and occasionally also with blood agar plates, and dialysed against phosphate buffered saline prior to concentration by ultrafiltration through a UM2 membrane (AMICON Ltd.). The tissue pieces were incubated for 10 min at 37° C with a solution of trypsin (Sigma Grade III, 0·25%) in a Hepes buffered balanced salt solution. The incubation mixture was centrifuged (2,000 g x 10 min) and the supernatant chromatographed on Sephadex G-25 to remove any free radioactive substrates.

3. Extraction of tissue with 3M potassium chloride

The procedure used was essentially that of Reisfeld et al. (1971) and typical yields of 70 μg protein/mg dry tissue were obtained.

4. Lymphocyte transformation assay (Fig. 2)

Lymphocytes, isolated by the Ficoll/Hypaque technique (Böyum, 1968) and washed three times in MEM (calcium and magnesium free)

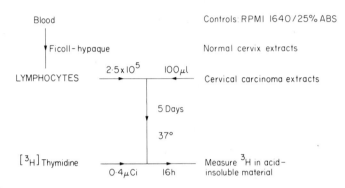

Fig. 2. Lymphocyte transformation procedure.

were re-suspended at 12·5 x 10⁶/ml in RPMI 1640 containing Hepes (20 mM), Glutamine (4 mM), Penicillin (100 units/ml), Streptomycin (0·1 mg/ml) and 25% AB serum, pooled from six male donors who had had no blood transfusions. The viability of the lymphocytes at this stage was always greater than 90% as estimated by Trypan blue exclusion. Cultures were set up in microtiter plates (Linbro 96 FB TC) such that each well had 2·5 x 10⁵ lymphocytes in 120 μl of RPMI 1640/25% AB serum dialysed and concentrated media from cultures of normal or carcinomatous cervical tissue, or 3M potassium chloride extracts of these tissues, at a protein concentration (Folin-Lowry assay—Lowry et al. 1951) of 100-250 μg/ml. Duplicate test wells and eight control wells per lymphocyte donor were used. Tritium incorporation into the TCA insoluble material was measured by scintillation counting in a Packard Liquid Scintillation counter using a Triton/Toluene/PPO/POPOP scintillant (Patterson and Green, 1965). A positive reaction occurs when the mean CPM of the test well pair is greater than that of the control wells (students "t" test p = 0·05).

C. Results and Discussion

The use of short term organ culture in the presence of radioactive substrates enabled us to extract labelled proteins/glycoproteins from normal and carcinomatous cervical biopsies. As (^{14}C)-glucosamine is incorporated mainly into the carbohydrate moieties of glycoproteins (and glycolipids) and (^{3}H) leucine is incorporated mainly into proteins we were able to follow these during gel and ion-exchange chromatography, with a far greater sensitivity than using colorimetric methods. Figures 3 and 4 show the elution profiles on Sephadex G100 of aliquots of the culture medium and trypsin released glycoproteins/peptides (supernatant fraction in Fig. 1) of a squamous cell carcinoma of the cervix. They reveal the presence of a complex mixture of proteins and glycoproteins across a wide molecular weight range.

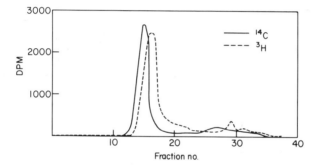

Fig. 3. Fractionation of the culture medium from a squamous cell carcinoma of the cervix on Sephadex G100 showing the activity in disintegrations per minute as a function of fraction number.

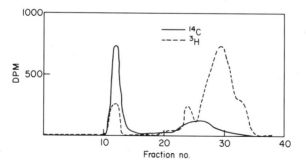

Fig. 4. Fractionation of trypsin released glycopeptides and peptides from a squamous cell carcinoma of the cervix on Sephadex G100.

In order to determine whether tumour associated antigens were present in both the culture medium (Fig. 1) which will contain cellular secretions and shed cell-surface components and in the 3M potassium chloride extracts, we examined the ability of these samples to induce blastogenic transformation of peripheral blood lymphocytes from cervical carcinoma patients. This assay has been used to demonstrate tumour associated antigens in a number of human tumours (Stjernsward *et al.* 1970; Jehn *et al.* 1970; Brooks *et al.* 1972; Gutterman *et al.* 1972; Mavligit *et al.* 1972; Mavligit *et al.* 1973). It is believed (Gutterman *et al.* 1972; Mavligit *et al.* 1972) to represent a secondary response of *in vivo* sensitised lymphocytes upon re-exposure to the appropriate antigen. The results of a preliminary series of experiments are shown in Fig. 5.

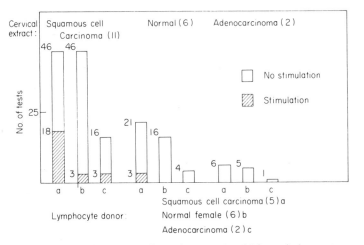

Fig. 5. Results of lymphocyte transformation tests in which cervical extracts were used to try and induce blastogenic transformation of peripheral blood lymphocytes. The highest percentage stimulation (39%) was obtained when both the cervical extract and the lymphocytes came from patients with squamous cell carcinoma.

The proportion of positive responses in lymphocytes from patients with squamous cell carcinoma tested against extracts of squamous cell carcinoma was 18 out of 46, i.e. 39%. This is higher than when lymphocytes from the normal female controls were tested (3 out of 46, i.e. 6·5%). This difference is considered to be consistent with the presence of tumour associated antigens.

That these responses are not due to transplantation antigens is shown by the low proportion of reactions obtained in the control groups of (1) normal lymphocytes versus normal cervix or tumour extracts, and (2) of lymphocytes from carcinoma patients versus normal cervix extracts. These control values make it unlikely that the observed reactions are due to bacterial antigens, unless the cervical bacterial flora of carcinoma patients is qualitatively different from that of the donors of normal cervical tissue and normal lymphocytes. Herpes simplex type II antigens have been detected in cervical carcinoma (Hollinshead *et al.* 1972; Aurelion, 1972) and an etiological role for this virus has been proposed (Aurelion, 1972; Rawls *et al.* 1968; Sabin and Tarro, 1973). Interpretation of our results leads us to the conclusion that we have shown the presence of a tumour specific antigen, though we cannot be categorical concerning the exclusion of Herpes virus involvement. The reactions of lymphocytes from patients with adenocarcinoma against squamous carcinoma extracts may imply the presence of a common tumour antigen. That a larger number of positive responses was not seen may be because too low a concentration of tumour associated antigen was present in some of the extracts. Further work is in progress to extend these results and to localise the antigen in chromatographic fractions.

D. CONCLUSIONS

An organ culture technique has been used which allows the incorporation of radioactive substrates into glycoproteins and proteins of biopsies of carcinoma of the cervix and normal cervix. The presence of incorporated radioactive label greatly facilitated analysis of gel chromatographic fractions.

Tumour associated antigens were demonstrated in extracts from the tumour in 18 out of 46 tests. Control groups showed much lower reactivity.

ACKNOWLEDGEMENTS

This work was supported by the Medical Research Council. Acknowledgements are due to Miss J. M. Huckle, Mrs. J. Edwards and Mrs. E. M. Whitehouse for skilled technical assistance.

REFERENCES

Aurelion, L. (1972). *Fed. Proc. 31*, 1651.
Böyum, A. (1968). *Scand. J. Lab. Invest. 21, Suppl.* 97, 77.
Brooks, W. H., Netsky, M. G., Normansell, D. E. and Horwitz, D. A. (1972). *J. exp. Med. 136*, 1631.
Byfield, J. E., Weintraub, I., Klizak, I. and Lagasse, L. D. (1973). *Radiology, 107*, 685.

Disaia, P. J., Rutledge, F. N., Smith, J. P. and Sinkovics, J. G. (1971). *Cancer*, 28, 1129.

Goldstein, M. S., Shore, B. and Gusberg, S. B. (1971). *Amer. J. Obstet. Gynaec.* 111, 751.

Gutterman, J. U., Mavligit, G. M., McCredie, K. B., Body, G. P., Freireich, E. J. and Hersch, E. M. (1972). *Science, 177*, 1114.

Hollinshead, A., Lee, O. B., McKelway, W., Melnick, J. L. and Rawls, W. E. (1972). *Proc. Soc. exp. Biol. Med. 141*, 688.

Jehn, U. W., Nathanson, L., Schwartz, R. S. and Skinner, M. (1970). *New Eng. J. Med. 136*, 1631.

Lowry, O. H., Rosebrough, N. J., Farr, A. L. and Randall, R. J. (1951). *J. biol. Chem. 193*, 265.

Mavligit, G. M., Gutterman, J. U., McBridge, C. M. and Hersch, E. M. (1972). *Proc. Soc. exp. Biol. Med. 140*, 1240.

Mavligit, G. M., Ambus, U., Gutterman, J. U., Hersch, E. M. and McBride, C. M. (1973). *Nature, Lond. 243*, 188.

Patterson, M. S. and Green, R. C. (1965). *Analyt. Chem. 37*, 854.

Rawls, W. E., Tompkins, W. A. F., Figueroa, M. F. and Melnick, J. L. (1968). *Science, 161*, 1255.

Reisfeld, R. A., Pellegrino, M. A. and Kahan, B. D. (1971). *Science, 172*, 1134.

Sabin, A. B. and Tarro, G. (1973). *P.N.A.S. 70*, 3225.

Stjernsward, J., Almgard, L., Franzen, S., VonSchreeb, T. and Wadstrom, L. B. (1970). *Clin. exp. Immunol. 6*, 963.

Vasudevan, D. M., Balakrishnan, K. and Talwar, G. P. (1970). *Int. J. Cancer, 6*, 506.

DISCUSSION

Kohorn suggested it might be useful to repeat this work allowing less time for blast transformation since even in the presence of non-cancer patient lymphocytes, target cells start being killed after a delay of about three days.

Brockas said if it were a non-specific reaction, a greater degree of reactivity between normal lymphocytes, which came from six donors, against the soluble extracts would be expected. Also certainly with transplanted antigens, the *de novo* reaction against solubilised antigens is less than against the antigen on an intact cell membrane.

Smets commented that depending on the type of trypsin used, as little as 40% of all the relevant material could be removed from the surface, so 10 min at 37°C might not be long enough to remove all the trypsin sensitive glycopeptide. On the other hand if enzymic treatment continued for a longer time the antigen might be destroyed.

Hallowes said it had been shown by Abraham at Oakland (personal communication, 1973) that collagenase will remove the surface antigen of mouse mammary tumours. Brockas said they had not used collagenase and asked if other proteases were present in the collagenase preparation used by Abraham. Hallowes continued that a crude extract of collagenase was used so the presence of protease cannot be excluded. On the other hand, this is not likely to release a virus-induced antigen as has been shown by other workers because virus is probably not excreted in this mouse strain.

3. Assessment of Ovarian Tumour Immunity by Blastogenic Responses to Crude Extracts of Ovarian Tumour Cells

L. Levin, J. E. McHardy, O. M. Curling and C. N. Hudson

We have investigated the cell mediated immune response of ovarian cancer patients by studies of the blastogenic response of cultured lymphocytes to an ovarian cancer cell membrane extract. These extracts were prepared from autologous and from allogeneic cells which came from patients with broadly similar histology.

The cell extract was prepared by rapid homogenisation of fresh tumour material, followed by rapid freezing in liquid nitrogen and finally by the addition of hypotonic saline solution (0·07 M followed by 0·035 M NaCl at 4° C). The pooled supernatants from each stage were centrifuged at 105,000 G and the protein content of the membrane extract estimated by the Lowry technique (Lowry *et al.* 1952). This technique is essentially similar to that developed by Oren and Herberman (1971).

10^6 lymphocytes (prepared by layering over Ficoll-Triosil) were set up in 1 ml cultures in 12% autologous or Foetal Calf Serum (FCS) and challenged with 100 μg of the cell membrane extract (CME). Blastogenesis was assessed by ^{125}IUdR (Iodo-deoxyuridine) incorporation after a 5-day culture. The blastogeneic response to CME was assessed in ovarian cancer patients in remission and relapse. The blastogenic responses in normal controls matched for age and sex were also assessed (Fig. 1).

We found that six out of twelve of the ovarian cancer patients in remission from disease had a blastogenic response to the tumour extracts. None of the patients in relapse demonstrated a blastogenic response to the extracts in autologous serum, but there were slight responses when the lymphocytes were cultured in FCS.

From this data alone, it was not possible to draw any conclusions about the nature of the antigen responsible for this effect and whether it was tumour associated, tumour specific or oncofoetal. The four autologous reactions however, led us to assume that there was an antigenic determinant on the cell membrane to which the patient was sensitised. The allogeneic reactions in the remission

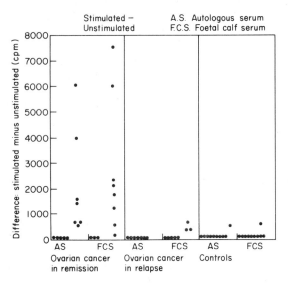

Fig. 1. Blastogenic response to 100 µg ovarian cancer cell membrane extract. The difference in ^{125}IUdR uptake between stimulated and unstimulated cultures is recorded in counts per min. AS = autologous serum; FCS = foetal calf serum.

group, which were not seen in normal controls, supported this hypothesis. It therefore seemed reasonable to attempt to boost this response by immunotherapy.

Accordingly, we initiated a pilot study 8 months ago into the immunotherapy of ovarian cancer and now have three patients in the study. Our protocol consists of innoculating once monthly with 2×10^7 irradiated ovarian cancer cells, stored at $-196°$ C, using BCG as an adjuvant. As we do not feel ethically justified in denying our patients chemotherapy, we are giving them monthly bolus intravenous cyclophosphamide or other appropriate drugs two weeks after each innoculation.

We have once again resorted to challenging cultured lymphocytes with CME to assess the patients' immune response to immunotherapy. The immune response is complicated by cyclophosphamide which is an immunosuppressive agent. To clarify interpretation of results, we have therefore assessed the blastogenic response to tuberculin purified protein derivative (PPD) in parallel with CME.

As shown in Fig. 2 the blastogenic response to both PPD and CME tails off two weeks after chemotherapy and rises two weeks after immunotherapy. The last cycle of this response was assessed using

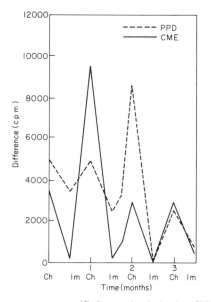

Fig. 2. Blastogenic response to purified protein derivative (PPD) and cell membrane extract (CME). The difference in ^{125}IUdR uptake between stimulated and unstimulated cultures is recorded in counts per min. Ch = chemotherapy (1 g cyclophosphamide (i.v.)); Im = immunotherapy (2×10^7 irradiated ovarian cancer cells + BCG). Interval between chemotherapy and immunotherapy is two weeks.

autologous CME and in the first two cycles an allogenic CME was used. Although the patients' response to the same allogenic CME was negative before immunotherapy, we have no way of proving whether there is true immunostimulation two weeks after immunotherapy, or whether this only reflects a "rebound" effect following the immunosuppression induced by cyclophosphamide. We will only know the answer to this when we are able to omit a course of immunotherapy or chemotherapy.

Using an autologous CME in the same patient, we have demonstrated no delayed skin hypersensitivity response to 0·25 mg of the extract during the immunosuppressed part of the cycle, and a positive response (7 mm in diameter) during the immunostimulatory part of the cycle; a punch skin biopsy of this reaction showed perivascular mononuclear cell infiltration.

We have demonstrated the immunosuppressive effect of cyclophosphamide on the response to what we presume to be a tumour antigen—this effect may be transient on intermittent pulsed I.V. therapy and we assume it is continuous on maintenance therapy.

The immunosuppressive effect could be very serious in patients whose tumours are resistant to the cytotoxic effect, and this emphasises the need for a good predictive test for the use of such drugs.

REFERENCES

Lowry, O. H., Roseborough, N. J. and Farr, A. L. (1952). *J. biol. Chem. 19*, 265.

Oren, M. E., and Herberman, R. B. (1971). *Clin. Exp. Immunol. 9*, 45.

DISCUSSION

Kohorn referred to their own study of the effect of chemotherapy and radiation therapy on cell mediated immunity and "blocking factor" in patients with ovarian carcinomas. He said Embleton had mentioned blocking factor and Hellström and Hellström (1974) had reported, particularly with melanoma, that there is a factor in the serum or plasma of patients which appears in association with relapse and prevents the killing of the target cells by the lymphocytes *in vitro*.

Unlike the Hellströms who used a mixed lymphocyte culture, Kohorn and colleagues have tried to remove most of the macrophages by placing the leucocytes, after isolation, into big glass bottles. All therapy with drugs has been by pulsed chemotherapy and even when patients have been given repeated courses of cyclophosphamide or melphalan over a long time, there is no net depression of cell mediated immunity. Also, there seems to be no correlation between the *in vitro* effect of the lymphocytes on the target cell and the total lymphocyte count in the patient.

In terms of blocking factor, about 8 patients have been studied from 4-18 months, very often until they died. On only two occasions has a correlation between the appearance of blocking factor and relapse or the disappearance of blocking factor and remission been demonstrated. One patient was particularly interesting, since she had a rectal ulcer from an ovarian carcinoma and was treated with chemotherapy. Her rectal ulcer healed and this was accompanied by the disappearance of blocking. Blocking factor reappeared some 14 months later with the reappearance of clinical symptoms. There is one other such patient, but Kohorn did not think there was a 100% correlation.

Many clinicians have expressed the fear that prolonged chemotherapy will interfere with the immune state. The only encouraging thing from this very preliminary data is that in so far as one can identify the immune state with cell mediated immunity measured in this way, chemotherapy does not appear to be significantly detrimental.

REFERENCE

Hellström, K. E. and Hellström, I. (1974). *Advances in Immunology, 18*, 209.

4. The Investigation of Host Factors Influencing the Growth of Leukaemia Cells using a New Liquid Microculture Technique

F. R. Balkwill, R. T. D. Oliver and D. Crowther

The short-term culture of myelogenous leukaemia cells has previously only been accomplished in semi-solid agar or in diffusion chambers (Sumner *et al.* 1972, Moore *et al.* 1973). The agar technique, although useful for morphological and differentiation studies, does not easily permit studies of kinetic factors influencing the growth of these cells, and the diffusion chamber is a rather cumbersome technique requiring large quantities of reagents.

We have developed a simple, reproducible technique for short-term liquid microculture of these cells, which requires no external stimulating factors, and can be used for both fresh and liquid nitrogen stored peripheral blasts.

The cells are suspended at 10^6/ml in Medium 199 and 10% foetal bovine serum. 0·2 ml aliquots of this are added to each flat-bottomed well of a microculture plate which is incubated at $37°C$ in a humid 5% CO_2 atmosphere. Under these conditions, the cells undergo a short-term proliferation, maximum at 3-4 days as measured by the incorporation of tritiated thymidine. A pulse of 0·5 μCi/ml of label is added 16 hr before harvesting on an automatic cell harvesting machine. The resulting activity in the filter paper discs corresponding to each well is counted in a liquid scintillation counter.

The results of an experiment to investigate the kinetics of proliferation can be seen in Figs 1 and 2. The peak of DNA synthesis is reached at the third day of culture with 10^6 cells/ml, as shown in Fig. 1, and during this time there is an increase in cell numbers, as shown in Fig. 2.

Cytocentrifuge preparations taken at the time of peak growth indicate that the majority of cells are primitive myeloid cells. Figure 3 shows one such preparation stained with May Grunwald Giemsa stain and Fig. 4 demonstrates that these cells have a weak sudan black positivity, indicating their myeloid origin. In autoradiographic studies, as illustrated in Fig. 5, it can be seen that it is these large primitive myeloid cells that are incorporating the label.

10*

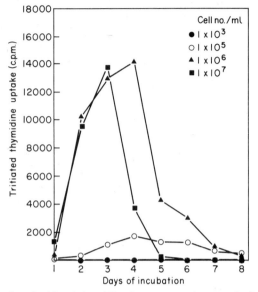

Fig. 1. The uptake of tritiated thymidine by acute myelogenous leukaemia cells (AML) during culture. ● 10^3 cells/ml; ○10^5 cells/ml; ▲10^6 cells/ml; ■10^7 cells/ml.

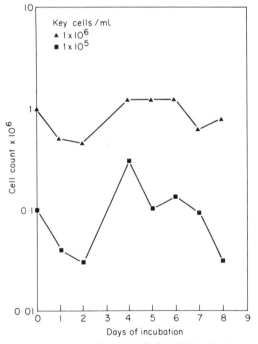

Fig. 2. Change in cell number during AML cell culture.

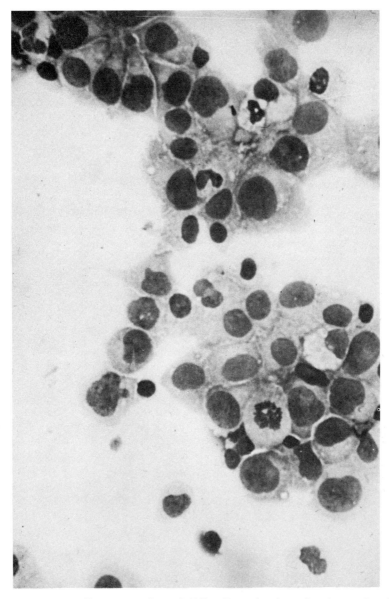

Fig. 3. Cytocentrifuge preparations of AML cells at the time of peak growth stained with May Grunwald Giemsa.

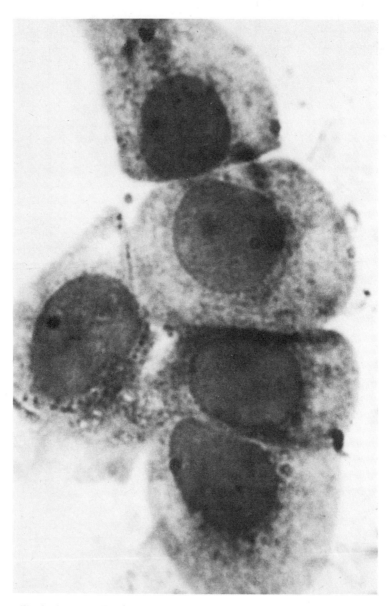

Fig. 4. Cells as in Fig. 3 at a higher magnification and stained with sudan black.

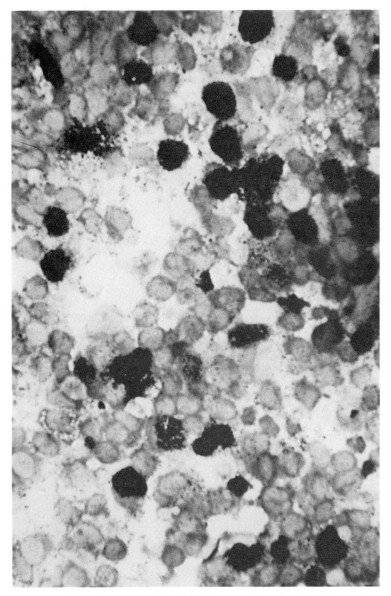

Fig. 5. Autoradiographic preparation of AML cells at the time of peak growth showing the incorporation of tritiated thymidine into the nucleus.

Thus we have a quantitative system for establishing a short-term proliferation of myelogenous leukaemia cells which may have applications to several fields of leukaemia research. However, our main interest has been in investigating host resistance to this tumour and some preliminary results obtained in this field will now be described. The material for these studies has been obtained from acute myelogenous leukaemia patients who have been treated by immunotherapy after drug induced partial or complete remission. This immunotherapy consists of the injection of allogeneic leukaemia cells with B.C.G. at weekly or three-weekly intervals.

The microculture technique can be used to study different manifestations of the host response against the tumour. Firstly, we have studied complement dependent activity in serum against leukaemic blasts. In this assay we add 10% heat inactivated test serum to the cell culture described above, and 3% weanling rabbit serum (w.r.s.) as a source of complement.

Our first observations were made in an allogeneic system and one example of alloimmune complement dependent serum inhibition of cell proliferation is shown in Fig. 6. Encouraged by this and other results, we have begun to investigate autologous inhibition in serum samples taken during various stages of the disease directed against liquid nitrogen stored pre-treatment peripheral blood cells in nine patients. A summary of the results we have obtained so far is shown

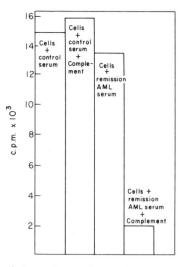

Fig. 6. Demonstration of allogeneic complement dependent activity against AML cells in microculture.

in Fig. 7. This demonstrated the resulting inhibition caused by the addition of complement to the cell/test serum mixture. In some of the controls, the w.r.s. showed toxicity and this value has been subtracted from the values obtained with the test sera where appropriate.

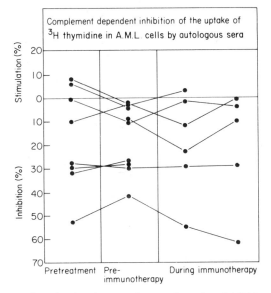

Fig. 7. Summary of results showing complement dependent inhibition of the uptake of tritiated thymidine by autologous serum.

In four of the nine patients we have found significant inhibition with autologous test serum that is complement dependent and gives inhibitions of between 30 and 70% of the controls. This inhibition is present prior to treatment and in two patients we can see that this remains approximately the same during treatment. In another patient it has diminished during treatment, and in the fourth, no further samples are available at the moment.

The number of patients in this study is far too small to draw any conclusions or relate results to the course of disease and prognosis, but new patient material is being obtained regularly and we hope to have a sufficient number of experiments to enable us to draw some firm conclusions.

Antibody which can activate non-sensitised lymphocytes to lyse target cells to which the antibody was directed was first reported by Moller in 1965 and characterised by Perlmann et al. (1972) and

Maclennan (1972). The technique is a very sensitive method of detecting low titre antibody and is of special interest to tumour immunologists.

The technique described above has been modified to allow investigation of this phenomenon. The cells are incubated at 10^5/ml in microculture plates with v-shaped wells for 60-72 hr, then antisera, and effector lymphocytes at a ratio of 10:1 to the target cells, are added, the contents of each well mixed thoroughly and incubated 6-8 hr. The plates are then labelled with "hotter" tritiated thymidine, so that they give counts of a similar magnitude to the previous experiments and incubated for 16 hr before harvesting. The v-shaped wells seem to be of key importance in this technique as this cell concentration will not proliferate in flat-bottomed wells. Also, there is greater target cell/effector cell contact which may be important.

Hersey *et al.* (1973) have demonstrated allogeneic cell-dependent antibody effect in sera from leukaemia patients directed against stored leukaemic blasts using a chromium release assay and we have been able to confirm this finding in our system as shown in Fig. 8. It

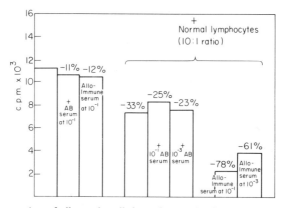

Fig. 8. Demonstration of allogeneic cell dependent antibody activity against AML cells.

can be seen from this figure that we are still obtaining a significant effect at 1:1,000 and, in some cell/antisera situations the titre is higher. Using the same serum in the complement system, the activity would titre out at about 1:20. Thus we have a very sensitive technique for looking at antitumour activity and autologous experiments are currently being carried out.

In summary, therefore, we have a simple technique which is potentially of importance in the study of host/tumour relationships in A.M.L. and has already shown some promising results. The technique has two advantages over the direct cytotoxicity micromethods, as pioneered by Tagasuki and Klein (1970). Firstly it is objective and secondly it is probably more sensitive because it is measuring cytostasis as well as cytolysis.

So far there is only circumstantial evidence that this autologous serum activity against leukaemic blast cells is antibody and no evidence that it changes during the course of immunotherapy, but further studies are being undertaken to investigate these points.

REFERENCES

Hersey, P., MacLennan, I. C. M., Campbell, A. C., Harris, R. and Freeman, C. B. (1973). *Clin. exp. Immunol. 14*, 159.
MacLennan, I. C. M. (1972). *Transplant Rev. 13*, 67.
Moore, M. A., Williams, N. and Metcalf, D. (1973). *J. Nat. Cancer Inst. 50*, 603.
Moller, E. (1965). *Science, 147*, 873.
Perlmann, P., Perlmann, H., Wigzell, H. (1972). *Transplant Rev. 13*, 91.
Sumner, M. A., Bradley, T. R., Hodgson, G. S., Cline, M. J., Fry, P. A. and Sutherland, L. (1972). *Br. J. Haemat. 23*, 221.
Takasugi, M. and Klein, E. (1970). *Transplantation, 9*, 219.

DISCUSSION

In reply to a question from Levin about the possibility of substantial macrophage contamination in the population, Balkwill made several points:

(1) The frozen cells are peripheral blasts taken from patients who have a very high white blood cell count, sometimes in excess of 200,000 so there is little prospect of having normal cells present.

(2) The normal cells will not grow in this system.

(3) There *are* macrophage-like cells when myelomonocytic leukaemia is grown, but evidence so far has shown that these too are tumour cells.

Asked to give details of immunotherapy, Balkwill said that the patients received weekly injections of 10^9 allogeneic AML blast cells intradermally/subcutaneously, divided between three limbs and BCG applied by a heaf gun onto the fourth limb. Using allogeneic blast cells does produce anti HLA antibodies (Klouda *et al.* 1975), but these cannot be the cause of activity demonstrated when testing autologous serum with the patient's own blast cells taken at the time of diagnosis.

In reply to Freshney, she said although it had not been investigated systematically, preliminary results suggested that the asparagine was not a critical factor in leukaemic cell cultures. Cell to cell contact might be critical as 10^5 cells will grow successfully in V-bottom wells, but fail to proliferate in a flat bottom plate. Probably somewhere between 5% and 30% of the cells are in cycle at the peak growth, with 1 to 2% mitoses. However all cycling must be very variable because ^{3}H counts after ^{3}H thymidine labelling of cells from different patients can vary from 2,000 counts per minute per cell to 60,000 counts per minute.

REFERENCE

Klouda, P. T., Lawler, S. D., Pawles, R. L., Oliver, R. T. D. and Grant, C. K. (1975). HL-A Antibiotic Response in patients with Acute Myelogenous Leukaemia treated by Immunotherapy. Transplantation (in press).

Chapter 7

CLINICAL USE OF CYTOTOXIC DRUGS ON THE BASIS OF TISSUE CULTURE TESTS

(Moderator: C. N. Hudson)

1. Individualised Chemotherapy of Ovarian Cancer by Means of the Tissue Culture Method

H. Limburg

The success of any form of treatment of ovarian malignancy with chemotherapy is very difficult to assess. For an evaluation free from subjective influence, it is indispensable to have a satisfactory system of tumour stage classification before the initiation of treatment. Kottmeier has called special attention to the fact that particularly in ovarian cancer the TNM classification of the U.I.C.C. (1966) is more precise for statistical purposes than the familiar classification of FIGO into 4 stages (Table 1). Another difficulty is the presence of 17 histologically distinguishable ovarian tumour types, with several of these having 4-6 sub-groups, whose precise diagnosis places the highest demands on the capabilities of the examining histopathologist. Under these are included the so-called borderline cases, that is to say proliferative cystadenomas or papillomas with continuing development in the region of the surrounding organs.

TABLE 1

Classification of primary ovarian cancer. (Comparison of FIGO and TNM)

Figo	TNM
Stage I	T1 NX MO
	T2 NX MO
Stage II	T1 NX M 1 a
	T2 NX M 1 a
	T3 NX M 1 a
	T4 NX MO
	T4 NX M 1 a
Stage III	T1 NX M 1 b
	T2 NX M 1 b
	T3 NX M 1 b
	T4 NX M 1 b
Stage IV	T1 NX M 1 c
	T2 NX M 1 c
	T3 NX M 1 c
	T4 NX M 1 c

Their classification with the true ovarian malignancies may improve many statistics of 5-year recovery rates and explain instances of so-called miracle recoveries. A further possibility for improving the statistics is offered by the disontogenetic tumours of the germinal epithelium, especially the granulosa cell carcinoma. This is unquestionably a true carcinoma whose diagnosis, particularly as cylindroma, is not easy and whose relatively favourable prognosis is well known. In any statistics on ovarian cancer a special group, including disgerminomas, as well as the group of borderline cases should be presented. Of course, the histological findings do not alter the T classification but represent important additional information. In order to avoid too many sub-divisions, the UICC accepted the following histopathological definitions:

G_1 —Tumours with low potential malignancy, i.e. serous or mucinous or endometrioid (highly differentiated) carcinomas.
G_2 —Predominantly undifferentiated solid, anaplastic carcinomas.

These definitions are the first step towards better criteria for the effectiveness of a cytostatic therapy. However, in our studies on ovarian carcinoma we have found not infrequently histological alteration of the tumour type during chemotherapy. Patients under observation for between 200 and 2,500 days developed undifferentiated, anaplastic carcinomas proven by second look operations, after a first diagnosis of tumours with low potential malignancy. The alteration of the tumour type may correspond with a secondary resistance against the cytostatics used following a clinically objective primary regression of the tumour under selective chemotherapy. This change of resistance is well known from work in animals. After successful retardation initially, new tumour cell lines can develop as early as the fourth week after the initiation of treatment and the cytostatic drug employed is then totally ineffective (Lettré, 1967).

The Cancer Unit of the WHO in Geneva inaugurated and sponsored in 1970 a new Committee on better diagnosis and treatment of ovarian cancer. Representatives from ten countries (Australia, Brazil, France, Federal Republic of Germany, Hungary, Switzerland, United Kingdom, Sweden, United States and Russia) are collecting randomised studies on prospective cases under the chairmanship of Professor Netchajeva and centralised evaluation and histological diagnosis of Professor Serov, both from the Cancer Centre of Leningrad. The collection of 2,000 histologically and clinically observed cases over more than 5 years, may improve our knowledge and therapeutic procedures for the disease with the worst prognosis in gynaecology.

In 1962 we started to prepare primary cultures of human cancer tissues (Limburg and Krahe, 1964) especially from ovarian tumors. The total material evaluated to date includes more than 3,000 explanted human tissues, the overall success rate being 80% and in ovarian carcinomas, 94%.

The sensitivity of the cancer tissue can be tested as a routine procedure against 8-10 cytostatics in common use to find the most effective carcinostatic drug. The dose of each cytostatic drug *in vitro* has to be adjusted to the conditions of the clinical treatment. (The activation of cyclophosphamide for example *in vitro,* is performed under standardised conditions by incubating the inactive transport form of the drug with slices of rat liver for 20 min). Morphological examination of cell proliferation under phase contrast microscopy in the chemotherapy-sensitivity test, allows classification *in vitro* from the completely resistant culture to the cytolytic destruction of the cell monolayer within 48 hr.

In cases where less than 20 gm tumour material is available, a diffusion chamber technique has been developed (Heckmann, 1968). Primary explants of human tissues were cultured in diffusion chambers in the peritoneal cavity of the rat and an initial growth rate of 100% was achieved. The rats can be treated with cytostatic agents from the fifth to eighth days after transplantation. The concentration of cytostatics employed always corresponds to continuous or intermittent therapy in man. The chambers are removed 48 hr after the last intraperitoneal injection of the drug, and cell growth in the transplanted tissue is assessed with the least possible delay, staining the cells by Papanicolaou's method directly on the membrane filters. This *in vivo* test for ascertaining the sensitivity of human carcinoma tissue to a wide spectrum of cytotoxic drugs, has proved of considerable value in supplementing the *in vitro* test.

In earlier studies (Limburg and Heckmann, 1968; Limburg *et al.* 1971) we demonstrated differences in the mean survival time of cases with undifferentiated, anaplastic stage T4 carcinomas of the ovary with the worst prognosis in this tumour type, under different therapeutic conditions. Fourteen patients without chemotherapy died with a mean survival time of 82 days. Fifteen patients with conventional (blind) chemotherapy died with a mean survival time of 283 days. The average duration of life span rose from 283 to 655 days for selective chemotherapy after the sensitivity test was employed. Out of 28 patients treated, 8 (28%) achieved excellent remissions with total regression of all palpable masses, pleural effusions and ascites, surviving from 1,250 to 2,100 days. Husslein *et al.* (1974) have recently published a 5-year cure rate of ovarian FIGO stage 3 carcinomas (corresponding to T4) of only 3·6%.

Since 1969 we have collected cases of ovarian carcinoma for the International reference centres of the WHO. In our series of 102 primary ovarian malignancies, 83·4% were in stage T4 or FIGO 3 and 4 (with epigastrical and extraperitoneal metastases), only 16·6% were in stages T1 to T3. It must be stated here that the casuistry, i.e. the subdivision of stages, differs in every part of the world from hospital to hospital.

Among the new series of 51 primary ovarian carcinomas, 9 were in stage T1-T3 (7 out of 9 alive) and 42 T4; No or Nx; Mla-c (28 alive and well, with survival times between 200 days and 3 years). Three of them survived 5 years and the longest remissions were for 2 patients who died after 2,365 and 2,583 days respectively. These cases were repeatedly treated by operations, irradiation, second looks and 6 to 8 different cytostatics because of secondary resistance. During the last stage of the disease, we could find no available cytostatic to which the tumour was sensitive. Until 3 months before their death the general condition of the patients was good. The histological picture of the tumours and secondaries changed slightly during the whole period from the differentiated to the anaplastic type of carcinoma.

In Tables 2-5 test results of *in vitro* sensitivity and resistance of ovarian carcinomas against cytostatic drugs for the primary tumour, solid metastases, ascites and pleural effusions are shown.

TABLE 2

In vitro *sensitivity of primary ovarian cancer against cytostatic drugs*

	Test Result	
Cytostatic Agent	resistant	sensitive
Endoxan (Asta)	74 (61%)	65 (39%)
Trenimon (Bayer)	83 (61%)	50 (39%)
Proresid (Sandoz)	26 (18%)	114 (82%)
Thio Tepa (Lederle)	120 (90%)	13 (10%)
Methotrexate (Lederle)	116 (91%)	11 (9%)
VM 26 (Sandoz)	27 (34%)	53 (66%)
Progesterone (Schering)	69 (63%)	35 (37%)
Norgestrel (Schering)	61 (88%)	17 (12%)
Velbe (E. Lilly)	15 (12%)	115 (88%)

TABLE 3

In vitro *sensitivity of ovarian cancer (solid metastases) against cytostatic drugs*

Cytostatic Agent	Test Result	
	resistant	sensitive
Endoxan (Asta)	17 (50%)	17 (50%)
Trenimon (Bayer)	19 (61%)	12 (39%)
Proresid (Sandoz)	7 (21%)	27 (79%)
Thio Tepa (Lederle)	24 (86%)	4 (14%)
Methotrexate (Lederle)	26 (72%)	2 (28%)
VM 26 (Sandoz)	4 (27%)	11 (73%)
Progesterone (Schering)	18 (78%)	5 (22%)
Norgestrel (Schering)	12 (80%)	3 (20%)
Velbe (E. Lilly)	3 (10%)	28 (90%)

TABLE 4

In vitro *sensitivity of ovarian cancer (ascites) against cytostatic drugs*

Cytostatic Agent	Test Result	
	resistant	sensitive
Endoxan (Asta)	26 (46%)	30 (54%)
Trenimon (Bayer)	33 (60%)	22 (40%)
Proresid (Sandoz)	7 (12%)	50 (88%)
Thio Tepa (Lederle)	55 (95%)	3 (5%)
Methotrexate (Lederle)	49 (95%)	3 (6%)
VM 26 (Sandoz)	16 (46%)	19 (54%)
Progesterone (Schering)	26 (59%)	18 (41%)
Norgestrel (Schering)	30 (83%)	6 (17%)
Velbe (E. Lilly)	2 (4%)	46 (96%)

TABLE 5

In vitro *sensitivity of ovarian cancer (pleural effusion) against cytostatic drugs*

Cytostatic Agent	Test Result	
	resistant	sensitive
Endoxan (Asta)	3	4
Trenimon (Bayer)	4	1
Proresid (Sandoz)	1	6
Thio Tepa (Lederle)	5	—
Methotrexate (Lederle)	5	1
VM 26 (Sandoz)	3	2
Progesterone (Schering)	5	1
Norgestrel (Schering)	3	—
Velbe (E. Lilly)	1	8

Many problems must still be solved. For example, it is nearly impossible to determine the exact cell cycle kinetics of the individual tumour growth. In animal tumours or HeLa cells, the generation time has been shown to be between 20 and 48 hr, but in some ovarian carcinomas it is between 14 and 45 days. Timing in relation to the cell cycle is of great importance during any cytostatic treatment and use of two drugs with different effects (e.g. vinblastine and cyclophosphamide) and an interval of 48 hr between the two combination partners, might be suitable with the combinations repeated weekly during the patient's treatment.

Finally, I would like to focus attention on the therapeutic application of nucleosides like thymidine, cytidine, uridine and guanosine in combination with cytostatics. The synchronising action of excess thymidine on cells in culture is well known (Bootsma *et al.* 1964; Petersen and Andersen, 1964). DNA synthesis is inhibited but the synthesis of other macromolecules continues, and there is a wave of mitoses when the inhibitor is removed (Cohen, 1967). More recently, Osswald (1970) has described a synergistic effect of the combination of thymidine and cyclophosphamide on the Ehrlich Ascites tumour. The chemotherapeutic action of cyclophosphamide on this tumour was enhanced when thymidine was injected 6 hr previously. Lengthening or shortening the time interval between applications of the two compounds, reduced their chemotherapeutic efficacy.

Since 1969 we have used cytidine and, more recently, thymidine in patients with recurrent mammary and ovarian cancers. Absolute tumour regression was achieved for a 45-year old patient, who presented with a papillary ovarian cancer stage T4 Nx Mlb with widespread liver and peritoneal metastases and ascites, after a monotherapy with 159 gr cytidine and 500 gr thymidine. The diagnosis was made after explorative laparotomy and removal of cancer tissue for histology without any other treatment. She is now alive at 5 years and in excellent condition. For the past 18 months we have used the following: weekly, 1 infusion over 5-6 hr of thymidine solution at 30 mg/kg bodyweight in 500 ml NaCl; 24 hr later cyclophosphamide 25 mg/kg bodyweight over 6 hr; and 12 hr later thymidine at the same dose as before. The cyclophosphamide therapy is only effective if the predictive test shows sensitivity of the tumour. A second schedule uses vinblastine under similar conditions. Weekly: 7·5-10 mg velbe as an infusion, followed 24 hr later by thymidine infusion at 30 mg/kg bodyweight over 6 hr. Using this schedule with no other treatment, two patients with ovarian cancer

T4 Nl Mlb and c with ascites, have had absolute remissions of palpable tumour masses, disappearance of ascites and are in excellent general condition 12 and 18 months after the beginning of treatment. Four other patients are receiving this treatment, but it is not yet possible to draw any conclusions. Therapy with nucleosides even at the highest doses has proved to be absolutely harmless for the patient (Limburg, Schmahl and Osswald, to be published).

Six out of 9 normal embryonic tissues were resistant to thymidine in culture, while proliferation of the other three was affected at a concentration of 42 μg/ml. Even higher concentrations of 2,100 μg/ml showed the same results. Cytidine concentrations of 60 and 3,000 μg/ml had no effect on 5 out of 6 cultures. However, the combination of 42 μg/ml thymidine with cyclophosphamide was very effective and cell proliferation stopped in 6 out of 8 cultures. Cytidine also increased the efficacy of cyclophosphamide, but no difference in effectiveness was seen between the two thymidine concentrations. These experiments will be continued with human cancer tissue cultures, so the conclusions must remain tentative until a larger number of specimens have been tested.

In summary we may say:

(1) The TNM classification seems to give better criteria than the FIGO classification. However, the presence of ascites and liver metastases are not specifically classified.

(2) Stages T1-T3 Nx Mo should be treated by radical surgery and radiotherapy. Prophylactic chemotherapy was not acknowledged to achieve better results.

(3) Radical surgery is not possible in the majority of patients with ovarian cancer—83·4% of our cases come to hospital for primary treatment with stages T4; Nx; Mo—Mlc. Nevertheless, as much tumour tissue as possible should be removed in order to get better basic conditions for cytostatic therapy. Experimental and clinical observations have proved that successful cytostatic treatment is closely correlated with the amount of tumour tissue removed.

(4) Experimental as well as clinical observations have shown that a rational combination chemotherapy with consideration of the time factor gives the best results.

(5) Ultra-high doses of a mono-therapy should be avoided.

(6) Only a small group of cytostatics can be recommended for the treatment of ovarian cancer. These are: Endoxan, Velbe (high doses should be avoided), VM 26, 5-Fluorouracil, Proresid, Trenimon and Progesterone.

(7) In a combination therapy 2 drugs with different effects should usually be employed. An interval of 48 hr between the two combination partners seems to be necessary, and combinations may be repeated weekly during the patient's treatment.

(8) Some authors find good results after treatment with testosterone or progesterone in combination with other cytostatics. No improvement could be demonstrated with oestrogens.

(9) In cases of progressive tumour growth the combinations must be changed after 4 weeks' treatment.

(10) It has been demonstrated clinically that selective chemotherapy after a tissue culture test result (oncobiogram as a predictive test) seems to get better results than blind chemotherapy.

REFERENCES

Bootsma, D., Budke, L. and Vos, O. (1964). *Exp. Cell Res. 33*, 301.

Cohen, L. S. (1967). *J. Cell comp. Physiol. 69*, 331.

Heckmann, U. (1968). "A New *In Vivo* Test for Assessing the Resistance of Human Carcinomas to Cytostatic Agents". Georg. Thieme Verlag, Stuttgart, Vol. XIII No. 5, p. 220.

Husslein, H. *et al.* (1974). *Fortschritte der Medizin vom 10.1.74, Jahrgang 92, No. 1.*

Lettré, H. (1967). *Mat. med Nordmark, 19*, 553.

Limburg, H. and Heckmann, U. (1968). *J. Obstet. and Gynaec. of Brit. Commonw. 75*, 12.

Limburg, H. and Krahe, M. (1964a). *Dtsch. Med. Wschr. 89*, 1938.

Limburg, H., Tranekjer, A.-S. and Heckmann, U. (1971). Chemotherapy of Gynaecological Cancer. *In* "Modern Radiotherapy Gynaecological Cancer", (Thomas J. Deeley, ed.). Butterworths, London (pp. 243-283.

Osswald, H. (1970). *Z. Krebsforsch. 74*, 376.

Petersen, D. F. and Anderson, E. C. (1964). *Nature, Lond. 203*, 622.

2. Studies on the Drug Sensitivity of Short Term Cultured Tumour Cell Suspensions

J. Mattern, M. Kaufmann, K. Wayss and M. Volm

For the past few years, we have been working on the sensitivity testing of tumours *in vitro*, using mainly the method shown in Fig. 1 (Mattern *et al.* 1972; Mattern *et al.* (in press); Volm *et al.* 1974*a*; Volm *et al.* 1974*b*; Volm *et al.* (in press); Wayss *et al.* (in press).

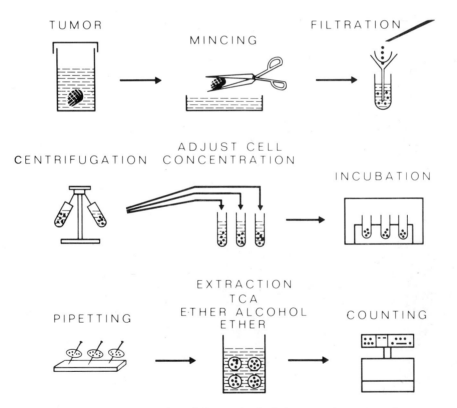

Fig. 1. Schematic representation of the standardised short term incubation of tumour cell suspensions.

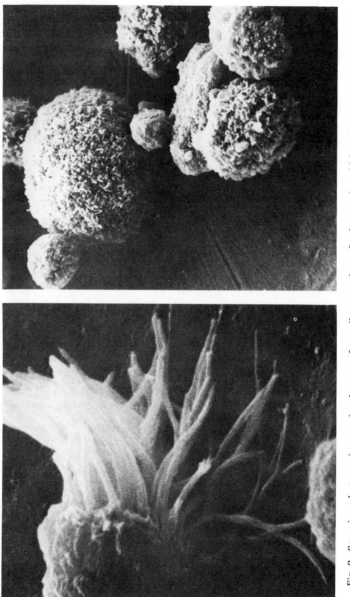

Fig. 2. Scanning electronmicroscopic pictures of a cell suspension of a human bonchial tumour.* Right: 3,000x; left: 10,000x, ciliated epithelial cell.

* We thank Dr. Paweletz (Deutsches Krebsforschungszentrum, Institut für Zellforschung, Heidelberg) for the scanning electronmicroscopic pictures.

The solid tumours are first mechanically disrupted and filtered through gauze. The cells are sedimented and subsequently re-suspended at a defined cell density. The suspensions are then incubated with the particular cytostatic agent to be tested in a water bath for 3 hr. The appropriate radioactive precursor is added during the third hour of incubation. Aliquots of the cell suspensions are pipetted on to filter paper discs, the acid soluble radioactivity is extracted and the incorporated activity measured by scintillation counting. This method is extremely simple and the results can be obtained in a few hours. In addition, all cell types present in the tumour are used in the test, since selection of particular cells can be excluded by the very short incubation time. All types of tumour can be tested by this method. Figure 2 shows that cells in suspension prepared in this way are largely intact.

In our test system, the appropriate radioactive precursor must be used to test each cytostatic agent (see Table 1).

TABLE 1

Radioactive nucleic acid precursors used in short-term tests

	Thymidine	Uridine	Deoxuridine
Cyclophosphamide	●	●	
Triaziquone	●	●	
Procarbazine	●	●	
Adriamycin	●	●	
Daunorubicin	●	●	
Methotrexate			●
5-fluorouracil			●
Dactinomycin		●	

The activity of cyclophosphamide, triaziquone, procarbazine, adriamycin and daunoubucin can be determined from either thymidine or uridine incorporation, whereas the activity of methotrexate and 5-fluorouracil can only be determined from deoxyuridine incorporation, and that of dactinomycin only from uridine incorporation. In order to compare this short-term method with the commonly used tissue culture, tumour cells from solid tumours were cultivated *in vitro,* incubated with the appropriate cytostatic agent for 48 hr and the activity of the substance evaluated morphologically. In Fig. 3, examples are given of the different activities of cytostatic agents on the mouse sarcoma 180 : procarbazine (N) exhibits, in comparison with controls (C), either no effect or a slight stimulatory activity, while 5-fluorouracil

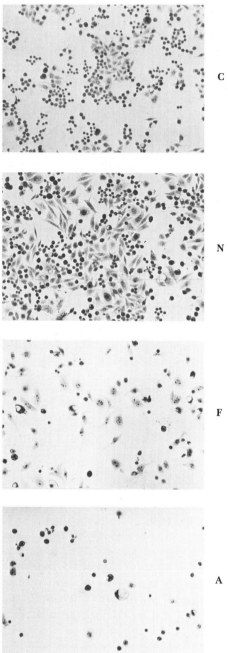

Fig. 3. Effect of different cytostatics on the mouse sarcoma 180 at
10 times therapeutic dose. Cells were
cultivated on cover slips and exposed
to the cytostatic substance for 48 hr.
C = control, N = procarbazine, F =
5-fluorouracil, A = adriamycin.

(F) causes moderate and adriamycin (A) very pronounced morphological changes in the cells. In order to make a quantitative estimate of the activities of the cytostatics, cell counts were determined using the coulter counter.

This procedure gave results similar to those obtained by morphological evaluation. The effects of different cytostatic substances on the cell numbers in cultures of the mouse sarcoma 180 and the adenocarcinoma of the rat were compared with their influence on ^{3}H-uridine incorporation in short-term incubated cell suspensions (Fig. 4). For both of these tumours the results obtained

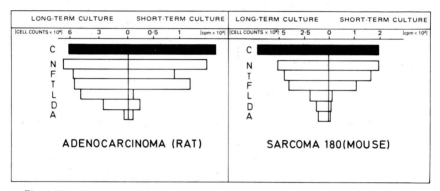

Fig. 4. The effects of different cytostatics on long term tissue cultures (cell counts per ml) after 48 hr exposure to the substance and on the incorporation of ^{3}H-uridine in tumour cell suspensions (cpm/0·1 ml) after 3 hr exposure to the cytostatic substance. Abbreviations: C = control, N = procarbazine, F = 5-fluorouracil, D = daunorubicin, T = triaziquone, L = dactinomycin, A = adriamycin.

using the two test systems are similar. It can therefore be said that the successes which can be obtained by cultivation of tumour cells and morphological evaluation after long exposure to cytostatics, can also be obtained using the method of short-term incubation of tumour cell suspensions, at least for the cytostatic agents tested here.

The usefulness of a test depends on the degree to which the *in vitro* results can be correlated with the results of therapy on patients. It is, however, extremely difficult to demonstrate such a correlation in the clinic. For this reason, we have attempted to test the correlation between *in vitro* and *in vivo* results using a simple system—the transplanted Walker carcinoma 256 of the rat.

Figure 5 shows the effects of various drugs which influence uridine incorporation, on tumour size *in vivo* (closed circles). The highest dose used corresponded to 4/5 of the LD 50. At the same time, the effects of corresponding doses on uridine incorporation in tumour

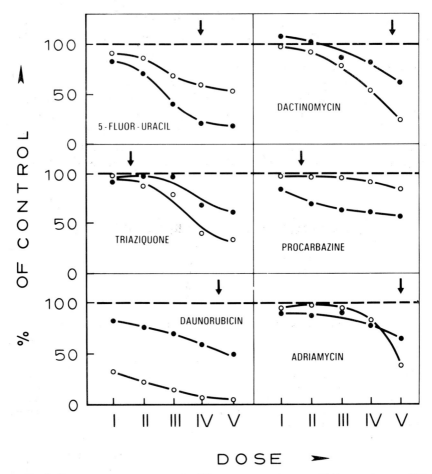

Fig. 5. Dose response curves of different cytostatics on Walker-carcinoma 256. Percentage effect on tumour size *in vivo* (•———•) and ^{3}H-Uridine (o———o) incorporation in cell suspensions *in vitro*. Abscissa: Doses I–V (log. scale). Maximum dose V = 4/5 LD$_{50}$.

cells *in vitro* were measured (open circles). The dose response curves show clearly that the results of therapy in animal experiments can be predicted using this simple *in vitro* test. The above tests were carried out using chemosensitive animal tumours.

Figure 6 shows a comparison of the effects of various doses of cytostatics on both animal and human tumours. It can be seen that the four animal transplanted tumours investigated show similar dose-dependent effects, whereas the human tumours respond differently to the agent tested. Some tumours exhibit responses

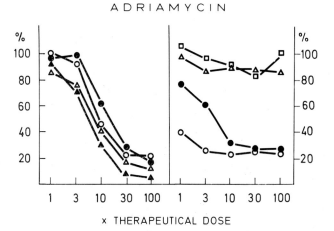

Fig. 6. Dose response curves for the effects of adriamycin at different doses (1x, 3x 10x, 30x, 100x, therapeutic dose) on 4 animal tumours (left) and on 4 human tumours (right) □———□ Rectum-carcinoma, △———△ Ependymoglioma, ●———● Rectum-carcinoma, ○———○ ovary-carcinoma.

similar to those of the animal tumours, while others do not react even to doses corresponding to 100 times the therapeutic dose. For human tumours, adriamycin at a concentration of 10 times the therapeutic dose can be conveniently used to distinguish between chemosensitive and non-sensitive tumours.

On this basis, one hundred human tumours from various organs (circles with numbers) were tested using adriamycin at ten times the therapeutic dose and the results were compared with those obtained on different chemosensitive transplanted animal tumours (filled signs) Fig. 7. Whereas this substance caused an inhibition of at least 50% with respect to controls in all animal tumours tested, the responses of the human tumours varied. Some human tumours are inhibited to the same extent as animal tumours, and the remainder exhibit either less or no response. Similar results were obtained using daunorubicin and dactinomycin. Roughly 30% of the human tumours tested could be inhibited by the three substances to the same extent as animal tumours.

Since we do not yet have the results of clinical therapy on the human tumours investigated, we decided to compare the results of the short term *in vitro* tests with the appropriate literature data on the responses of human tumours to clinical therapy, in order to see whether in principle a correlation exists (Table 2).

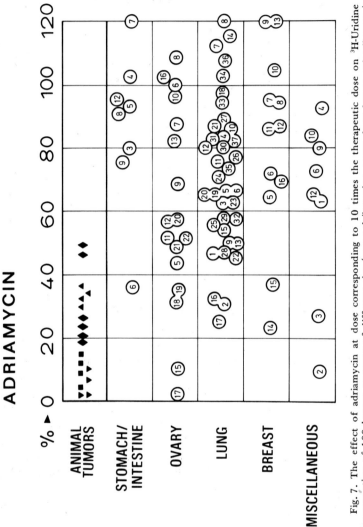

Fig. 7. The effect of adriamycin at dose corresponding to 10 times the therapeutic dose on ^{3}H-Uridine incorporation of 100 human tumours of different site (stomach/intestine, ovary, lung, breast, miscellaneous) compared with various transplanted animal tumours. Inhibition of incorporation is given in % of controls (= 100%). Each point represents 4 measurements on one tumour. Numbers in the open circles indicate the individual human tumour. Animal tumours: ▼——— DS-carcinoma, ▲——— plasmocytoma, ◆——— melanoma Fortner III, ■——— Walker-carcinoma 256.

TABLE 2

Comparison of the in vitro *results with the literature data*

Tumours	In vitro response (%)	In vivo response (%)	References
Ovary	50	46	Rozmann *et al.* 1972; Smith *et al.* 1972; Barlow *et al.* 1973
Breast	18	27	Livingston and Carter, 1970; O'Bryan *et al.* 1973; Gottlieb *et al.* 1974
Lung	27	22	Kenis *et al.* 1972; Selawry, 1973
Stomach/intestine	22	11	Livingston and Carter, 1970; O'Bryan *et al.* 1973

Only the substances adriamycin, daunorubicin and dactinomycin are shown. It can be seen that the *in vitro* test results are comparable with the effects described in the literature. The responses of individual tumour groups in patients treated with the same cytostatics are of the same order of magnitude as the responses involved *in vitro*. For example, tumours of the ovary, which are known to be relatively chemosensitive, also exhibit *in vitro* a large response to the cytostatics. *In vitro* 50%, *in vivo* 46% inhibition. The other tumours, lung, breast, stomach/intestine, are less sensitive both *in vivo* (11-27%) and *in vitro* (18-27%). It can therefore be said that the results of the *in vitro* tests on human tumours in no way contradict the literature data on clinical therapy.

At the present moment, clinical studies are being carried out in Heidelberg to see whether the responses of patients to therapy really correspond to the results of the tests described.

REFERENCES

Barlow, J. J., Piver, M. S., Chuang, J. T., Cortes, E. P., Ohnuma, T. and Holland, J. F. (1973). *Cancer, 32,* 735-743.

Gottlieb, J. A., Rivkin, S. E., Spigel, S. C., Hoogstraten, B., O'Bryan, R. M., Delaney, F. C. and Singhakowinta, A. (1974). *Cancer, 33,* 519-526.

Kenis, Y., Michel, J., Rimoldi, R., Israel, L. and Levy, P. (1972). *Europ. J. Cancer, 8,* 485-489.

Livingston, R. B. and Carter, S. K. (1970). "Single Agents in Cancer Chemotherapy". IFI/Plenum Press, New York.

Mattern, J., Volm, M. and Wayss, K. (1972). *Arzneimittel-Forsch. 22,* 1721-1722.

Mattern, J., Kaufmann, M., Hinderer, H., Wayss, K. and Volml, M. (1975). Z. Krebsforsch. 83, 97.

O'Bryan, R. M., Luce, J. K., Talley, R. W., Gottlieb, J. A., Baker, L. H. and Bonadonna, G. (1973). Cancer, 32, 1-8.

Rozman, C., Camps, E. S., Mundo, M. R., Solsona, F., Dantart, I., Raichs, A. and Giralt, M. (1972). Clinical trial of Adriamycin In "International Symposium on Adriamycin" (S. K. Carter, A. Di Marco, M. Ghione, I. H. Krakoff and G. Mathe, eds.), pp. 188-194. Berlin, Heidelberg, New York: Springer 1972.

Selawry, O. S. (1973). Cancer chemother. Rep. 4, 177-188.

Smith, J. P., Rutledge, F. and Wharton, J. T. (1972). Cancer, 30, 1565-1571.

Volm, M., Mattern, J. and Wayss, K. (1974). Arch. Geschwulstforsch. 43, 137-144.

Volm, M., Kaufmann, M., Wayss, K., Goerttler, Kl. and Mattern, J. (1974). Dtsch. med. Wschr. 99, 38-43.

Volm, M., Kaufmann, M., Mattern, J. and Wayss, K. (1975). Z. Krebsforsch. 83, 85.

Wayss, K., Mattern, J., Kaufmann, M., Hinderer, H. and Volm, M. Korrelation von In-vivo-Testung und Therapieergebnis bei tierischen Transplantations-tumoren nach Cytostatika-Behandlung. Arzneimittel-Forsch. (in press).

3. Detection of Acquired Resistance to Cytotoxic Drugs *In Vivo* by Short Term *In Vitro* Cultures of Human Tumours

H. M. Warenius

The development of resistance to a cytotoxic agent which has initially been successful in inducing some degree of remission in human malignant disease and the subsequent recurrence of that disease, is a not infrequent clinical observation.

Such acquired resistance is probably due to the selection of a small proportion of cells which have the necessary biochemical factors to resist the action of the drugs (Ball, 1969). These biochemical factors have been demonstrated and investigated in both clinical and experimental situations.

Djerassi *et al.* (1967) recognised clinically acquired resistance to methotrexate in childhood acute lymphoblastic leukaemia which could be overcome by giving much larger doses of the same drug. They felt this could be explained by the resistance to methotrexate being due, at least in part, to decreased permeability of the resistant cells to the drug. Defective methotrexate entry into the cell has been implicated in resistance to this drug by human cell lines (Fischer, 1962, Kessel, 1965) and an increase in the level of dihydrofolate reductase, the target enzyme for methotrexate has also been demonstrated as a further possible mechanism (Stock, 1966).

With regard to purine antimetabolites, resistance to 6-thioguanine associated with an increased level of the enzyme responsible for its degradation to 6-thiouric acid has been shown experimentally (Sartorelli *et al.* 1958). A similar resistance to 6-mercapto-purine due to loss (Ball, 1969) or change in specificity, of the enzyme responsible for its activation by conversion to the 6-mercaptopurine ribonucleotide has also been shown (Brockman *et al.* 1959).

Similar mechanisms have been demonstrated for pyrimidine antagonists such as 5-fluorouracil (Skold, 1963) and resistance to the alkylating agents has also been studied in human cell lines (Chun *et al.* 1967).

Recently Skipper (1974) has shown, using the sensitivity to cytosine arabinoside of the L1210 leukaemia in mice, that detection of drug resistance to a single agent may depend on the number of cells used in the inoculum and that combining cytosine arabinoside with a second agent, 6-thioguanine, resulted in a lower incidence of such drug resistance.

Though we have not so far investigated human tumours in such specific biochemical detail, we have some evidence of acquired resistance developing in patients on chemotherapy as shown by *in vitro* short term cultures of human tumour material (for methods see earlier papers by Dendy and Wright and Dawson *et al.*) and the selected cases which follow demonstrate this.

First with regard to treatment with the single agent Trenimon (triaziquone). Figure 1 compares 15 patients who had received no prior treatment with Trenimon, to 8 patients treated with this drug for varying periods up to the time of testing.

Though there is overlap between the two groups, 12 of the cases who had not received Trenimon are definitely very sensitive lying well below the 10% ^{125}IUdR uptake line with only 3 more resistant cases above. Only two out of the 8 cases in the group previously treated with Trenimon are in the sensitive range, while the others are above the 10% level and three in particular are very resistant.

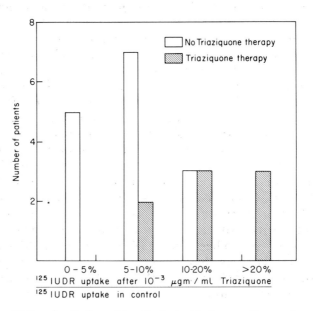

Fig. 1. Sensitivity of cells from 23 patients to triaziquone. The specimens from 15 patients who had not been treated with triaziquone were markedly more sensitive *in vitro* than those from patients who had been given triaziquone therapy.

Further information can be obtained by longitudinal study of the few well-documented cases who have had repeated tissue culture tests. Usually, this has been possible because of the development of recurrent ascites giving readily available material for culture.

Figure 2 shows the time course of a patient who by morphological assessment of tissue culture in July 1971, was very sensitive to Trenimon which she had not at that time received, having been on chlorambucil for the preceding month. She was started on a course

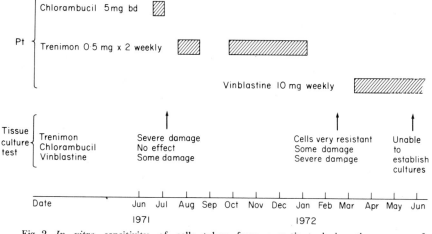

Fig. 2. *In vitro* sensitivity of cells taken from a patient during the course of chemotherapy.

of Trenimon and apart from a break of approximately one month due to haematological depression by the cytotoxic agent, she continued until the first week of January 1972. Tissue culture testing one month later, on cells grown from ascitic fluid, showed severe resistance to Trenimon, but she also appeared to have developed concomitant sensitivity to vinblastine and possibly to chlorambucil. This may be an illustration of how tumour cell populations change during a course of chemotherapy. Her therapy was thus changed to vinblastine but her disease continued to advance clinically. Unfortunately, two further attempts to establish tissue cultures from subsequently recurring ascites failed, so that we could not obtain

HTSTC—12

evidence as to whether or not she had become resistant to vinblastine.

The patient in Fig. 3 had a bilateral salpingo-oophorectomy in October 1972 for ovarian carcinoma which had penetrated the ovarian capsule. There was no ascites and no tissue culture test was

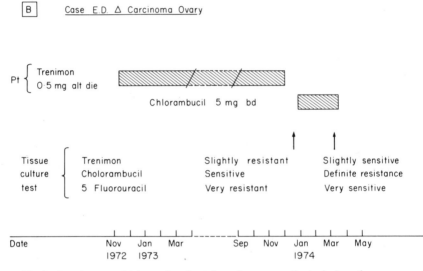

Fig. 3. *In vitro* sensitivity of cells taken from a patient during the course of chemotherapy.

performed at that time. She had had no previous chemotherapy and was commenced on a course of Trenimon which was continued for over a year. She did very well until December 1973, when ascites developed and was drained yielding cells for tissue culture; these showed only slight resistance to Trenimon, despite her previous one year's exposure to this drug. The cells were, however, clearly sensitive to chlorambucil and her Trenimon was therefore stopped and chlorambucil started.

Two-and-a-half months later a repeat tissue culture test on a further growth of cells from ascitic fluid showed that resistance to chlorambucil had developed. There was little to no change in sensitivity to Trenimon. Clinically, her disease had advanced whilst she was on Tenimon and it would have been expected that during the year in which she was receiving this drug, resistant clones would have had time to emerge if they were going to do so. Nonetheless, in this case the tissue culture test failed to demonstrate any resistance *in vitro.* A concomitant change in sensitivity to a drug not being used in the patient as with vinblastine in the first case, is again observed, this time with 5-fluorouracil.

The third patient (Fig. 4) treated with single agent chemotherapy, was discovered at laparotomy in April 1972 to have widespread

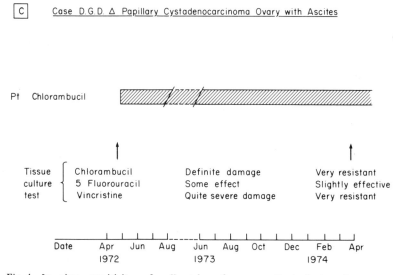

Fig. 4. *In vitro* sensitivity of cells taken from a patient during the course of chemotherapy.

omental secondaries and ascites from a papillary cystadeno-carcinoma of the ovary. She was started on chlorambucil at the end of April 1972 and maintained on this drug with occasional two- to three-week breaks because of low blood counts up to the present. The tissue culture test on the original tumour obtained at laparotomy showed definite damage by chlorambucil developing slowly morphologically. 5-fluorouracil produced slight damage and vincristine quite severe damage.

Two years later after almost continuous single agent chemotherapy with chlorambucil, a further tissue culture test, this time on cells from ascitic fluid, was performed and showed these cells to be very resistant to chlorambucil and slightly sensitive still to 5-fluorouracil. In this case, however, concomitant resistance to vincristine had apparently occurred, although the patient had not been exposed to this drug.

One of the stated advantages of combination chemotherapy is that

TABLE 1

Effect of combination chemotherapy on acquired drug resistance measured in vitro

Patient	Diagnosis	Type of chemotherapy	No. of courses	Drug tested	^{125}IUdR uptake as % of control after this no. of courses
D.L.S.	Carcinomatosis with ascites. Primary site unknown	5 fluorouracil 500 mg + vincristine 1 mg every 2-3 weeks	6	Vincristine 0·01 μgm/ml 5 fluorouracil 1·5 μgm/ml	13·8% 2%
J.M.T.	Carcinoma of breast. Malignant ascites	Cyclophosphamide 500 mg +5 fluorouracil 500 mg + vincristine 1 mg + methotrexate 50 mg every 3-4 weeks	4	Vincristine 0·1 μgm/ml 5 fluorouracil 1·5 μgm/ml	9·1% 14·2%
M.P.	Stage IV carcinoma of ovary	Cyclophosphamide 500 mg + methotrexate 40 mg + vincristine 1 mg + 5 fluorouracil 400 mg every 3-4 weeks	3	Vincristine 0·01 μgm/ml 5 fluorouracil 1·5 μgm/ml	7% 9%
E.A.	Carcinoma of breast with recurrent pleural effusion	5 day CRC regimen using: cyclophosphamide 300 mg + vincristine 1 mg + 5 fluorouracil 500 mg + methotrexate 20 mg	1	Vincristine 0·01 μgm/ml 5 fluorouracil 1·5 μgm/ml	3·2% 18·6%

by using two or more cytotoxic agents at the same time, the development of acquired resistance is prevented. We have a small amount of information on patients receiving more than one drug at the same time and in these few cases drug resistance is not evident. Table 1 shows four cases, all of whom have had treatment with vincristine and 5-fluorouracil. In the first case these two drugs only were used together, and in the other three cases they were combined with methotrexate and cyclophosphamide. The percentage of [125] IUdR uptake for vincristine and 5-fluorouracil for each patient is shown in the end column. All these percentage uptakes fall within the sensitive range of the appropriate histograms (for 5-fluorouracil see Fig. 4, p. 145) so that there is no indication of resistance to either of the drugs used in combination.

Only the first of these patients has had consecutive tissue culture tests performed and these results are shown in Fig. 5. This

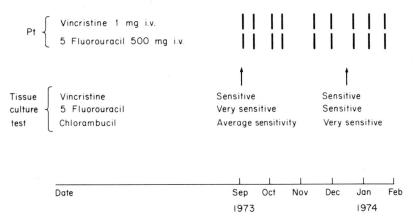

Fig. 5. *In vitro* sensitivity of cells taken from a patient during combination chemotherapy.

middle-aged woman presented with malignant ascites secondary to an unknown primary. Cells from her ascites grew well in tissue culture and were sensitive to both vincristine and 5-fluorouracil. She was treated with these two drugs in combination as intermittent pulsed therapy, administered intravenously at intervals separated by one to three weeks as haemotological tolerance permitted. A repeat tissue culture test after she had received 6 courses of treatment in a period of 4 months, showed no change in the *in vitro* sensitivity of short term culture of tumour cells from ascitic fluid to vincristine; and very little change in sensitivity to 5-fluorouracil.

Interpretation of the preceding results in these patients is, of course, subject to the known hazards of *in vitro* short term cultures, such as difficulty in controlling conditions and reproducibility of results. However, Table 2 illustrates that consecutive tests can be

TABLE 2

Sensitivity of cells from different patients to Oncovin (vincristine)

Patient	Site of Primary Tumour	$\dfrac{^{125}IUdR \text{ uptake after Oncovin \%}}{^{125}IUdR \text{ uptake in control}}$		Notes
		0·3 µgm/ml	0·1 µgm/ml	
GG[1]	ovary		5	7/8/72
GG[2]	ovary	1	2	8/8/72
DD	ovary		7	
AB	ovary		12	
EA [1]	ovary		21	8/5/72
EA[2]	ovary		20	31/5/72
EA[3]	ovary		16	27/6/72
NP	melanoma		45	
JB	glioma		54	
RM	uterus	27 (16)	31 (34)	Results for two patients after
GE	ovary	47 (52)	68 (67)	treatment with Oncovin. Figures in brackets show sensitivity to Velbe

capable of giving consistent results. Here the sensitivity of *in vitro* cultures of human ovarian tumours to Oncovin (vincristine) is measured by expressing ^{125}IUdR uptake in the drug-treated cultures as a percentage of the uptake in controls (see Dawson *et al.,* p. 144). The first two results are independent tissue culture tests on two consecutive days on the same tumour sample from one patient and can be seen to be very consistent. The next three results are for tests on samples taken from the same patient on different dates, and again can be seen to give closely consistent results.

It is obviously not possible to draw any definite conclusions from these few clinical examples selected retrospectively and chosen to illustrate that acquired drug resistance may be studied in the human as well as in the experimental situation. There is much scope for further investigation of acquired resistance however, with regard to predictive tests of chemotherapeutic sensitivities in the human clinical situation and to the subsequent techniques of clinical administration of drugs recommended by such tests. Thus from the chemotherapeutic viewpoint, combination therapy may be made more rational using two or more drugs to which the tumour is shown to be most sensitive in tissue culture and omitting drugs to which resistance is shown. Another possibility is for two or more single agents, predicted as being possibly effective against the tumour by in vitro testing, to be given alternately for periods of one to two months each. It may prove possible to delay the onset of acquired drug resistance by this method which might also carry the benefit of less toxic side effects, than the large multiple drug regimes presently used.

Such an approach may possibly also be used to adapt the development of acquired resistance to the clinician's advantage by modifying the tumour population with one agent, so that an almost homogeneous population sensitive to a second agent is produced, allowing the latter to exert a high cell kill. One such method has been described by Tattersall et al. (1973).

Fundamental to all these approaches is the need to repeat tissue culture testing at regular intervals wherever clinically possible, in order to check on the changing population of tumour cells. In this respect a further reference should be made to the work of Skipper (1974) with L1210 leukaemia in mice, mentioned at the beginning. He has suggested that tissue cultures established from only small numbers of tumour cells may not detect a potentially resistant clone; thus it is important to obtain as large a number of cells as possible from the tumour specimen at the outset.

I conclude by suggesting that more attempts should be made to look at the problem of acquired resistance in the clinical situation by in vitro short term cultures, and that for this suitable protocols should be drawn up. Probably the most ideal cases to study are those with ovarian carcinoma and malignant ascites which are capable of yielding repeated plentiful samples for growth in tissue culture. The cases should have previously received no cytotoxic therapy and tissue culture testing should be performed prior to starting drug treatment. Many clinicians are still happy to use single agent chemotherapy where possible, because of its simplicity and low toxicity, and acquired resistance to these agents could be studied systematically by regular tissue culture at monthly intervals. If resistance is detected, then the resistant clone may be selected by encouraging growth of the cells in low concentrations of the agent to which resistance is shown. Once such cells have been isolated, their mechanism of resistance may be examined more specifically by biochemical methods and further drugs tested against the resistant clones to determine what concomitant changes in sensitivity may also have occurred, with a view to exploiting these in the clinical situation.

REFERENCES

Ball, C. R. (1969). *In* "Scientific Basis of Cancer Chemotherapy" (George Mathe, ed.), Heinemann Medical Books Ltd., London; Springer-Verlag, Berlin, pp. 26-40.

Brockman, R. W., Sparks, C., Simpson, M. S. and Skipper, H. E. (1959). *Biochem. Pharmacol. 2*, 77.

Chun, E. H. L., Gonzales, L. J., Lewis, F. S. and Rutman, R. J. (1967). *Fed. Proc. 26*, 872.

Djerassi, I. (1967). *Cancer Res. 27*, 2561.

Fischer, G. A. (1962). *Biochem. Pharmacol. 11*, 1233.

Kessel, D., Hall, T. C., Roberts, D. W. and Wodinksy, I. (1965). *Science, 150*, 752.

Sartorelli, A. C., Le Page, G. A. and Moore, E. C. (1958). *Cancer Res. 18*, 1232.

Skipper, H. E. (1974). Cancer Chemotherapy Reports Part 2, Vol. 4, p. 137.

Skold, O. (1963). *Biochem. Biophys. Acta, 76*, 160.

Stock, J. A. (1966). *In* "Experimental Chemotherapy", Vol. 4 (R. J. Schnitzer and F. Hawking, eds.), Academic Press, New York and London.

Tattersall, M. H. N. (1973). *Br. J. Cancer, 27*, 406.

GENERAL DISCUSSION

Limburg questioned if it was possible to study inhibition of mitotic index as quickly as described by Mattern since one must be sure before starting a cytotoxic test that the cells are alive and capable of division. Furthermore, there is no need to have a test result within 24 hr because patients can certainly wait 2-3 days for treatment or even a little longer. MacNally added that the differences noted by Mattern between the effect of adriamycin on an established animal tumour and some human tumours (Fig. 6, p. 307) might be a reflection of the fact that with human tumours it may take very much longer for the cells to grow well when put into the petri dish system. Three hours may not be long enough for them to be in a condition where they are comparable with respect to precursor uptake to the animal tumours which after transplantation may establish quicker.

Mattern said the inhibition of DNA or RNA synthesis depends on the proliferating state, and human tumours and animal tumours in the same proliferating state showed the same inhibition.

(The dangers inherent in equating DNA synthesis during or immediately after radiation or drug treatment with cell survival are considered in greater detail on pages 156-7.)

Freshney asked if the ascites samples which appear periodically and are used for tissue culture analysis, are representative of the solid tumour. He also wondered if cells found in the ascites during ovarian carcinoma are destined to die anyway, since some of their cultures prepared from ascites had very short *in vitro* lives, whereas the cultures from solid tumours seemed to last longer.

Warenius said that from a scientific point of view studies would be important. Tumours tend to become more anaplastic as the disease progresses and metastases are frequently more anaplastic than the primary tumour, so it would not be surprising to find that the biological behaviour was different. Clinically, it may not matter, because when treating a patient with ascites who is developing a resistance to drugs, one assumes the cells obtained from the ascitic fluid are closely related to the development of the ascites and it is reasonable to grow these cells and examine them.

Dendy said of the ten specimens analysed in Fig. 3 and Table 3, pp. 94-95, one was a pleural effusion and two were ascitic fluid. These abnormal cells were certainly still capable of cell division.

Laing and Hudson both supported the use of cells from the ascitic fluid. They have had better sucess with malignant cells from ascitic fluid than from the solid tumour. Hudson added that in patients under treatment with cytotoxics, the character of the cells may change as a result of the treatment, not merely as a result of being in ascites. Furthermore, one may get an increased proportion of mesothelial cells and chronic inflammatory cells which may still grow in tissue culture.

Twentyman drew attention to the phenomenon of potentialy lethal damage (Hahn *et al.* 1973). Cells left in their original environment following treatment with radiation or cytotoxic drugs, often have the ability to repair some of the inflicted damage. If they are removed from that environment, some of the potentially repairable damage can become fixed ,and kill the cells. For an established cell line 'in *vitro*, cells in plateau phase which are crowded have more ability to repair potentially lethal damage than exponentially growing cells.

Twentyman and colleagues have studied several drugs and find for example that if 4 mg/kg bodyweight bleomycin is given to a mouse, the tumour is taken out 1 hr later and a cell suspension is made and cloned, the surviving fraction may be 1%. If sub-culture is delayed for 6-8 hr the surviving fraction may rise to 70-80%. If the tumour is left in the mouse and serial measurements are made as the tumour grows, there is no deflection in the growth curves at all. They conclude that by leaving the cells *in situ* in the solid tumour for this extra period, virtually all the damage has been repaired. This means that from the clinical end point one is looking at least as much at the ability of cells to repair damage caused by the drug, as at the initial response to the drug itself. When cells are taken out of the tumour environment to study their response *in vitro*, one is not looking at this very important factor of ability to repair potentially lethal damage.

REFERENCE

Hahn, G. M., Ray, G. R., Gordon, L. F. and Kallman, R. F. (1973). *J. Nat. Cancer Inst. 50*, 529.

4. Management of Patients During Chemotherapy based on an *In Vitro* Predictive Test

T. K. Wheeler

There has been increasingly successful use of cytotoxic regimes in the treatment of advanced malignant disease, but all the reports on treatment of advanced carcinoma of the ovary by a standardised approach reveal few remissions and these are of short duration. Wiltshaw (1965, 1967) reported treatment of carcinoma of the ovary with chlorambucil, obtaining remissions of at least two months duration in 38 of 62 patients (61·4%). Kottmeier (1968) reported a 5% 5-year survival rate using thio-tepa for advanced ovarian cancer. Decker *et al.* (1968) achieved 10% 2-year survival with cyclophosphamide therapy for advanced ovarian carcinoma. Frick *et al.* (1968) advocated melphalan and reported 6% survival at 2 years. Rutledge (1968) also reported the use of melphalan. Greenspan (1968) reported combined therapy using thio-tepa and methotrexate in cases of patients with advanced ovarian carcinoma.

Combined chemotherapy in standard schedules is the practice for chorionic carcinoma, the acute leukaemias and the advanced reticuloses. Constanzi and Coltman (1969) proposed treatment of advanced solid tumours with a combination of cyclophosphamide, methotrexate, vincristine and 5-fluouracil. The dosages were modified by Hanham, Newton and Westbury (1971) (see Table 1) because toxic side effects were found to be unacceptable. Out of 75

TABLE 1

Combination Chemotherapy used at the Westminster Hospital

	Day	1	2	3	4	5
Cyclophosphamide 300 mg		●				●
Methotrexate 0·25 mg/kg		●			●	
Vincristine 0·015 mg/kg			●			●
5-Fluorouracil 7·5 mg/kg		●	●	●	●	●

(After Hanham *et al.* 1971)

patients who were treated for a variety of advanced malignant diseases, 40 patients underwent objective remission but the four patients with carcinoma of the ovary failed to respond. Price and Goldie (1971) used combinations of cyclophosphamide, 5-fluorouracil, actinomycin-D, vincristine, methotrexate and cytosine arabinoside given intravenously for periods not exceeding twenty-four hours (see Table 2). They also reported the use of four of these agents only. Partial or complete tumour regression was observed in 20 of the 40 patients treated, but no response was observed in the three patients with carcinoma of the ovary in the series.

TABLE 2

Combination Chemotherapy used at the Royal Marsden Hospital

Schedule 1	
Cyclophosphamide	600 mg/m^2 (maximum 1 g)
5-fluorouracil	500 mg/m^2 (maximum 750 mg)
Actinomycin D	0·25 mg/m^2 (maximum 0·5 mg)
Vincristine	1 mg/m^2 (maximum 2 mg)
Methotrexate	400 mg/2 litres normal saline/24 hr.
Cytosine arabinoside	100 mg x 4
Schedule 2	
Omits vincristine and cytosine arabinoside	

(After Price and Goldie, 1971)

Dendy's group has studied a large number of tumours by an *in vitro* test first reported in detail in 1970 (Dendy *et al.* 1970). This paper reports 63 patients all of whom had ascites at the time the tissue culture test was performed. In 40 cases drug sensitivities were reported on the basis of results obtained with malignant cells from ascitic fluid; in 10 cases solid tumour removed at the time of diagnosis was cultured, and in 13 cases information was obtained from both solid and fluid specimens. Of the 63 patients reported, 49 had carcinoma of the ovary, 34 in Stage III (FIGO), 9 in Stage IV, 5 in II and 1 in Ic, 8 had carcinoma of the breast in Stage IV, and the remainder had primaries in the colon (2), the bronchus (1), stomach (1), body of uterus (1) and in one patient the primary could not be identified. The malignant diagnosis was confirmed in every case by independent histological examination. Thirty-one of the 63 patients were alive one year after the date of the test, 13 were alive at two years, 9 are still alive. The drugs tested are shown in Table 3.

TABLE 3

A list of the drugs used in these studies together with the number of times each was prescribed on the basis of tissue culture predictions in the management of 52 patients with advanced carcinoma of the ovary

Trenimon	28
Cyclophosphamide (Endoxana)	14
Prednisolone 21 phosphate (Codelsol)	7
Vinblastine sulphate (Velbe)	8
Progesterone (Micryston)	4
Chlorambucil (Burroughs-Wellcome)	4
ThioTEPA (Lederle)	3
Proresid	2
Stilboestrol diphosphate (Honvan)	2
Norethisterone acetate (Schering)	2
Mustine hydrochloride (Boots)	2
Oxymetholone (Anapolon)	1
Melphalan (Alkeran)	1

TABLE 4

Distribution of number of patients alive at 1 year as a function of the number of drugs used in treatment

Number of drugs used	Number of patients	Number alive at 1 year
1	15	5 (33%)
2	18	9 (50%)
3	13	6 (48%)
more than 3	17	11 (56%)

Table 4 shows that survival at 1 year was not strongly dependent on the number of drugs used. Since over 75% of these patients had ovarian tumours, the results tend to confirm that "blind" multiple chemotherapy is of little value for this disease.

In 32 patients treatment followed the recommendations of the *in vitro* test closely. In the other 31 patients, treatment varied from the test predictions because the patients were only given one of the recommended drugs and were usually also given drugs which had not been recommended or, in some instances, not even tested.

At one year 22 of the 32 patients treated strictly in accordance with the test were alive (Group A) whilst only 9 of the 31 other patients were alive. The one-year survival figures have been analysed

TABLE 5

The survival of patients with advanced carcinoma of the ovary matched for age, stage and histology

Group A	Age/Stage/Histology	Survival (Months)	Group B	Age/Stage/Histology	Survival (Months)	Survival at one year Group A	Group B
EF	59/III/D	17	LB	59/III/D	30*	+	+
GP	85/III/D	5	EJ	78/III/D	4	–	–
GLD	70/III/U	13	DB	76/III/U	9	+	–
AD	66/III/U	12	ET	56/III/U	5	+	–
KL	48/III/D	43	SP	49/III/D	3	+	–
DC	33/III/D	13	NH	37/III/D	4	+	–
HS	41/III/U	18	RD	45/III/U	41	+	+
VM	45/III/U	5	PH	52/III/U	33	–	+
MT	61/III/D	12	EP	61/III/D	21	+	+
KH	52/III/D	19*	AJ	50/III/D	13	+	+
FC	46/III/D	5	FT	47/III/D	8	–	–
BL	65/III/D	14	EM	68/III/D	11	+	–
OB	63/III/D	6	HG	62/III/D	3	–	–
GF	60/III/D	14	DB	60/III/D	3	+	–
NW	75/IV/D	12	GM	71/IV/D	3	+	–
EJ	54/IV/D	29	MT	50/IV/D	3	+	–

D = differentiated; U = undifferentiated; * = still alive.

Adapted from Wheeler et al. (1975).

in a 2 x 2 contingency table, with Yates correction for continuity to allow for the small numbers. χ^2 is 8·4 and P = 0·004.

Thirty-two patients with advanced carcinoma of the ovary could be matched for age, stage of disease and histological grade of differentiation (Table 5). The survival times are highly skew and must be examined by non-distributional statistics. If the results are examined by a sign test, survival in Group A exceeded survival in Group B for 11 pairs, while survival in Group B exceeded survival in Group A for 5 pairs. These figures show the same 2:1 ratio in favour of Group A noted earlier but the figures are not significantly different on a 2-sided test, now that the degrees of freedom are greatly reduced, assuming a binomial distribution about a mean value of 8 pairs in each group (P = 0·21).

However, making full use of the data, survival at one year may be examined in a paired test. The 16 pairs can be classified as shown on the extreme right of Table 5. There are 7 tied pairs where either both patients survived or both patients failed to survive one year. The untied pairs favour Group A in the ratio 8:1. On the null hypothesis that there is no difference in survival between Groups A and B, then assuming a binomial distribution, these figures are significant on a 2-sided test (P = 0·039).

Two years after the tissue culture test there is no difference in the surviving ratios for the two groups—7/32 for Group A and 6/31 for Group B. This result can readily be explained in terms of acquired drug resistance during chemotherapy (see p. 311) and indicates that either sequential *in vitro* testing is required or that the problem of acquired drug resistance must be attacked some other way.

This paper presents the results of treatment on the basis of an *in vitro* predictive test of patients with advanced carcinoma particularly of ovarian primaries, where the results are known to be disappointing. In spite of the fact that this is a retrospective analysis the limitations of which have been discussed in detail elsewhere (Wheeler *et al.* 1975), the Cambridge group considers that the results are sufficiently encouraging to justify a prospective clinical trial (see p. 333).

REFERENCES

Constanzi, J. J. and Coltman, F. J. (1969). *Cancer*, 23, 589.
Decker, D. G., Mussey, E. and Malkasian, G. D. Jr. (1968). *Clin. Obstet. Gynaec.* 11, 382.
Dendy, P. P., Gabrielle Bozman and Wheeler, T. K. (1970). *Lancet*, Jul. 11, 68.
Frick, H. C., Tretter, P. and Tretter, W. (1968). *Cancer*, 21, 568.

Greenspan, E. M. (1968). *J. Mount Sinai Hosp. NY, 35,* 52.
Hanham, I. W. F., Newton, K. A. and Westbury, G. (1971). *Br. J. Cancer, 25,* 462.
Kottmeier, H. L. (1968). *Clin. Obstet. Gynaec. 11,* 428.
Price, L. A. and Goldie, J. A. (1971). *Br. Med. J. 4,* 336.
Rutledge, F. (1968). *Clin. Obstet. Gynaec. 11,* 354.
Wheeler, T. K., Dendy, P. P. and Dawson, M. P. A., (1974). *Oncology, 30,* 362.
Wiltshaw, E. (1965). *J. Obst. Gynaec. Br. Commonw. 72,* 590.
Wiltshaw, E. (1967). *Br. Med. J. 2,* 142.

Editor's Note. Since these manuscripts were prepared several papers relating to the culture of human tumour biopsies either *in vitro* or in animals have been published. Much of this work is related either directly or indirectly to the management of patients with chemotherapy. Among the more important papers published recently and not referred to elsewhere in this book are:

Beeby, D. I., Easty, G. C., Gazet, J-C., Grigor K. and Neville, M. (1975). An assessment of the effects of hormones on short term organ cultures of human breast carcinomata. *Br. J. Cancer, 31,* 317.
Berry, R. J., Laing, A. H. and Wells, J. (1975). Fresh explant culture of human tumours *in vitro* and the assessment of sensitivity to cytotoxic chemotherapy. *Br. J. Cancer, 31,* 318-226.
Berenbaum, M. C., Sheard, C. E., Reittie, J. R. and Bundick, R. V. (1974). The growth of human tumours in immunosuppressed mice and their response to chemotherapy. *Br. J. Cancer, 30,* 13.
Holmes, H. L. and Little, J. M. (1974). Tissue culture microtest for predicting response of human cancer to chemotherapy. *Lancet,* October, 26, p. 985.
Knock, F. E., Galt, R. M., Oester, Y. T. and Sylvester, R. (1974). *In vitro* estimate of sensitivity of individual human tumours to anti-tumour agents. *Oncology, 30,* 1-22.
Lickiss, J. N., Cane, K. A. and Baikie, A. G. (1974). *In vitro* drug selection in antineoplastic chemotherapy. *Europ. J. Cancer, 10,* 809-814.
Volm, M., Kaufmann, M., Mattern, J. und Wayss, K. (1975). Möglichkeiten und Grenzen der prätherapeutischen Sensibilitätstestung von Tumoren gegen Zytostatika im Kurzzeittest. *Schweiz med. Wschr. 105,* 74-82.

5. General Discussion on the Use of a Predictive Test in the Management of Gynaecological Cancer

Hudson opened a discussion on the particular clinical problems in the evaluation of laboratory tests for chemotherapeutic sensitivity. He said the reason gynaecologists had been particularly chosen for this panel was that in gynaecology we have perhaps two of the outstanding examples of solid tumours in which chemotherapy can be either a major or an important part of the treatment. First, there is malignant trophoblastic disease in which chemotherapy has completely revolutionised the prognosis. What was previously an almost invariably fatal disease is now one concerning which, if treated promptly and adequately, it is reasonable to talk in terms of cure. The other disease is carcinoma of the ovary which in this country causes more deaths than any other cancer arising in the female genital tract, excluding of course, the breast. Deaths from this disease almost equal those from cancer of the cervix and the body of the uterus combined, and it is one in which we have probably made the least progress in the last twenty years. One of the reasons is that such a high proportion of the patients present with disease which is already disseminated. It is, however, only those patients for whom all other forms of treatment can make no significant contribution who are available for the evaluation of variations in chemotherapeutic treatment.

Hudson then outlined the methods we have for controlling the use of chemotherapy, besides the tests which have been described. The management of malignant trophoblastic disease depends upon the production of a hormone by the malignant tumour tissue. It is possible to monitor the use of chemotherapy by quantitative assay of a tumour indicator substance which is excreted in amounts roughly dependent on the surviving tumour cell population (Bagshawe, 1969). This same system is very occasionally available for cancer of the ovary, but only in certain specific and rather unusual tumours. Certain malignant teratomata secrete chorionic gonadotrophin and other substances which have been found and used are 5-hydroxytryptamine and alpha feto protein. This type of control is not, however, available for the vast majority of the common epithelial tumours which do not secrete a detectable indicator substance. Future research may result in the identification of ectopic or inappropriate hormones and hopefully this may become relevant to the use of chemotherapy in this type of patient. There is also the possibility that the development of specific tumour antigens might be identified and the assay of tumour specific antibodies could form part of the diagnostic service.

When these tumour indicator substances are available, they may help by telling us whether the treatment being used is efficacious long before there are measurable clinical criteria. The presence of recurrent ascites which is valuable as evidence that the disease is progressing, has been referred to previously. When the disease is fully controlled, ascites should be controlled as well and this must be remembered when advocating the chemotherapy sensitivity test on ascites as a progressive event, since persistence of ascites does signify that full control has not yet been achieved.

Among other criteria which are available, is radiological evidence of metastases but lung metastases are relatively uncommon in this disease and are not a very helpful method of providing objective measurement of response. Sometimes pelvic or abdominal examination can detect a lump which is amenable to crude measurement and diagnostic ultrasound may provide a more objective and finer judge of whether our treatment is successful. But in the final analysis, follow up until death is the only end point about which there can be no argument; provided of course that death is due to the disease. This is one reason why ovarian cancer provides a good model for study in this type of work because the majority of patients, in due course, die of their disease, so for any statistical group there is only a relatively small wastage from inter-current causes.

Hudson concluded that the problems we have to consider are the ways in which we should choose which drug, or group of drugs, to use. We must also consider the duration, dosage regime and route of treatment. Further considerations are whether combinations of drugs should be used and how should the development of resistance be detected and managed?

Robinson said that in applying an *in vitro* predictive test a better correlation was required between the level of drug effective in tissue culture and the drug level that may be used in the patient. Kohorn suggested this might not be necessary. If we can demonstrate convincingly that the *in vitro* test will help us choose a drug that kills the tumour cells, this drug should be used as long as there are no adverse effects. The dosage to the patient is then limited by the amount we can administer safely to the patient, and this applies particularly to drugs like cyclophosphamide and vincristine which definitely have patient toxicity limitations.

Kohorn continued that evidence is mounting to show that multiple drug regimes have no superiority over single drugs in ovarian carcinoma (Gynaecological Oncology Group 1975). Evidence from the M. D. Anderson Hospital shows that AcFuCy (actinomycin, fluorouracil, cytoxan) has no superiority over phenylalanine mustard alone. A combination of MOFuCy (methotrexate, vincristine, fluorouracil, cytoxan) also shows no superiority over single agents. The Gynaecological Oncology group in the United States (1975 report) coordinates 26 centres doing prospective studies in various stages of ovarian cancer. For Stage III, radiation is being compared with melphalan alone, melphalan with Fu, and AcFuCy. (AcFuCy may be dropped following the results from M. D. Anderson.) So perhaps use of multiple agents should await more information from chemotherapy sensitivity testing. When there is reliable information from prospective clinical trials, and one must emphasise that there have been virtually no worthwhile prospective clinical trials in gynaecological cancer, then the effects of drugs in combination can be studied. In the meantime, we should explore various methods of cytotoxicity testing like those presented in previous papers. The advantages may not be immediately apparent. In the leukaemias, it took many years before clinical benefit was achieved and we may be at a stage in ovarian cancer where leukaemia was ten years ago.

Wheeler said another parameter relevant to the choice between one drug or multiple drugs, was that in using one drug the patient is treated continuously. The problem raised by four-drug therapy is not simply that four agents work along different metabolic pathways, but that the treatment is pulsed. In certain diseases, and this is now widening the discussion beyond ovarian cancer, the interval between drug treatment when an immunosuppressive effect may be released, is as important as the moment at which cell kill is attempted by administering the drugs. Patients with ovarian carcinoma who come to chemotherapy, are already so overwhelmed by their disease that whatever has been previously holding the disease in check can no longer be released. The failure reported by the Royal Marsden Hospital and by the Westminster Hospital with combination chemotherapy when one might suppose it would have worked, was because host defences were exhausted. Combination chemotherapy is worthwhile when the therapeutic ratio is high as in trophoblastic disease and in acute leukaemia where it is known that drugs exhibited to the point of maximum toxicity produce lengthy remissions or even cures. In ovarian carcinoma, maximum exhibition may do nothing except produce iatrogenic problems and exhaustion.

Kohorn agreed that this disease is diagnosed late when there is a tremendous tumour load, and said there were numerous animal experiments in which this was a very important factor. Once the tumour load reaches a certain significant size, no immune mechanism can cope with it. Surgically excisable tumor, or small tumor loads, can be dealt with and in offering chemotherapy to patients, we must aim to eradicate residual tumour loads left behind after surgery but so disseminated as to be unreachable by effective radiation therapy. There is evidence (Kohorn *et al.* 1974) that pulsed chemotherapy does allow continued cell mediated immunity over a prolonged period but antibody release has not been measured. The humoral antibody factor is probably at risk with continuous chemotherapy, because it is continually suppressed so in gynaecology as in other chemotherapeutic disciplines, we must look to pulsed therapy and continuous therapy should be discouraged.

Hudson said gynaecologists had frequently been criticised for exhibiting an alkylating agent in continuous low dose therapy, but the situation is now under reappraisal. In particular with myeloma where the progress of the tumour can be studied accurately, there is some evidence that melphalan given continuously is more effective than when pulsed. The action of alkylating agents may be distributed through different parts of the cell cycle and has not yet been fully understood. Dendy and Hudson have surveyed patients who had responded to chemotherapy based on the *in vitro* test and an alkylating agent was one of the drugs used and recommended in very nearly all cases. There is little evidence of good responses in patients with a regime containing no alkylating agent.

Kohorn said the question of a second-look operation before

stopping alkylating agents in patients who have no clinical sign of disease, is most important. In a recent survey of 28 cases where melphalan had been stopped after a second look, half showed clinical disease. Although there is a risk of lymphoma and leukaemia, it is really difficult to stop the drugs without knowing there is no disease. Robinson found it impossible, having embarked on single drug therapy, and achieved one or two years apparently disease-free, to stop treatment if there is no evidence of recurrence.

Laing agreed that we do not know if multiple agents are any better than a single agent. In Oxford there is a prospective trial comparing multiple agents with a single agent. In this context it is important when dealing with a fatal disease not to judge "success" by the time a patient survives, because this is an extremely poor parameter of success or failure. What really matters is the quality of life for that patient during the time remaining and it may be that with a single agent, although the patient lives a slightly shorter time, the quality of survival may be better. Hudson suggested that instead of talking about a test of sensitivity, most benefit might come from the tissue culture work as a test of resistance. We may be able to spare patients from unpleasant agents, particularly epilating ones and those with neurotoxicity, which really can add considerable misery to the last days of a disease which itself is very unpleasant.

Hudson continued that a working party has been set up by the Cancer Committee of the Medical Research Council to study the treatment of ovarian cancer and one of its first duties will be to identify questions which are the essential basis for any prospective trial about the control of chemotherapy. For example, it is most important to correlate with pathologists to ensure uniform staging and histological grading without which the whole concept becomes meaningless. An admirable booklet on the histopathology of carcinoma of the ovary is now available, but it may be a long time before this has percolated through to the innumerable pathologists throughout this country who have to report this multifarious disease. Unless organisation can be arranged on a central basis through a few centres with common pathology, the information collected may be of no value whatsoever.

Kohorn said ovarian cancer was not one disease but a multiplicity of diseases, and when we talk about cure rates and good results with continuous drugs or with intermittent drugs, we have to specify the stage of the disease in more detail than even the TNM classification implies. Anatomical description specifying where there is disease and where there is no disease is vital to objective reports. Frequently, omental biopsies are not done, lymph node biopsies along the aorta are not done, and very few people do a washing of the peritoneum to see if there is cell positive fluid. Furthermore, we know very little about the cell cycling pattern of this disease and all the details which have been worked out for HeLa cells are really needed for the different histological grades and different histological patterns before we can start treating this disease scientifically.

Limburg said another question which should be incorporated into such trials, is whether one should use prophylactic chemotherapy for early stages of carcinoma of the ovary (FIGO stage 1 or 2; or T1 to T3 in the TNM classification) after operation and radiotherapy. Also for a FIGO stage 3 or 4; or T4 what should be done clinically when the patient is released and goes home? It is necessary to compare high dose intravenous therapy with continuous low dose therapy and the possibility of infusion therapy followed by at least 2 years low dose therapy at home should also be considered.

Robinson thought a prospective survey of the value of *in vitro* testing was essential. Without any form of tissue culture whatsoever, drugs have been used, and sometimes used very effectively, in the treatment of ovarian carcinoma. Patients sometimes become apparently disease-free for a considerable period of time. Since predictive testing is very time consuming and difficult, we must examine it extremely critically to see if its continued use is justified.

Dendy said a prospective, controlled clinical trial for very advanced carcinoma of the ovary, had started in Cambridge to find out if treatment based on the results of a tissue culture predictive test is more beneficial than treatment selected without any knowledge of the behaviour of the patients' tumour cells in culture. Patients are considered for the trial where there has been incomplete removal of an ovarian tumour at laparotomy and there is extensive malignant disease. Cases where radiotherapy is planned as post-operative treatment, are not included.

After the tissue culture test three types of report are issued:

(1) "Test successful" with full details
(2) Test successful but details withheld
(3) Test failed.

Patients are randomised between groups (1) and (2) after the report has been written but before it leaves the tissue culture laboratory.

For report type (1) treatment is based on the tissue culture recommendation as closely as possible. For report type (2) there is complete freedom of treatment. It is hoped that follow-up until death of groups (1) and (2) will give valid information on the usefulness of the *in vitro* test. Examination of group (3) may give information about the types of tumour which fail to grow in culture and about their prognosis.

Hudson said the very large amount of material Limburg had analysed, some 3,000 explants, showed that the number of *in vitro* tests from which it is possible eventually to draw conclusions, because the patient has in fact been treated in a valid way with one of the drugs which has been adequately tested, is extremely small. In preliminary discussions with Dendy, it was agreed that this was probably no more than 25% of all the cultures which grew and were tested successfully. Making allowance for laboratory failures, the wastage of laboratory time and material is very considerable.

In conclusion, he said Limburg had reported that of some 200 patients, 83% were in the advanced group of ovarian cancers so it is probably in this group that we must concentrate when looking for objective evidence for evaluation of the *in vitro* test. He hoped very much that it would be possible to include in forward planning a prospective analysis which would permit this. If it can be done in parallel with patients who are put on different regimes according to a national study, it will be a most valuable by-product of this much needed work.

REFERENCES

Bagshawe, K. D. (1969). "Choriocarcinoma", Arnold, London.

Kohorn, E. I., Davis, J. M., Mokyr, M. B. and Mitchell, S. M. (1974). *Gyn. Investigation*, 5, 44.

Report Gynaecological Oncology Group, Buffalo, New York, January 1975.

6. Some Problems Associated with Clinical Co-operation

M. V. Bright

My interest in the study of *in vitro* methods for growing human tumours, particularly those arising in the ovary, and in the use of these techniques to assess the relative sensitivities of such tumours to different chemotherapeutic agents originated some 6 years ago while I was a Registrar in Gynaecology in Cambridge. Even then I was very conscious of the painstaking nature of the work and how frequently the laboratory efforts were wasted by the clinicians who provided the tumour material. Whether through carelessness or apathy, good specimens were on many occasions slow to arrive and, if from other centres, poorly packed and not infrequently infected.

In 1969 I moved to London and hoped to start similar work at St. Mary's Hospital, but it soon became apparent that this was not feasible because of lack of finance and technical help. Instead I became involved in an attempt to find evidence of host immunity in patients with ovarian carcinoma. In this project I undertook a small part of the scientific work myself but was chiefly concerned with the provision of tumor material. This naturally led to clinical involvement outside my own unit and I soon realised the wide gulf that separated the practising clinician from the true scientist. It was relatively easy to generate interest from different clinicians in the project, but on the whole such interest tended to be short-lived and required constant stimulation. Clinicians wanted quick results whereas the scientist's attitude was much longer-term, requiring painstaking analysis of data to try and achieve some significance.

Simple communication and arrangements for transfer of tumour material are always a problem. Almost all clinicians claim to be overworked and this may even be true in some cases, so methods for despatch of specimens must be very simple. Thought has to be given to the problem of material that is obtained out of working hours. Nothing is more irritating to a clinician who has troubled to obtain a specimen than to find that those who should be receiving it have gone home, or that it is impossible to find anyone who can give instructions for proper storage until the laboratory re-opens. This problem is particularly true for the rarer tumours where specialists in smaller peripheral units may be involved for the first time.

In his efforts to contribute to major scientific advance, the aspiring clinician may well tread on sensitive pathological toes. Thought should therefore be given in advance to achieving sensible collaboration with the pathologists thus avoiding the embarrassment of finding, too late, that there is no histological proof to support the original clinical diagnosis.

In some situations obtaining tumour material for research, or using the results of new work to treat patients, causes ethical problems. Relatively few scientists appreciate the dilemma that may confront the clinician. The latter has to ensure that his patient's interests always come first, that procedures resulting in the provision of material for scientific research do no harm to the patient in question and that any treatment devised as a result of such research is likely to do more good than harm. Most patients are very willing to help, but many are equivocal, ultimately acquiescing to the persuasive doctor who, by emphasising the potential benefit to other patients, makes the individual patient feel rather guilty if he or she refuses to take part.

On the other hand, the scientist has a dilemma when attempting to guide the clinician with regard to treatment. Using the techniques of *in vitro* testing for chemotherapeutic sensitivity of ovarian carcinoma as an example, the clinician prefers a wide choice of chemotherapeutic agents so that he can tailor his treatment for the individual. The scientist, however, may prefer to concentrate his efforts on a fuller understanding of a few agents. There is no easy answer to this problem but on balance fundamental progress will only be made by studying fewer agents in depth, rather than by a more superficial approach. This divergence of attitudes usually reflects the control of such research in any centre and whether it is clinically or scientifically orientated. Furthermore, the scientist will usually prefer to delay results until statistical significance has been achieved, whereas the clinician is naturally impatient where his patient's welfare is concerned. The scientist then becomes subject to pressure to produce results which may be invalid and this is not helped by awareness that the money for his research may come from clinical sources.

I have implied so far, that it is relatively easy to achieve some correlation between the results of *in vitro* testing for drug sensitivity and clinical response, but even if the clinician knew that a particular drug would be of benefit to his patient he would be bound by limitation of dosage due to toxicity, length of treatment due to anticipated side effects such as bone narrow suppression, and sometimes drug idiosyncrasies in the individual patient. This clinical barrier must be of prime concern to the scientist, for it is quite useless to recommend to a clinician a particular drug which shows a good *in vitro* response at a dosage which, when extrapolated for the human, would be potentially lethal.

Even if the problems of drug concentration and toxicity are within safe bounds, there still remains the difficult question of clinical response. The patient's general sense of well-being or otherwise may be a guide, but this is so often obscured during treatment by minor but depressing side-effects; for example nausea, diarrhoea, loss of hair; that a reasonably reliable objective assessment may not be possible. From the clinician's point of view, gross deterioration with weight loss, loss of appetite and progressive dehydration and anaemia, are all too obvious, and with the ultimate death of the patient there is a possibility to correlate treatment with response using survival rates of treated patients against controls. This does, however, require many patients, a long-term follow-up and also a consistency in treatment which may be difficult to achieve in the light of new advances and ideas.

Assessment of the results of treatment in patients with less advanced cancers may be exceedingly difficult. With ovarian carcinoma in particular, the rate of recurrence of ascites may give a guide, but this may only reflect the effect of the drugs on a small proportion of the original tumour population. Clinical examination to detect solid 'tumour recurrence is a very unreliable way to determine tumour mass. Operations to visualise the tumour are open to the same objection and sometimes ethical considerations, although one could argue that further tumour material could thus be obtained to check that no secondary resistance to drugs had been acquired during treatment (but this perhaps begs the question of correlation with *in vitro* tests).

It is not easy for the research scientist to become clinically involved but it is quite common for the young clinician, as part of his training, to be directly concerned in scientific research. He thus has an incentive to provide material, maintain good clinical records and reliable follow-up data in relation to the project in question and to keep open efficient channels of communication. He may share in publications as well as widen his experience and is unlikely to forget his scientific associations in his future more clinically orientated career. The underlying theme of this paper has thus been one of communication and co-operation. As Louis Pasteur once said "Science and the application of science go together like the fruit and the tree"! I hope this will cease to be wishful thinking in the not too distant future.

INDEX

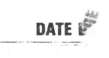

DATE

SE